T0176943

Forensic Science Education and Training

Forensic Science Education and Training

A Tool-kit for Lecturers and Practitioner Trainers

Edited by

Anna Williams
School of Applied Sciences, University of Huddersfield, UK

John P. Cassella
Department of Forensic Science and Crime Science, Staffordshire University, UK

Peter D. Maskell
School of Science, Engineering and Technology, Abertay University, UK

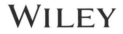

Registered Offices
John Wiley & Sons, Inc., 111 River Street, Hoboken, NJ 07030, USA
John Wiley & Sons Ltd, The Atrium, Southern Gate, Chichester, West Sussex, PO19 8SQ, UK

Editorial Office
The Atrium, Southern Gate, Chichester, West Sussex, PO19 8SQ, UK

For details of our global editorial offices, customer services, and more information about Wiley products visit us at www.wiley.com.

Wiley also publishes its books in a variety of electronic formats and by print-on-demand. Some content that appears in standard print versions of this book may not be available in other formats.

Library of Congress Cataloging-in-Publication Data

Names: Williams, Anna, (Forensic anthropologist), editor. | Cassella, John P., editor. | Maskell, Peter D.
Title: Forensic science education and training : a tool-kit for lecturers and practitioner trainers / edited by Anna Williams, John Cassella, Peter D. Maskell.
Description: Chichester, UK ; Hoboken : Wiley, 2017. | Includes index.
Identifiers: LCCN 2016049894 | ISBN 9781118689233 (hardback) | ISBN 9781118689165 (Adobe PDF) | ISBN 9781118689158 (epub)
Subjects: LCSH: Forensic sciences–Study and teaching (Higher)–Great Britain. | BISAC: MEDICAL / Forensic Medicine.
Classification: LCC HV8073 .F 2017 | DDC 363.25071/141–dc23 LC record available at https://lccn.loc.gov/2016049894

Cover design: Wiley
Cover images: (top) courtesy of Kris Thomson; (inset images) courtesy of John P. Cassella

Set in 10/12pt WarnockPro by Aptara Inc., New Delhi, India
Printed and bound in Malaysia by Vivar Printing Sdn Bhd

10 9 8 7 6 5 4 3 2 1

This book is dedicated to Dave Rogers who sadly passed away before the publication and never got to see the fruits of his efforts.

Contents

List of Contributors

Luke Bracegirdle
School of Physical Sciences
and Geography
Keele University, Keele
Staffordshire, UK

Graham Braithwaite
Cranfield University
Shrivenham
Swindon, UK

Sue Carney
Ethos Forensics
Manchester, UK and
University of Central Lancashire, UK

John P. Cassella
Staffordshire University
Department of Forensic Science
and Crime Science
Faculty of Computing
Engineering and Science
Science Centre
Stoke on Trent, UK

Peter Cross
University of Central Lancashire
Preston, UK

Claire Gwinnett
Staffordshire University
Department of Forensic Science
and Crime Science
Faculty of Computing
Engineering and Science

Science Centre
Stoke on Trent, UK

Christopher Hargreaves
Cranfield University
College Road, Cranfield
Bedfordshire, UK

Karl Harrison
Cranfield University
Cranfield Forensic Institute
College Road, Cranfield
Bedfordshire, UK

Benjamin J. Jones
Abertay University
Dundee, UK

Janice Kennedy
University of West Scotland
School of Science and Sport
Hamilton Campus
Hamilton, UK

Peter D. Maskell
Abertay University
School of Science
Engineering and Technology
Dundee, UK

Colleen Morgan
University of York
Centre for Digital Heritage Research
King's Manor
York, UK

Anna-Maria Muller
Swindon
Wiltshire
UK

Jackie A. Potter
School of Physical Sciences
and Geography
Keele University, Keele
Staffordshire, UK

Richard D. Price
Faculty of Computing
Engineering and Science
University of South Wales, UK

Jamie K. Pringle
School of Physical Sciences
and Geography
Keele University, Keele
Staffordshire, UK

David Rogers＊
Staffordshire University
Department of Forensic Science
and Crime Science

Faculty of Computing
Engineering and Science
Science Centre
Stoke on Trent, UK

Mark Roycroft
University of East London
University Way
London, UK

Luke Taylor
University of Kent
Canterbury, UK

Kris Thomson
Anatomage
San Jose
California, USA

Anna Williams
University of Huddersfield
School of Applied Sciences, Queensgate
Huddersfield, UK

＊ David is deceased.

Foreword

I am particularly pleased to write the Foreword to this book, because it addresses the crux of the whole scientific investigative process. The effectiveness of that process is completely dependent on education and knowledge, simply because it's a truism that 'you do not know what you do not know.' So if you have no idea that pond water contains diatoms you would never see the significance of their absence in a drowning victim. If you do not know that the diatom population changes from month to month, you would never see the possibility of determining how many months ago a person drowned in a river. Nor would you be able to produce the analytical diatom results in the first place unless you knew how to retrieve and analyse the samples.

This book is a comprehensive and authoritative treasure trove of how to teach both principles and practice.

Of course one change in forensic science education over the last 15 years has been the greatly heightened profile of the subject due to the popularity of TV programmes such as CSI – which in turn has led to an almost exponential increase in the number of courses and students. I have no reservations about saying this is a very good thing—indeed it raises the public understanding of science and has the major advantage of increasing the number of undergraduates studying science. It also provides a feed of excellent students into forensic science research in academia, a role which they have taken over from the Forensic Science Service (FSS). Of course, there are hardly any jobs available as court going forensic scientists, but this is not a new problem—it was exactly the same when I started in the early 1970s. And in fact this is not a problem at all, as it turns out that forensic science graduates possess the very attributes sought by employers of all types—logic and assessment, using a scientific method, communication skills and of course scientific skills.

At school, I always wanted to be Sherlock Holmes, although my initial interest simply lay in the delight of solving logical puzzles. Of course, Sherlock Holmes had the serious advantage that he knew the solution in advance, so that the logic simply involved assembling the building blocks of an already known solution; however that advantage was not immediately apparent to a fascinated ten-year-old.

Towards the end of a long career in forensic science I eventually became a forensic investigator as head of physical evidence at National Crime Faculty (NCF), and my overall aim was still very Sherlock Holmes like, but the process was indeed completely opposite. My job was to think of all the possible explanations for the facts, thus creating multiple hypotheses, which often confused matters further as far as the investigators went. By then analysing the micro-sequence of events, that is the actions and interactions between the offender and victim and environment that must have taken place, we could use physical evidence to prove or disprove that particular hypothesis: pretty well back to Sherlock Holmes and his 'when you have eliminated the impossible etc., etc.'

At Crime Faculty my primary role was to review undetected and cold case murders and rape series. The initial casework experience was horrific, a word I use advisedly. Crucial observations and inferences that would have detected crimes simply (and cheaply!) were being overlooked. It quickly became apparent that the main problem in using forensic science effectively in the United Kingdom was simply a lack of shared knowledge. The scientists thought in terms of evidence and simply did not appreciate the value of intelligence to investigations–the potential impact of their observations and results over the dozens of investigative lines of enquiry. Equally the police could define their problems but had insufficient knowledge to see which of the myriad techniques available would be most appropriate. The situation was compounded because forensic science is inherently context dependant–often investigators would demand inappropriate tests simply because they had worked previously, under different circumstances.

Progress was made–NCF and the FSS introduced specialist advisors, generalist scientists attached to the investigative team, a role designed to enhance the thinking process in investigations. And the UK Parliamentary Select Committee (PSC) Report on Forensic Science (2004) stated unequivocally that the real benefit of forensic science lay in the provision of intelligence during the investigative phase, not hard evidence for use in court.

That overarching view of techniques and processes is particularly necessary because as new scientific instrumentation expanded throughout the 1970s and 1980s, forensic scientists themselves became more and more specialised. By the 1990s it became increasingly unreasonable to expect the police to second guess all the scientific solutions, and thus counterproductive for investigators to choose items to send to the laboratory to answer specific questions, as they traditionally had. The questions were still fine but the laboratory increasingly had more and more and better and better ways of answering them–or answering completely different, and more useful questions, which were completely unknown to individual detectives.

The Chair of the Association of Chief Police Officers (ACPO) (now National Police Chiefs Council) Homicide once described my NCF role as 'asking stupid questions.' He meant (I hope!) asking questions that had not occurred to the specialist scientists or investigators. However, forensic science (and forensic intelligence) is not really about DNA or other clever test results but about the significance of those analytical results and observations in any particular context. So forensic science educators need to teach scientific techniques, process and logical thought and apply these skills across a wide range of instrumental techniques and crime types. A glance down the chapter list will demonstrate that this aim has been admirably fulfilled.

Less easy to define and engender are attributes such as a questioning approach and especially the need to encourage a 'Bayesian thinking' mind-set, which will lead students to think automatically 'what other possible explanation can there be for that result.' Undergraduate courses will provide a bedrock of factual information as well, but students really need to link that questioning mind-set to a wide breadth of factual knowledge of their own. As an example, scientists all know that you just cannot ignite petrol with a cigarette end, but the public who watch films and TV don't. This means the criminals don't either, and giving an impossible explanation for criminal events is often quite a good clue!

If only this book had been available when I was giving evidence in Court! Because whilst it is designed as a resource for educators and trainers, it provides a wealth of information that should also underpin our discussions with lay audiences, whether in Court or when trying to convince a Senior Investigating Officer (SIO) to authorise tests s/he believes irrelevant. Or to explain anything remotely scientific to members of the legal profession…

In summary, it is impossible to provide effective forensic science without a good knowledge of the known context, and an excellent and broad education as to the methods and processes available to clarify that context and to assess significance. That educative resource is exactly what is provided by this book, and I commend it to you unreservedly.

Dave Barclay
Fellow of the Forensic Science Society
Honorary/Emeritus Professor
November 2016

Acknowledgements

The Editors would like to thank Anna-Maria Muller for all her hard work and dedication at the beginning of the journey towards completion of this book.

We would also like to express our thanks to all the contributors whose expertise, experience and diligence has made this book possible, and to the students who have inspired us to produce this text. We hope that the knowledge, experience and enthusiasm accumulated in these pages will benefit forensic science lecturers and trainers and in turn, generations of future students and forensic scientists.

Anna Williams would like to thank her husband Graeme for his unwavering support.

John P. Cassella would like to thank those staff and students who have inspired him to be a better teacher.

Peter D. Maskell would like to thank his family Dawn, Imogen and Caitlyn for keeping him sane in the exile years.

1

Forensic Science Education – The Past and the Present In and Out of the Classroom

John P. Cassella,[1] Peter D. Maskell,[2] and Anna Williams[3]

[1] Staffordshire University, Department of Forensic Science and Crime Science, Faculty of Computing, Engineering and Science, Science Centre, Stoke on Trent, UK
[2] Abertay University, School of Science, Engineering and Technology, Dundee, UK
[3] University of Huddersfield, School of Applied Sciences, Queensgate, Huddersfield, UK

Introduction

This chapter aims to reflect upon and to consider the 'where are we now' aspect of forensic science education and training. Despite the rhythms and reflective cycle that academia requires, it is surprising how little time the *on-the-ground* academics and practitioners involved in education and training get to truly reflect upon the curriculum and assessment of what they deliver. Of course what is specifically taught depends upon many variables; the interests, skills and experiences of those academics delivering the material coupled with the requirement of the industry to teach it. Whilst such criteria are of importance to say 'art' colleagues in their curriculum design, they are not as crucial as they are to a subject such as forensic science. This offers limited latitude for what is taught and requires industry professionals and accreditation boards to drive the expectations of the curricula to a greater degree. What is apparent over the coming pages is the change and the rate of change that has taken place in the forensic science profession at all levels, technical, practical and academic and its use within the Courtroom is now greater than ever, demanding higher and higher levels of skill, competence and understanding of what is useful in a police investigation and criminal trial.

> Forensic science is a 'critical and integral part' of any judicial system in the 21st Century because forensic science is one of the primary means through which 'democratic governments fulfill one of the most fundamental obligations to their citizens: public safety insurance in a just manner'.
>
> *Houck, 2006*

Well over a decade ago, in 2000, in the United Kingdom (UK), the educational landscape for forensic science was very different to today's current situation.

The changes that have occurred in the past decade not only in the forensic science area but also within policing (Neuroyd, 2011) are the greatest since either forensic science or indeed policing came into being. A number of key national and international events have occurred and documents have been published that have aimed to examine the status quo and to offer direction for future developments within forensic science and hence its delivery and education. Some of these early key events and the documentation resulting from them include:

- The report by the UK House of Commons Science and Technology Committee – Forensic Science on Trial, published in 2005.
- The UK SEMTA Report (Science, Engineering, Manufacturing Technologies Alliance (SEMTA) Sector Skills Council, Forensic Science: Implications for Higher Education 2004, UK) of 2004 on the forensic science implications for Higher Education institutions.
- The UK Skills for Justice Report in 2009 for the Forensic Science Occupational Committee in 2009 into the provision of forensic science degree programmes in UK Higher Education institutions (HEIs).
- The National Academy of Sciences (USA) report (2009) into strengthening forensic science in the United States.
- The publication of the Silverman report on UK Forensic Science Research published in 2011.
- The 'paradigm shift for UK Forensic Science' (Royal Society Meeting) in 2015 ... and the list could go on.

As a result of the field's prominence and popularity (Mennell, 2006), the number of education providers offering forensic science courses and the number of students enrolling in these courses increased exponentially (Engber, 2005; NIFS, 2006) but the subjective observation is that there is now a downward trend in recruitment in forensic science courses in favour of policing based education.

The expansion in forensic science education worldwide driven by university consumer forces and popular demand, in addition to the inconsistency and lack of clarity in the huge range of forensic science courses on offer, have led to inconsistencies in skills and competencies acquired by the graduates seeking employment in the field. Whilst this has clearly been addressed through accreditation by the laudable attempts of learned societies in their host countries (such as the UK Chartered Society of Forensic Sciences) to harmonise the content of delivery, this has worked within countries to some extent, but less so across countries, which reflects the relationship of forensic science with the law and the wider Criminal Justice System within that particular country.

In 2004 that may have been the case, but the situation is now somewhat improved. The question concerning the variety and the value of the many publications and reports on this topic into forensic science provision and education and the legacies and the recommendations that they have offered will be considered further within this chapter and indeed as a paradigm throughout this book. There is, however, much still to be done as forensic science education enters the second decade in the UK HEIs. As Samarji (2012) observed, forensic science academic programmes are still characterised by a great deal of randomness and uncertainty.

Burnett *et al.* (2001) had argued that little research has been undertaken and published on forensic science education; it is reasonable to surmise that this issue of a paucity of literature at the turn of the twenty-first century has long since been redressed with a myriad of documents, investigations and recommendations at national and international level into all levels and aspects of forensic science. Four years later, Lewis *et al.* (2005) concluded that the random expansion in forensic science education worldwide, in addition to an inconsistency and lack of clarity in the wide range of forensic science courses on offer, led to variations in the skills and the competencies acquired by trainees and graduates seeking employment in the forensic field. Moreover, forensic science education departments still lack formal arrangements with practitioners and employers to discuss course content, delivery and assessment. Currently in the HEI sector, at best there is a 'Memorandum of Understanding' but more often there is a reliance upon the good will of management level staff from both the academic and practitioner organisations involved. Instead 'what exists is a series of *ad hoc* arrangements' (with a couple of notable exceptions), which occur on an individual basis between employers or individuals and UK universities through which 'employers liaise with universities about particular courses' (SEMTA, 2004) and how they should or could develop their courses.

Forensic science suffers a non-consensus within the academic community on whether it is a stand-alone and distinct applied field of knowledge, an associate field of study, or merely a technical derivative of existing arenas. Moreover, some scholars and practitioners argue in the public domain in the extreme as to whether or not forensic science education is a necessity *at all* within Higher Education.

Despite this dialogue, criticisms by potential employers (Lewis *et al.*, 2005) abound more than a decade after the first courses were introduced. Forensic science (education) departments still lack formal arrangement or requirements with employers and national level organisations, for example, the College of Policing (CoP), Chartered Society of Forensic Sciences (CSFS) and Skills for Justice (SfJ), offering endorsement programmes to discuss course content in a meaningful fashion and certainly not at a national, European-wide or international level.

These inconsistencies have resulted, particularly in forensic science education courses because of the lack of dialogue between the various contexts, cultures and mind-set, in a field of shifting but unconfirmed reigning paradigms. This lack of dialogue, compounded by the lack of Quality Assurance Agency (QAA) guidance (until 2012), had resulted in a set of competencies determined to a large degree by the skill set of the academics from the university at the time that the course was first designed. This has been offset in part by up-skilling of HEI academics in the realisation, from advice given by forensic practitioners from industry when attending university forensic science course 'validation events', that the course *must* be more than 'forensic' in name. Whilst this has been achieved to varying levels across the HEI sector, most, if not all institutions involved, are guilty (in part) of not fully entering into dialogue with legal or policing colleagues. The closure of the UK Forensic Science Service (FSS) in 2012 had one positive effect upon HEIs as an industry, in that it offered a willing pool of highly qualified individuals who could join the academic teams. Previously, such individuals had only entered this pool at retirement on a visiting lecturer basis.

Despite the prominence and high stature that forensic science has gained within the general public consciousness and the consequent expansion it has achieved within Higher Education institutions, forensic science 'has not enjoyed a similar rise in stature within the academic community' (Jonakait, 1991). Garrison (1991) asserted that forensic science identity is complex because it is the 'product of an uneasy and unholy mating of science, the objective seeker of truth and knowledge, and forensics, the argumentative persuader of courtroom advocacy'; competency compounded by its association with the Police Service in the UK undergoing one of the most radical changes in over 100 years (Neyroud, 2011).

Forensic science remains a relatively new and developing field in terms of its education, practice and stature. It is the proverbial Cinderella to chemistry, physics and biology and is likely to be so for the foreseeable future, until its importance in both an educational and employment context are fully recognised and appreciated. The reasons for this are still being debated, however, the relative youthfulness of such educational courses may in part explain the attitudes of employers to such courses when compared with the much more established sciences such as physics, chemistry and biology.

Therefore, complexity and uncertainty issues are experienced at the epistemological level of forensic science, in the nature of the actual practice and within a wide grasp of images, profiles, impressions, expectations and perceptions that attempt to shape the identity of this field.

In the eyes of the media, UK educational establishments that were given university status in 1992 (and beyond) are criticised as being only devoted to responding to either government's wishes or fulfilling businesses' obsession with income, whilst giving up their historic fundamental role as a 'civilising force' and a source of moral development (Cullingford and Blewitt, 2004). Forensic science education has sometimes been used by universities for business reasons, where the word 'forensic' is used as a popular term to attract enrolments and polish the perceived less attractive conventional subjects, such as chemistry and physics, which are subject to closure (SEMTA, 2004).

Despite the levelling-off (in fact a clear decline) of the number of HEIs validating forensic science based courses, the initial rapid growth in forensic science education over the last decade continues to raise concerns about the quality of many of the forensic science programmes offered (Daéid and Roux, 2010; Quarino and Brettell, 2009; Mennell, 2006). This rapid growth is argued to be the cause of the inconsistencies and the lack of clarity reflected in the huge range of forensic science courses on offer (Lewis *et al.*, 2005). This inconsistency in education has resulted in the lack of agreement on the 'appropriate' competencies acquired by forensic science graduates, which have led to further criticisms from potential employers (Lewis *et al.*, 2005; Hanson and Overton, 2010). The CSFS accreditation process has done much to level the playing field in terms of quality and content but as this is still not a requirement for course delivery it has not been taken up by all HEI providers.

Reviews have been conducted to study the current status of this education and establish some recommendations for the future (Daéid and Roux, 2010). With this in mind, the following studies are pertinent to consider.

The Sector Skills Council for Science, Engineering and Manufacturing in the UK conducted a study on forensic science (2004) which recommended that: (1) forensic science degree content be monitored for quality assurance and be set-up in close cooperation with the forensic industry; (2) professional technical/laboratory skills training programmes should be established; (3) pure science disciplines (e.g. chemistry) in Higher Education should receive more government funding (SEMTA, 2004). This study was supplemented by a study in 2009 presented in a 'Skills for Justice' report in response to the on going debate and concerns of the UK Government about the employability and postgraduate 'value' of many of the forensic science courses offered within the UK (Daéid and Roux, 2010). The Skills for Justice's report observed that a number of the issues raised years previously in SEMTA's 2004 report remain a concern over a decade later, including the failure of large numbers of forensic science graduates to secure employment in the forensic sector. At the time of the SEMTA report in 2004, the forensic landscape was very different for both practitioner and educators, and it was indeed very different for students within a university environment; the questions remain as to the success or not of the levels of employment of forensic science graduates.

The USA National Institute for Forensic Science (NIFS) criticised the United States educational establishments in 2006, in that forensic content was present sometimes 'by name only' in their US curricula, in order to add or associate the adjective 'forensic' with the title of the offered courses; hence, the courses became more attractive and enrolled more students.

We now have the UK Forensic Science Regulators' role in Quality Assurance (Codes of Practice and Conduct) (https://www.gov.uk/government/uploads/system/uploads/attachment_data/file/118949/codes-practice-conduct.pdf) within the industry and their role in related areas in practice that is well entrenched within the Home Office and Criminal Justice structures. The closure of the Council for the Registration of Forensic Practitioners and the Skills for Justice, Skillsmark process, has since been initiated. The CSFS 'Education and Industry Liaison Forum' was formed to facilitate forensic practitioners engagement in a more structured manner with education and research in HEIs.

This development represents a landmark shift in the way that practitioners and HEIs engage – this is something that has taken a decade to bring to fruition and demonstrates the significant changes in the attitudes of stakeholders, practitioners and drawbridge keepers that has made this possible with HEIs.

The R v T, where in October 2010, the English Court of Appeal overturned a murder conviction on the basis of, as it saw it, severe flaws in the generation and presentation of the prosecution's forensic shoe-print evidence (see Hamer, 2012) report and the closure of the Forensic Science Service in the UK in 2012, was a stern wake-up call to the whole forensic industry, not just in the United Kingdom but indeed globally. Equally, the United States National Academy of Sciences (the national research council of the national academies), report make very clear statements about directions for moving forward for their forensic science community and sent a Tsunami warning to the United Kingdom in terms of policy and practice in 2011, and yet the FSS closure went ahead with little or no published plan of what would replace the void it left behind.

Hannis and Welsh (2009) published the 'Skills for Justice – Fit for Purpose – Research into the provision of forensic science degree programmes in UK HEIs' and reported that 'a number of areas of forensic education needed improving to be truly fit for purpose.'

In 2006 the United Kingdom Forensic Science Education Group (UKSFEG) was established as a forum in part to provide careers information and more general career advice to potential and current forensic science students. It comprised a number of highly influential and high-ranking individuals and groups including: the Association of Chief Police Officers (ACPO), the Home Office Forensic Science & Pathology Unit, Forensic Science

Service, Scottish Forensic Science Service, Northern Ireland Forensic Service, Laboratory of the Government Chemist (LGC) Forensics, Centrex NTC, Metropolitan Police Service, Strathclyde Police, Derbyshire Police, Cleveland Police, the Chartered Society of Forensic Sciences, UK Higher Education Academy and a number of UK universities in which forensic science degrees were delivered. Part of its remit was to encourage links with forensic science employers and academia. The group's aim is to continue to promote recognisable and relevant degrees in 'forensic practice'.

Its wider remit has been to establish forensic science employer Higher Education (HE) requirements and priorities for new and existing staff by agreeing a framework for forensic science users and providers to work collaboratively with HE to influence the design, content and delivery of courses, to ensure graduates are well equipped to meet the needs of the forensic science community. For a time, UKSFEG assisted in influencing forensic science degree courses and working with forensic science users and providers to identify key priority areas for the future, such as Crime Scene Science and Digital Forensics. Through this, it facilitated providers with a pool of high quality graduates to recruit from; it produces undergraduates and postgraduates with realistic career expectations and opportunities and a framework of Higher Education professional development activities for forensic practitioners. In achieving these aims, the group complemented the work of existing organisations such as the Chartered Society of Forensic Sciences, Higher Education Academy and the Association of Chief Police Officers 'Forensic Science Sector Training Strategy Group'.

At a meeting of UKSFEG in 2011, a representative of the National Policing Improvement Agency (NPIA) gave an overview of the Association of Chief Police Officers (ACPO) remit regarding research in forensic science into the next decade. Building on the publication of the 'Science and Innovation Strategy for Policing' document, published in 2011 (https://connect.innovateuk.org/documents/3144739/3824722/Live-time+Forensics+brochure(draftv6LR).pdf/a65350a2-683d-4476-9a1e-99c1883ae33e), this presentation outlined the ACPO Forensic Strategy as a framework for national research, with the more immediate timescale of 2011–2015. Arising from this framework, three work streams were to be commissioned to provide an initial focus for the needs of the Police with respect to developments in forensic science. These work streams were:

(a) Improving the custody process with respect to forensic evidence and database information.
(b) Digitising crime scenes, both with respect to recording the crime scene and using on-site tests.
(c) Personal identification.

What became clear was the discordant understanding between the policing and HEI forensic aims and objectives for research into the next decade. The 2012 ACPO document 'Harnessing Science Innovation for Forensic Investigation in Policing' (https://connect.innovateuk.org/documents/3144739/3824722/Live-time+Forensics+brochure(draftv6LR).pdf/a65350a2-683d-4476-9a1e-99c1883ae33e) has offered the opportunity for dialogue and development of research plans between HEIs and organisations such as the UK Home Office 'Centre for Applied Science and Technology'.

In 2011 the 'Lowering the Drawbridges' report (McCartney *et al.*, 2011) into the inter-relationship of education between the legal and scientific communities demonstrated the desperate need for pedagogic harmonisation for those entering into a criminal justice framework in education as students or in practice as graduates. The imperative is for law educators and science educators to 'lower their drawbridges' and seek mutually beneficial solutions to common educational problems, not only to reap benefits for students, but also to contribute towards developing the legal/forensic science professions of the future, and ultimately, assist the Criminal Justice System in realising its ideals and objectives.

In part, this issue is confirmed by an earlier report by Samarji (2012), who suggested that forensic science education is arbitrarily organised, as the forensic science courses considered in his study possessed no clear pattern(s) of:

(a) The knowledge fields that should be incorporated (e.g. chemistry, biology, mathematics, physics, law and/or forensic subjects).
(b) The place and extent of practice, the non-consensus on the academic level at which forensic science education should start (non-award, undergraduate and/or postgraduate).

In the United States, the American Academy of Forensic Sciences (AAFS) website revealed over 155 undergraduate forensic science programmes, nearly 70% of which lead to bachelor's degrees in forensic science or in forensic science associated with other disciplines such as chemistry, biology, criminal justice, anthropology and/or psychology (AAFS, https://www.aafs.org/).

The non-award programmes (~30%) distribute between associate degrees, certificate programmes and training programmes mainly in forensic DNA profiling. In the United Kingdom, forensic science education is no less popular. The number of students studying forensic science degrees increased from 2191 in 2002–2003 to 5664 in 2007–2008 (Skills for Justice, 2009).

At one point in time there were over 500 listed combinations of undergraduate courses with 'forensic' in the title being offered by over 70 British universities (Daéid and Roux, 2010).

The picture that emerges from what has been described from forensic science and its education is a long way from 'rosy.' The changing climate of the introduction of student fees, the increased pressure upon academic staff with the industrialisation of their roles and the burdens of ever increasing administrative responsibilities being placed upon them do nothing to foster a climate of enthusiastic experimentation and innovation to change the status quo in the arena of forensic Higher Education in the United Kingdom.

The bleakness of the forensic and general sciences job market globally, the expectations of students, increasing student numbers and increasing pressure upon the academic community generally, have led to a rethink of *who, what, why, when and how* we do our jobs as educationalists.

A quote from Woods (2010), a former CEO of Science for Justice, demonstrates the recognition of the requirement for HEI–practitioner partnerships:

> …lead the way globally in the delivery of higher education in forensic science… bringing together the universities and forensic science employers to work in partnership.
>
> *Woods, 2010*

In June 2011, Professor Bernard Silverman (Silverman, 2011) the Chief Scientific Adviser to the Home Office reported that:

> There are several factors, in addition to the managed closure of a major provider (the FSS), which make it timely to carry out this review. These include the distributed nature of forensic science provision, the rapid pace of scientific and technological advances in various areas, and the changing nature of public sector research funding and accountability.
>
> Overall the research landscape [in forensic science research] that has developed is varied and in some ways fragmented, and improvement in the degree of linkage and communication would drive forward innovation most effectively.
>
> *Silverman, 2011*

Whereas in the past academia concerned themselves mainly with science and the law, there are now courses inculcating policing and policing science into the equation.

This strengthens, not dilutes, what we have to teach, but we now have to be mindful of the changing landscape of policing and of intelligence and evidence gathering. The changing manpower structures as outlined in the Neuroyd report (2011) require a more efficient and transparent police service at a much cheaper cost, and this adds a new layer to what academics have to deliver on many of the HEI courses, for example, business protocols, budgetary awareness, working with constraints, systematic and strategic thinking.

There has, to date, been no single place in which all of these changes have been recorded, dialogued or even vignetted, so that those new to the profession, interested in the subject, or just plain 'nosey' about CSI-UK, can come and drink from the huge well of knowledge that has been created since forensic science undergraduate degrees exploded on the educational landscape in the mid-1990s. Now over two decades on, it is time for a retrospective and a prospective dialogue to map-out and to create a 'road map' of the way forward for the next decade.

It is also very important to be able to educate and prepare teachers and instructors to deal with teaching in an area such as this, requiring non-traditional methods. Some excellent classroom instructors and teachers struggle adjusting to the use of computer-based teaching, virtual formats and social networking tools, because the dynamics between the instructor and the student are very different and require more forethought and create different challenges than traditional teaching methods. All of these changes have taken place in the face of social changes in learning style and structure impacted upon by technology. 'Clicker technology' and Twitter, Instagram, Snapchat, Skype, Facebook, tablet technology and indeed perniciously invasive mobile phone technology have changed the way students engage with each other and with academics in their teaching and learning strategies. We will look to the **best aspects** of these to determine how we can more fully engage with students to facilitate their autonomous, deep and self-directed learning without damaging the pedagogic experience to produce forensic scientists with a continuing drive to learn and develop once in forensic practice.

Innovative teaching methods are required to deal with increased numbers of students, diverse student populations and the demand for value for money, as well as increased competition with other HEI educational providers. In order to understand and therefore to fully appreciate the current status of forensic science in the United Kingdom, the recent history of forensic science in its educational context should be considered. The 'science' behind forensic science cannot simply be discussed in isolation but must be done cognisant of government policy, policing requirements and initiatives and the politics and business practices that pervade every aspect of the science that is designed to assist the pursuit of justice into the twenty-first century.

Neumann observed that when he began his undergraduate degree in Switzerland, no one wanted to work in forensic science and only a small number of training programmes existed worldwide (Neumann, 2011). By the early 1990s there was a global proliferation of courses 'churning-out' forensic scientists. This visibility was clearly fuelled by forensic science-based television dramas, which to date have increased and appear likely to do so for the foreseeable future.

Over the past two decades, forensic science has begun to emerge as a field of study in which academia worldwide has literally hundreds of universities offering forensic science programmes (Quarino and Brettell, 2009; NIFS, 2006).

Such a need urged the expansion of these laboratory services, which in turn created new forensic science positions to be filled by individuals with the essential skills and science education, specifically in the areas of chemistry, biology and biochemistry (Quarino and Brettell, 2009).

According to Smallwood (2002) the popularity of forensic science is now such that 'every third person on the planet has expressed an interest in becoming a forensic scientist.'

However, as indicated by Robertson (2012), media representations are argued to have created an influence of unrealistic perceptions of forensic science in the public in relation to what a forensic practitioner can in reality do and the timeframe it takes to obtain results and answers. As a senior forensic colleague of mine regularly recounts in lectures 'on the television, crimes are solved in 60 minutes including commercial breaks – in my job it can take years!' (Dr Roger Summers, retired UK head of forensic services Derbyshire Police, personal communication).

Forensic science programmes were often housed within a university chemistry department and treated educationally as a chemistry derivative (Smallwood, 2002) although it could include other sciences and applications that can be invited to solve cases pertaining to law (Inman and Rudin, 1997). Well over a decade later the situation remains ostensibly the same, particularly in the United Kingdom, but not exclusively; there have been *no* new undergraduate (or postgraduate) forensic science departments created in either the post-1992 universities (once known as polytechnics) or indeed in any of the more traditional and long-established (red-brick) universities. In fact departments of Forensic Medicine are closing in the UK, with London being the only capital city in the world without a university department of Forensic Medicine. There may be many reasons for this, but clearly one of them has to be the cost of setting up the correct educational environment. The laboratories and equipment, although expensive, are a small cost in comparison with employing staff with experience and credibility. Those who are the UK leaders in forensic science educational provision have achieved this staff critical mass over a decade or more.

Since the 1990s, the number of Higher Education providers that offer forensic science courses/programmes have steadily increased in the United States, United Kingdom,

Australia and many other countries (Mennell, 2006; NIFS, 2006). A second example is Australia, where there are currently around 23 forensic science programmes covering various specialisations and academic levels (NIFS, 2006). A third example is the forensic programme at West Virginia University in the United States, where the programme grew from four students in year 1997 to more than 500 students in 2006 (Houck, 2006).

One line of current thinking is that the large number of forensic science programmes are randomly organised, where the curricula of these courses are unstructured, content is delivered in isolation from industry and graduates are not sought after by forensic science agencies. There a number of concerns associated with this increase in demand for student places on forensic-based courses. The first is that there are no forensic science jobs for them to go into as graduates, the second is that the content of the degree courses does not fit with the requirements of the job they would enter as a forensic scientist. However, there is a third and more worrying concern being expressed by a number of *interested parties*, and that is one of maintaining the highest possible standards in the industry.

There is also the tension created by what industry expects a graduate to have in terms of skills for immediate employability and the limitations created by a curriculum in terms of depth and breadth, and also one of content. One of the concerns that employers have voiced relates to the variations in forensic content from one university to another.

Surely a degree is a starting point for further study in the job, and as a newly graduated practitioner, years of study and research lie ahead in order to fully qualify for the title of 'forensic scientist.' There appears to be a blindness within the industry with the newly graduated students being labelled as 'not fit for purpose.' This observation has been unfairly levied; they are indeed fit for further training and for personal development, as indeed the well seasoned forensic practitioners should be if *they* are self-reflective and are themselves to remain competent in a forensic science arena. In order to improve the employability of forensic science graduates the CSFS introduced the pre-employment assessment of competence (PEAC) in 2015. The PEAC award demonstrates the evidence of a candidate's knowledge, skills, reasoning and problem-solving abilities through industry approved assessment (https://www.csofs.org/PEAC).

Universities have been criticised for seizing upon the growing interest of forensic science as a money-making opportunity; this is a bold statement with suggestions of a somewhat unprofessional attitude. However, as with any other 'business' driven venture (despite universities holding 'charitable' status), all UK universities have to survive in a financially constrained environment and it would be naïve, if not negligent to have not seized upon the market opportunity to develop forensic science courses in UK HEIs. That is not to suggest that a multitude of forensic-based courses were simply thrown together. This would be frankly impossible due to the internal and external quality assurance mechanisms that monitor and regularly check the quality of courses and the elements (modules) within those courses in HEIs. Any new programme of study goes through a rigorous process of documentation and validation meetings involving both internal and external panel members – usually from the industry at which the proposed course is aimed.

All documentation is available for scrutiny and auditing. Once the course is running, the programme is then monitored annually by external examiners who are drawn from similar courses or indeed from industry in the United Kingdom. Therefore, the criticisms directed at the quality of educational delivery are ill founded and erroneous. The issue that follows this is one of inappropriate content for the workplace. In 2004, the SEMTA report evidenced concerns that there were only *ad hoc* arrangements through which employers could liaise about the content of courses. Issues such as these have in the main been removed by virtue of having practitioners (both current and retired) on the academic staff and through the dialogue that has occurred through employers forums, closer liaison with regional Police Services and the engagement of the Chartered Society of Forensic Sciences by initiatives such as the accreditation process for universities. It must also be appreciated that academics aim to deliver the most appropriate and up-to-date knowledge and practice to students for the industry in which they are entering.

Again, many of these courses are created by drawing upon the advice from within the forensic industry – indeed it is a requirement of any university programme to demonstrate it has scanned the market place horizon for appropriateness of content and elicited feedback in writing from a suitable spectrum of individuals within that industry.

Welsh and Hannis (2011) reported that employers had commented upon the excellence of some of these forensic graduates, but also that some employers remarked that a number of graduates were not of the quality employers were looking for. Deficiencies such as a 'poor attitude' to the workplace professionalism and poor communication skills were cited as issues by employers.

However, surely this is the nature of any employment sector, some applicants will be excellent and some will not; hence the interview and selection process is a filtering mechanism in any employer's armoury.

In 2004 a report was prepared by SEMTA to consider the implications for Higher Education of the proliferation of forensic undergraduate degree course containing elements of forensic science. Why should such a report have been commissioned? There were, at that time, concerns about the increasing numbers of degrees in relation to the number of jobs available in the forensic science sector and a concern about the quality of skills delivered (SEMTA, 2004). Perhaps a catalyst for this was also the huge public interest and perception as forensic science being one of the most fascinating areas of science within our modern society (Richard Smith – SEMTA, 2004). In the years since the publication of the SEMTA report, forensic science continues to capture the imagination of millions of television viewers, radio listeners and readers.

The high profile of TV crime shows utilising forensic science and its spectrum of specialisms continues to dominate the television ratings and this shows no signs of abating. Indeed the expanding 'bubble' of student interest, which was anecdotally observed in 2002 to have offered forensic science degrees a 'shelf-life' of five years, showed no real evidence of a decline in interest amongst prospective students (the 'bubble' has yet to burst) in UK universities until the last year or so.

Clearly, forensic science has attracted young people to study science who would otherwise not have gone to university or who would, perhaps, have chosen a totally different subject of study. In addition, forensic science attracts a high proportion of female students (Houck, 2009) compared with other comparable science subjects.

The challenge for HEI educators has been for them to up-skill from their particular science specialisms, as many universities started from 'scratch' in terms of forensic educational provision, with respect to equipment and laboratories as well as subject-specific trained staff. Over a decade after this standing-start, most university departments delivering forensic science do so with a staff cohort comprising: academics, forensic scientists, scenes of crime officers and, in some cases, former police officers with 30+ years experience as part of the permanent teaching teams. This staffing development has arisen in part due to the concerns voiced by employers and high profile individuals (from both the police and forensic) communities questioning the skills base and appropriate experience of the academics teaching these degrees.

This situation has presented challenges in two directions. Firstly, the practitioners have had to develop new skills in terms of teaching, learning and assessment and become embedded in the academic world of assessment and award policy and practice – which is quite different to the forensic and policing world from which they came. Secondly, it has required academic staff to up-skill and either develop or indeed learn new forensic skills and techniques. This has facilitated a demand for the change to existing teaching and assessment materials from their 'pure' science context into one of an applied forensic context. It must be remembered that forensic science – 'science in the pursuit of justice' is *still* science but the context of the materials (the physical evidence) being investigated and the data it produces (the scientific evidence) must be evaluated in that context, wherein one key consideration is the statistical validity of such evidence.

The educational landscape in the second decade of the twenty-first century for forensic science remains far from clear.

The report by Welsh and Hannis (2011) presented a picture that forensic science degree programmes offered by UK universities were of a 'good' quality and that they provided the students with a positive learning experience. Yet the industry still reports dissatisfaction with this education and many forensic science graduates struggle to secure employment in the sector.

This book is designed to be a reflective of the current standpoint as to the position of forensic science education in the United Kingdom and beyond. Hopefully, this text will, in part, act as a nucleating medium to initiate, improve and direct dialogue about what forensic science does, how forensic science is taught and conducted and how it can be made more robust and pedagogically fit for purpose.

The national level changes seen in the last few years have had a profound effect upon the way that forensic science is perceived, conducted and indeed taught. The miscarriages of justice, the closure of the UK Forensic Science Service and the rise of independent forensic providers, the introduction of student fees in HEIs, the changes to policing and its education of police officers (Neyroud, 2011) and the changes to UK secondary (high school) examinations all serve to change the landscape in which forensic science and science in general is taught in the United Kingdom. This text will hopefully inform upon and stimulate discussion on future strategic directions to better serve the end users and ultimately the Criminal Justice System.

Although little research on forensic science education has been undertaken or published (Burnet *et al.*, 2001; Fookes, 2003) the benefits and outcomes of such research will facilitate improved insights into how forensic science education could possibly be organised and how such courses could be structured to lead to the graduation of more knowledgeable and more competent forensic practitioners fit for the twenty-first century crime scene, for the forensic laboratory and for the courtroom.

It is an unspoken truism that UK universities have prospered from forensic science educational provision over the last decade in terms of student recruitment, the finances that follow such a rich mine of students and in the reputations that have been built upon such a high (media) profile course. Whilst academics within such institutions have championed their new roles and striven to gain forensic science employer engagement and to develop relationships for both teaching and research opportunities, the rate of progress has been, quite frankly, painfully slow, with the reasons behind this being multi-faceted. A paradigm and step-change in attitudes and levels of engagement are required especially in the light of the closure of the UK Forensic Science Service in order to develop more employable students who have had the opportunities to engage more fully and deeper with the practitioner forensic and legal communities in which they will work. It is at this early educational stage of a scientist's career that they develop the essential skills of good laboratory practice, of ethical conduct in practice and research and the essential communication skills within and without their communities. Thus when is there a better time for young forensic scientists to become encultured into the multi-layered of policing and legal colleagues? To reiterate McCartney *et al.* (2011):

> This need for an improved dialogue between law and science is clear: educational boundaries need to be attenuated if forensic science is to deliver real benefits for the criminal justice system, with attendant risks minimised.
>
> *McCartney et al., 2011*

The exponential expansion in forensic science education since 2000 has attracted both authentic and inauthentic investments in such education by HEIs and more recently investment by colleges in foundation degrees. This investment in forensic science education can only be considered authentic when a course can emphasise the four zones of forensic science knowledge, reflect the ontological and epistemological nature of forensic science and manage the complexities that face forensic science education (Samarji, 2012).

There is a risk in such an educational expansion that a course will be 'inauthentic' if such a course fails to properly emphasise these four zones of forensic science knowledge and is unable to manage forensic science complexities, and perhaps most worryingly, is run in isolation from industry stakeholders (the forensic science power groups).

As Samarji (2012) eloquently remarked, an opportunity emerges from a critical integration of Maxwell's view of science as aim-oriented empiricism (AOE) with the notions of Bernstein, Kuhn and Pinar. Maxwell's notion of AOE raises questions about 'whose aims orient forensic science empiricism? Are they the aims of the legal practitioners, police forces, and/or scientists?' Such questions are mainly based on Maxwell's AOE notion, but they ultimately invite and critically integrate with:

- Bernstein's notion of power and control: How can the 'aims' of various power groups orient forensic science empiricism into the one direction or the other?
- Kuhn's notion of the paradigm shift: How can a paradigm shift within forensic science be promoted by certain 'aims' (avante-gardes) and be opposed by other aims (conservative-gardes)?
- Pinar's notion of the curriculum as a conversation: How can a conversation between various groups and stakeholders map various aims and orient forensic science empiricism?

Therefore, within forensic science, there currently exist both authentic and inauthentic forensic science courses in the United Kingdom (Samarji, 2012). Whilst the authentic forensic science courses emphasise the nature of forensic science and respond to its ontological and epistemological complexities, the inauthentic forensic science courses will fail to do so, and in not doing so they will fail to furnish forensic scientists to meet the shifting educational horizons within forensic practice.

One aspect not yet considered here has been the feedback from students: the consumers and customers of this knowledge and experience in HEIs. Whilst internal quality assurance mechanisms (staff–student liaison groups, module monitoring, programme monitoring, periodic review and the External Examiner) are firmly entrenched and tested methods of quality assurance, there is again little in the literature considering students perspectives. Hanson and Overton (2010) conducted a survey for the UK Higher Education Academy into the skills required by new forensic science graduates and their development in degree programmes (see also Fowler *et al.*, 2013; Turner and Yates, 2012).

The aim of the survey was to identify which areas of the forensic science curriculum (including generic skills) were particularly useful for new graduates and to evaluate how well they are developed within undergraduate forensic science degrees. The survey questionnaire aimed to determine which areas of knowledge and skills developed in the degree programmes had been of most use since graduation and how well they had been developed within the degree programmes. Completed survey forms were received from a total of 147 graduates from seven universities (78 from Chartered Society of Forensic Sciences accredited courses, 69 from non-accredited), an overall response rate of 33%. The areas and knowledge included in the survey are shown in Table 1.1 and demonstrated that core skills were considered highly valuable, with the forensic specific activities showing a similar level of importance.

Intriguingly, students reported that they would have liked greater opportunity to develop areas of knowledge and skills; see Figure 1.1. This offers a starting point for development of teaching and assessment to take these aspects further – such as quality assurance, health and safety issues and trace evidence recovery.

It is anticipated that the future of forensic science will experience migration of more science into forensic field practices (Samarji, 2012). This migration will result in further shifts of the current reigning paradigm towards the explicitly scientific reigning paradigm.

Table 1.1 Areas of knowledge and skills included in questionnaire

A	Crime scene management
B	Crime scene investigation
C	Crime scene evidence interpretation
D	Location and recovery of trace materials
E	Forensic analysis techniques
F	Instrumental methods of analysis
G	Interpretation of analytical results
H	Safe working procedures
I	Quality assurance
J	Planning of casework related experiments
K	Understanding relevant legal procedures

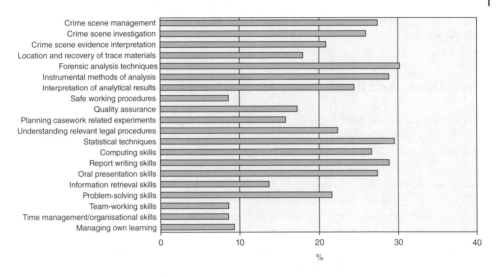

Figure 1.1 Percentage of all graduates indicating they would have liked more opportunity to develop the areas of knowledge/skills in their degree.

This will create research opportunities in forensic field areas and will facilitate stronger and more flexible partnerships between education providers and law enforcement agencies. These anticipated changes in forensic science will support the sustainability of the authentic forensic science courses on the one hand, whilst challenging that of inauthentic forensic science educational courses, and as such it will question their existence within the UK HEI sector.

Forensic science is a field of contention between various contexts, cultures and mindsets (scientific versus police/judicial). It is a field of an unconfirmed reigning paradigm but confirmed complexities associated with the paradigm. Hence, educational decisions related to forensic science may best be approached through a Pinarian conversation that maps the various complexities within the field and negotiates the distinct interests, preferences and concerns of various forensic social groups and forensic science students.

However, there is scant evidence that the present difficulties with specialisation within UK universities will be overcome soon. Inertia within the regulatory bodies for forensic science and Higher Education institutional management is a sufficient deterrent for those who may entertain thoughts of tinkering with the status quo. Perhaps, until the political classes and the public demand a more transparent and better linked forensic science–legal–police service, miscarriages of justice will be the inevitable outcome of the on going 'dialogue of the deaf' between forensic stakeholders in the UK.

There are many aspects not covered in this introductory chapter; we have left aspects relating to the 'here and now' and to the future until the final chapter to allow the reader to assimilate some of the work from the current educational landscape. Some essential aspects to consider are the closure of the UK Forensic Science Service, the UK House of Commons Science and Technology Select Committee reports on the current position of UK forensic science and the current practices involving (ISO) Accreditation, Quality Assurance and the Universities Research Excellence Framework Exercise. The effect these will have upon forensic science and its likely directions over the next 5–10 years will be discussed.

Conclusions and Implications for Teaching and Practice

It is important for the future development of forensic science education that the future direction includes the three groups of key participants, namely, educators, practitioners and users of forensic science (Police Services and Courts), all critical in approaching the nature of forensic science and forensic science education through different lenses. This triangulation practice is also essential in identifying the various social groups existing within forensic science and in representing their preferences in organising forensic science education and ensuring it is fit for purpose in the real world using competencies and accreditations strategies. The Forensic Regulator (who is a public appointee whose function is to ensure that the provision of forensic science services across the criminal justice system is subject to an appropriate regime of scientific quality standards) is in on going discussion with HEIs through appropriate educational forums, such as the CSFS, UKSFEG and independent organisations, such the Forensic Institute Research Network and the QAA. The educational impact of the UK Government Forensic Regulator recommendation that all providers of forensic science services gain accreditation from the United Kingdom Accreditation Service (UKAS), is still percolating through HEI curricula.

The pedagogy and adrogogy of teaching, learning and assessment (TLA) have been discussed by numerous workers and researchers across all the subject specific disciplines, yet there remains a paucity of literature to contextualise this within a forensic science teaching environment. Race (2014, 2003) has published widely on TLA and paraphrased Einstein's comment that 'It is simply madness to keep doing the same thing, and expect different or improved results.' If this is true for forensic science (and therefore for policing based studies), this book hopes to deal with some of these issues by addressing this paucity of literature and using the experiences of those academics and practitioners in the field. This provides the opportunity to share their experiences with other colleagues to facilitate assessment, reflection and development of their methods, manners and mechanisms of teaching, learning and assessment in a forensic context.

References

Burnett, A., Brand, J. and Meister, M. (2001) Forensics education? How the structure and discourse of forensics promotes competition. *Argumentation & Advocacy*, **38** (2), 106–115.

Cullingford, C. and Blewitt, J. (2004) The Sustainability Curriculum: The Challenge for Higher Education. Earthscan, London. ISBN 9781853839481.

Daéid, N.N. and Roux, C. (2010) Section IV: Education in forensic sciences, in *Fifty Years of Forensic Science: A Commentary* (ed. N.N. Daéid), Wiley-Blackwell, West Sussex, UK.

Engber, D. (2005) It's a killer course (West Virginia University), *The Chronicle of Higher Education*, **51** (24).

Fookes, B.G. (2003) Forensic science program research information. Forensic Science Program, Department of Chemistry, University of Central Florida, Personal Communication (18 June 2003) in, Samarji, A.N. (2010) *Mapping the complexity of forensic science: implications for forensic science education.* PhD thesis, Victoria University. http://vuir.vu.edu.au/17880/ (accessed 27 November 2016).

Fowler, M., Brawn, R., Marriott, A., Roy, P.L., Scott, N., and Patterson, H. (2013) *Addressing the Employability Needs of Forensic Science Graduates.* Available at: https://www.heacademy.ac.uk/resources/detail/resources/detail/STEM/conf-proceedings-2013/Phys/Addressing_employability_needs#sthash.efp2CUuJ.dpuf(accessed June 2015).

Garrison, D.H. (1991) Bad science, *Midwestern Association of Forensic Scientists Newsletter*, Oct. 1991.

Hamer, D. (2012) The R v T controversy: forensic evidence, law and logic law. *Probability and Risk*, **11** (4), 331–345.

Hannis, M. and Welsh, C. (2009) *Fit for Purpose? Research into the Provision of Forensic Science Degree Programmes in UK HEIs.* Sheffield, UK: Skills for Justice. http://www.skillsforjustice.com/websitefiles/Skills%20for%20Justice%20Forensic%20Science%20HE%20Report(2).pdf (accessed 8 May 2010).

Hanson, S. and Overton T. (2010) Skills required by new forensic science graduates and their development in degree programmes. *The Higher Education Academy Physical Sciences Centre*, 978-1-903815-30-4.

Houck, M.M. (2006) CSI: Reality. *Scientific American*, **295** (1), 84–89.

Houck, M.M. (2009) Is forensic science a gateway for women in science? *Forensic Science Policy & Management*, **1** (1), 65–69.

House of Commons Science & Technology Select Committee (2005) *Forensic Science on Trial.* Seventh Report of Session 2004–2005. The Stationery Office Ltd, London, 2005–2004-05 HC 427.

Inman, N. and Rudin, K. (1997) *An Introduction to Forensic DNA Analysis*, 2nd edn, CRC Press Boca Raton, Florida

Jonakait, R.N. (1991) Forensic science: the need for regulation, *Harvard Journal of Law & Technology*, **4** (109), 1–72.

Lewis, S., Brightman, R. and Roux, C. (2005) *Forensic Science Tertiary Education in Australia.* Melbourne, Australia: Royal Australian Chemical Institute. http://www.raci.org.au/chemaust/docs/pdf/2005/CiAApril2005p4.pdf (accessed 11 February 2007).

McCartney, C., Cassella, J. and Chin, P. (2011) *'Lowering the Drawbridges' Legal and Forensic Science Education for the 21st Century.'* Available at: http://www.ukcle.ac.uk/projects/past-projects/mccartney/ (accessed June 2015).

Mennell, J. (2006) The future of forensic and crime scene science. Part II. A UK perspective on forensic science education. *Forensic Science International*, **157** (1), 13–20.

National Academy of Sciences (2009) *Strengthening Forensic Science in the United States: A Path Forward*, Committee on Identifying the Needs of the Forensic Sciences Community; Committee on Applied Theoretical Statistics, National Research Council. ISBN: 0-309-13131-6, (2009) http://www.nap.edu/catalog/12589.html 9 (accessed 17 August 2015).

National Institute for Forensic Science (NIFS) (2006) *Australian Forensic Science: Education and Training for the Future, a Review of the Current Status of Forensic Science Education and Training in Australia and Options for the Future.* Docklands, Australia:

NIFS. http://www.nifs.com.au/Report% 20Final%20August%20Part%20A.pdf (accessed March 2012).

Neumann, C. (2011) Forensics: The call of the crime lab. *Nature*, **473**, 409–411.

Neyroud, P. (2011) *Review of Police Leadership and Training*, Home Office, London, April 2011. Available at: http://www.homeoffice.gov.uk/publications/consultations/rev-police-leadership-training/ (accessed 27 November 2016).

Quarino, L. and Brettell, T.A. (2009) Current issues in forensic science higher education, *Analytical and Bioanalytical Chemistry*, **394**, 1987–1993, Springer, published online, Available [pdf format] at: http://www.springerlink.com/content/u7067m4317502727/fulltext.pdf (accessed 6 September 2010).

Race, P. (2003) *Designing Assessment to Improve Physical Sciences Learning.* Available at: https://www.heacademy.ac.uk/sites/default/files/ps0069_designing_assessment_to_improve_physical_sciences_learning_march_2009.pdf(accessed 17 August 2015).

Race, P. (2014) *Making Learning Happen*, 3rd edn, Sage, London.

Robertson, J. (2012) Forensic science, an enabler or dis-enabler for criminal investigation? *Australian Journal of Forensic Sciences*, **44** (1), 83–91 http://dx.doi.org/10.1080/00450618.2011.595736.

Samarji, A. (2012) Forensic science education: Inquiry into current tertiary forensic science courses, *Forensic Science Policy & Management*, **3**, 24–36.

Science, Engineering, Manufacturing Technologies Alliance (SEMTA) Sector Skills Council, (2004) *Forensic Science: Implications for Higher Education 2004, UK* [pdf format], p. 88. Available at: <http://www.physsci.heacademy.ac.uk/Publications/ForensicScience/ForensicScienceReport2004.pdf> SEMTA Forensic Science: Implications for Higher Education 2004, Training Publication Ltd, ISBN 1 84019 189 9 (accessed June 2015).

Silverman, B. (2011) *Research and Development in Forensic Science: a Review* www.homeoffice.gov.uk/.../fsr/forensic-science-review/forensic-science-review-report?view=Binary (accessed June 2015).

Skills for Justice (2009) *Forensic Science Degree Programmes - Are They up to Scratch?* Available at: http://www.skillsforjustice.com/template01.asp?pageid=718 (accessed June 2015).

Smallwood, S. (2002) As seen on TV: "CSI" and "The X-Files" help build forensics programs. *Chronicle of Higher Education*, **48** (45).

Turner, G. and Yates, P. (2012) *NSS Report for Physical Sciences* https://www.heacademy.ac.uk/resource/nss-report-physical-sciences (accessed 17 August 2015).

Welsh, C. and Hannis, M. (2011) Are UK undergraduate forensic science degrees fit for purpose? *Science and Justice*, **51** (3) 139–142.

Woods, A. (2010) Guest Editorial. *Science & Justice*, **50** (2), 53–54.

Further Resources

Education and Training in Forensic Science. *A Guide for Forensic Science Laboratories, Educational Institutions, and Students*, https://www.ncjrs.gov/pdffiles1/nij/203099.pdf (accessed 17 August 2015).

Higher Education Academy – Knowledge Hub, https://www.heacademy.ac.uk/search/site/forensic (accessed 17 August 2015).

2

Forensic Anthropology Teaching Practice

Anna Williams

University of Huddersfield, School of Applied Sciences, Queensgate, Huddersfield, UK

Introduction

Forensic anthropology has become highly popular as a subject for both undergraduate and postgraduate courses. It is, in many ways, a victim of its own success. As its popularity in popular culture goes from strength to strength, and forensic anthropologists become household names, more people are viewing it as a viable career choice and wanting to gain qualifications in the subject. In order to cope with this increase in demand, and to capitalise upon the popularity of the subject, more universities and further education (FE) institutions are designing and delivering programmes that offer forensic anthropology courses. Some are adapting existing courses and using existing staff, whilst some are bringing in new expertise to create new courses.

Student numbers are increasing, as are student (and parent) expectations and demands, fuelled by rising tuition fees and maintenance costs, not just in the UK but in the global educational market. The portrayal of forensic anthropology and its experts in television drama and popular science programmes, as well as in literature, has, to some extent, encouraged students to form exaggerated and often unrealistic expectations of the capability of the subject and the prowess of its practitioners. As a result, teaching staff are under growing pressure to deliver high quality forensic anthropology teaching with limited resources.

Forensic anthropology teaching practice is a broad subject that could include everything from student recruitment to graduation and employability. This is beyond the scope of this chapter, and so it focusses on some of the most pertinent, practical issues facing teachers, lecturers and trainers of forensic anthropology today. It covers matters such as: organisation and design of practical sessions; how to teach forensic anthropology with a small skeletal reference collection; the nature of spotter examinations and their value as assessment tools; and the importance of students experiencing postmortem examinations in a forensic anthropology context. The aim of this chapter is to collate the most appropriate approaches from current forensic anthropology teaching practices from around the United Kingdom and internationally. This should provide

Forensic Science Education and Training: A Tool-kit for Lecturers and Practitioner Trainers, First Edition.
Edited by Anna Williams, John P. Cassella, and Peter D. Maskell.
© 2017 John Wiley & Sons Ltd. Published 2017 by John Wiley & Sons Ltd.

eager and resourceful teachers of this subject with inspiration and possible solutions to well-known and frequently-felt problems and issues with teaching, learning and assessment of this burgeoning subject.

Practical Teaching Methods

While in many sciences, the *lecture* is still the main method of delivering 'content' (Overton, 2003), laboratory and practical classes contribute significantly to the education of scientists or engineers (Boud, 1986), and most academics view this type of activity as essential and non-negotiable.

Forensic anthropology is a highly vocational discipline, which demands a high level of practical content. Practical laboratory sessions are the environment in which forensic anthropologists will develop the skills necessary for professional practice and employment. However, practical sessions are expensive in terms of staff time, consumables, support staff and equipment, and so it is vital that the experience is as effective as possible (Overton, 2003). In forensic anthropology, this is particularly relevant because the raw material for a laboratory practical is often human skeletal remains.

Practical laboratory classes have explicit and implicit aims. Apart from furnishing students with the valuable hands-on experience they need to become professionals, the sessions also provide many basic transferrable skills. Ostensibly, the classes enable students to learn how to implement the basic techniques of forensic anthropology practice, such as estimation of age at death, or determination of sex, or estimation of ethnic ancestry for example. It gives them practice evaluating the skeletal evidence and interpreting the observations they make. However, in addition to these overt learning objectives, there are other, more tacit aims, such as: gaining familiarity with the necessary equipment or tools; testing hypotheses; developing safe working practices; using judgement; and developing communication skills and independent thinking.

In forensic anthropology teaching, practical laboratory sessions can be used at every stage of the learning process. In fact, they are particularly valuable at the beginning, as a way to 'level the playing field' if there is a range of student abilities and experience within the cohort.

Basic Anatomy Teaching

Before a student of forensic anthropology can expect to master the techniques of building an osteological profile of unknown remains, s/he has to gain a thorough knowledge and familiarity with human skeletal anatomy. The objective of teaching human skeletal anatomy is to allow students to become familiar with touching and handling bone, recognising bone from non-bone material, distinguishing between human bone characteristics and that of non-human bone, and becoming conversant with human bone shapes and sizes, or general morphology.

The best method for teaching anatomy is widely debated (Kerby *et al.*, 2011), but forensic anthropology teaching practice can learn from extensive research that has been conducted into new and innovative anatomy teaching methods for medical and biomedical sciences students. The study by Kerby *et al.* (2011) has shown that, for students at least, hands-on dissection of cadavers and demonstrations of dissection and prosection by teachers, is the most 'fit for purpose' method for imparting anatomical information, providing a three-dimensional appreciation of the body and an appreciation of anatomical and biological variation. However, recent updating of medical school curricula has led to traditional, didactic methods of teaching anatomy, based solely on cadaver dissection and prosection, being branded as outmoded (Kerby *et al.*, 2011), and a move towards problem-based teaching and the use of advanced interactive technology.

Anatomy teaching for forensic anthropology students is no different. Some universities place a heavy emphasis on gross anatomy teaching for their forensic anthropology students, and are lucky enough to have facilities for receiving donated cadavers and large dissecting laboratories. This is arguably an ideal situation, but not all universities are in the position to offer such resources. Fortunately, human skeletal anatomy can be taught in a range of ways, incorporating traditional methods such as dissection, or using advanced interactive technology, and even with relatively low-tech and inexpensive equipment, without necessarily compromising teaching quality.

There are many hundreds, if not thousands, of inexpensive teaching aids readily available on the internet for teaching human (and faunal) anatomy. A generous sprinkling of these activities within anatomy sessions can help to lift a traditionally dry subject, increase learner enthusiasm and participation and make it more enjoyable for students and teachers. The American Association of Anatomists (www.anatomy.org) has a multitude of resources available for members and non-members, including links to anatomy image databases, educational animations and videos, apps for anatomy revision and digital libraries.

It is also possible to enthuse and excite learners through using a variety of teaching techniques that encourage deep learning (see later). Human skeletal anatomy need not be a boring subject, characterised by rote learning of Latin names. Just a few suggestions of ways to make anatomy teaching more fun, for learner and teacher, which can be adapted for the class, topic, or experience of the learners, are as follows.

Quizzes

- These can be competitive or non-competitive, and can involve students working in groups or independently.
- Flash cards with pictures of bones or bony landmarks that students have to name and describe against the clock.
- Unlabelled diagrams that students have to label correctly in competition with other groups.
- 'Buzzer round quiz', where students are issued a buzzer and have to answer quick-fire questions, either in groups or as individuals. These can be adapted to follow well-known quiz formats such as '*Who Wants to Be a Millionaire?*', '*University Challenge*' or '*Blockbusters*', to name a few. Questions could be tailored for the knowledge base of the students. Examples include: 'Name the three ossicles', or 'Which part of which muscle originates at the superior surface of the acromion process?' Questions can also include pictures or reference specimens. Individual students or groups accumulate groups and prizes can be awarded to the group that answers most questions correctly.

Activities

- Drawing around one member of the group lying down on a large piece of paper and then placing bones and appropriate labels in the correct anatomical position on the template. This can be used for very early familiarisation with skeletal anatomy, and is ideal for complete beginners. It is advisable to use plastic replicas of bones for this activity.

- Black and white diagrams that students colour in during class time or at home as a revision aid. Websites such as Biodidac (http://biodidac.bio.uottawa.ca/) (Morin, 1995) offer suitable diagrams.

Games

- 'Hand Bone Bingo' can be played to encourage identification of the carpals. Each student is given a bingo card and a handful of carpals. Names of bones are called out and a student who correctly identifies the bones at his/her station and has a row or a column on the bingo card shouts 'Bingo!' to win. This can obviously be applied to other groups of bones (Beckett, Cranfield University, UK, personal communication, 2011).
- Dentition '*Guess Who?*' This is an innovative game invented by Beckett (personal communication, 2011), which requires students to eliminate possible identities for a mystery tooth by discussing tooth characteristics. For example, the answer to the question 'Does the tooth have a double root?' eliminates several possibilities.
- Bone 'Botticelli/20 questions'. A sticky note with the name of a bone (or muscle, etc.) is placed on the forehead of each student, who cannot see it. Using only 'yes' or 'no' questions, up to a limit of 20 questions to fellow students, s/he must work out the identity of the bone on the sticky note.

Anatomy colouring books such as Kapit and Elson (2001) are always popular with students, as a learning and revision aid. Photocopies of the pages relevant to the course can be given to the students to take home.

Reciprocal peer teaching with students demonstrating dissection or anatomical structures to their peers is also very effective (Krych *et al.*, 2005). Not only does it assist the students who are demonstrating to learn (about a tenth of the class), with 100% of students in the study by Krych *et al.* (2005) reporting that the experience increased their understanding of the topics they taught, but it is also beneficial to the students being taught by their peers. In this study, 68% of students felt their retention as learners had increased. In addition, reciprocal peer teaching also fosters development of transferrable skills that can help employment, such as oral presentation, team work, communication, decision making and instils confidence (Krych *et al.*, 2005). From the teacher's perspective, it offers an alternative to didactic or individual teaching, and keeps the students engaged.

Forensic Anthropology Basic Techniques

Practical teaching of the basic techniques of biological anthropology can be difficult to do without access to real human skeletons. As it is fundamentally an analysis of human skeletal variation, it is necessary to gain an appreciation of the wide spectrum of skeletal morphology through examination of as many skeletons as is possible. Gaining such comprehensive knowledge is a life-long task, and cannot be imparted through a single Higher Education course, no matter how long it is. However, universities and HEIs can do their best to expose students to a range of skeletal material in an attempt to demonstrate the continuum of many skeletal features. For example, an interesting activity to propose in a practical class about sex estimation is to choose one skeletal feature (e.g. the greater sciatic notch), and then ask all the students in the class to bring forward the left ilium from the skeleton they are working on, and to arrange the notches in ascending order of width. Ask the class to draw the arbitrary line that we might use to differentiate between male and female greater sciatic notches, or the two lines that delineate the 'indeterminate' category.

In an ideal situation, a large number of skeletons in reasonable state of preservation would be used, to familiarise students with the individual variation visible on the skeleton. Of course, the teaching of the standard biological anthropology techniques, such as estimation of sex, estimation of age at death, stature estimation and estimation of ethnic ancestry, can be supplemented with the use of plastic casts and reference material. In fact, it is very difficult to do so without the use of reference casts, unless the department has access to a huge skeletal collection with examples of all ages, sexes, ethnicities and so on. France Casting Ltd (www.francecasts.com) have an excellent range of ageing and sexing standards, providing 'classic', archetypal models of each feature.

Taphonomy

Practical taphonomy exercises can take many forms, and many rely on the presence of, or regular access to, a taphonomy research facility (see Chapter 4). Small scale taphonomy exercises can be set up by depositing chicken carcasses or pork belly pieces in plastic boxes, which can be left in different environments (e.g. outside, in a refrigerator, underwater) for varying lengths of time, dependent on available resources. Students can then be tasked with describing the extent of decomposition present, charting the temperature and accumulated degree days and calculating rate of decomposition. This can tie in well with entomology exercises where students identify species of insect colonising the carcasses, monitor the development of maggots and calculate post-mortem (or in this case, post-deposition) intervals.

Comparative Faunal Osteology

Comparative faunal osteology exercises are an important ingredient for forensic anthropology courses, as practising forensic anthropologists need to be able to reliably and accurately distinguish between human and animal bone. Such classes should furnish the students with the tools to begin an identification of species by recognising features that allow vertebrate classification into broad Class categories such as bird, reptile, fish, amphibian, mammal, and then further into Orders such as Carnivora or Artiodactyla. Specimens of non-human animal skeletons can be viewed in natural history museums. Some museums host activity days and allow visitors to handle specimens, and some offer visits by curators and experts who bring a collection of specimens to the university. It is also a good idea to create a 'defleshing laboratory', where animal specimens brought in by staff or students can be cleaned and presented for teaching use. The relative value and ease of the most common defleshing methods are discussed by Mann and Berryman (2012) and McGowan-Lowe (2014).

Teaching Equipment

Equipment such as osteometric boards and callipers can also be sourced relatively cheaply. For example, good quality, hardy plastic osteometric boards that are perfectly adequate for use by undergraduate and masters' students are available from Wards Scientific (www.ward-sci.com). However, they are missing the notch for the tibial measurements from both condyles, but this can easily be created using a hacksaw. Good quality Vernier callipers and spreading callipers are not cheap, but adequate ones can be purchased from the UK company DIYTools (www.diytools.com). Mandibulometers can be made relatively cheaply from templates available on the internet.

Use Of Human Skeletal Material For Teaching Purposes

The use and retention of human remains, be they skeletonised, mummified, fossilised, frozen, embalmed or plasticised, for teaching and educational purposes is a controversial subject, and one that has been the object of debate for centuries. Once viewed as just another type of artefact, and the property of the intrepid collector, human remains are now rightly recognised as culturally, politically, socially and educationally valuable (Cassman *et al.*, 2007), and deserving of special measures to ensure and enshrine their protection and respect. It is incumbent on those who work with human remains to act together to promote improved care and management of human remains and to practice and teach appropriate curation and handling methods for research and teaching specimens (Cassman *et al.*, 2007).

Collections of human remains in United Kingdom and United States cultural and educational institutions are more ubiquitous than commonly thought (Cassman *et al.*, 2007). A survey by the Working Group on Human Remains (2003) discovered that approximately 61 000 human remains are housed in the United Kingdom currently. It has been estimated that, in the United States, approximately 200 000 Native American remains are held in US cultural institutions (Cassman *et al.*, 2007).

Although it is possible to provide quality forensic anthropology teaching without access to real human skeletal remains (see next section), the use of real human material is undeniably preferable for the majority of courses, for a variety of reasons. Access to real human material can be used to engender a climate of respect for the deceased amongst the next generation of forensic scientists, allow the visualisation and appreciation of a myriad of anatomical relationships and interactions that cannot be grasped from casts or replicas, as well as allowing the appreciation of the nuances of human variation within certain populations, which is not represented fully by the reproduction of select specimens. Of course, the use of real human skeletons by universities and HEIs is not to be taken lightly, and they must adhere to specific codes of practice written to protect the dignity of the human remains and their descendants. There are several published Codes of Ethics and Standards of Practice to choose from, but those from the British Association of Biological Anthropologists and Osteoarchaeologists (BABAO, 2010) and the American Association of Physical Anthropologists (2003) are particularly useful.

Access to Skeletal Collections

It is recommended that those Science/Anthropology departments wishing to house human remains incorporate the storage and curation of human skeletal remains into a mission statement, which expressly states the reasons for the retention of human remains, and eliminates ambiguity about their use, who has access to them and who is responsible for their curation (Cassman *et al.*, 2007).

In the UK adherence to the Human Tissue Act (HTA) (2004) and the application for a licence from the Human Tissue Authority are necessary if the intended remains are less than 100 years old. If documentary evidence is provided that proves antiquity of over 100 years, it may be possible to hold and retain human remains collections without such a license.

Forensic anthropology courses that spring up in Archaeology, Human Biology or Anatomy departments are at an advantage over those starting from scratch, because it is likely that the university will already have access to, or even hold their own, reference collections of skeletons or even donated cadavers. Radiology and Podiatry or Nursing departments may also be able to donate bone specimens to Anthropology courses. The retention of such specimens should not necessitate the acquisition of a Human Tissue Licence under the Human Tissue Act (2006), as long as the remains can be proven to be more than 100 years old.

Ideally, every department teaching forensic anthropology would have a comprehensive reference collection of skeletons, encompassing several (at least 20–50) human skeletons in a good state of preservation. This collection should preferably include adult skeletons and infant and sub-adult skeletons, with close-to-intact skulls, long bones, vertebrae, pelves and hands and feet, as well as a collection of skeletons or skeletal elements exhibiting a wide range of pathological and traumatic conditions. This skeletal material could be gathered from donations or from archaeological collections either excavated by the department or borrowed from another institution on a long-term loan. However, in light of the recent rapid growth of demand for forensic anthropology courses, there are currently many university departments building their reference and teaching collections from scratch, and starting from nothing.

In the United Kingdom, there are many museums and educational institutions that are willing to loan skeletal collections to universities without their own collections for teaching, reference or research. Several professional organisations (e.g. The British Association of Biological Anthropologists and Osteoarchaeologists) act as coordinators between institutions willing to donate skeletal collections and university departments desperately seeking them. This 'dating agency' approach can work well, especially for short-term loans. For longer term loans and research, it is worth building a good rapport with a local museum or archaeological unit that might have a reasonably steady stream of skeletal material, and is willing to donate it in exchange for written osteological reports about each individual represented by the assemblage. In particular, museum storage facilities run by local councils (such as the Oxfordshire Museum Service, run by Oxfordshire County Council), may be interested in long-term loans of skeletal material to Forensic Anthropology departments in order to release much needed space.

If the university or HEI conducts its own archaeological excavations, it is usually possible to apply to the Ministry of Justice for permission to retain any excavated human remains for the purposes of research and teaching. Usually, the period allocated for research is limited to two years before reburial is stipulated, but in some cases it may be possible to apply for an extension (Ministry of Justice, 2014). If the remains excavated are known to be less than 100 years old, compliance with the Human Tissue Act

(2006) is necessary. Otherwise, it may be possible to retain them within the university or HEI without an HTA licence.

Health and Safety Considerations

The use of human skeletons for teaching purposes is accompanied by a suite of ethical approvals and Health and Safety considerations that require adherence.

It is imperative that the appropriate Risk Assessments for any laboratory-based practical session using skeleton be carried out, to abide by the Health and Safety Guidelines of the university/HE/FE institution.

A detailed analysis of the risks to HEI staff and students when handling skeletonised human remains is beyond the scope of this chapter, but a thorough account of safety procedures and policies can be found in Arriaza and Pfister (2007).

Handling of dry archaeological skeletal material is associated with minimal risk, but precautions should be taken to avoid and minimise dust inhalation. Latex or non-latex gloves can be worn, and hands must be washed after bone handling. Laboratory white coats are also an appropriate addition to personal protective equipment. It is imperative that no food or drink is allowed in the laboratory.

Additional Health and Safety precautions become necessary when dealing with fleshed, decomposing, mummified remains, or skeletons found in lead coffins, or when undertaking fieldwork in exotic climes. For more details, see Arriaza and Pfister (2007) and Cox *et al.* (2008).

Correct Handling and Storage of Skeletal Remains

Much has been published about safe measures and precautions that should be taken to prevent breakage or damage of human skeletal remains, particularly in the comprehensive *Human Remains: Guide for Museums and Academic Institutions* (Cassman *et al.*, 2007), and the BABAO Code of Practice (BABAO, 2010). This section will crystallise the salient points from the point of view of the academic institution wishing to comply with current standards.

Human remains kept at a university or college should be curated by a dedicated member of staff, preferably one with suitable osteoarchaeological and conservation training. A university's skeletal collection should ideally be housed within a dedicated room or secure location, locked with controlled access and authorised personnel. Storage areas should include racking or shelving for the skeleton boxes, and boxes should be stored off the floor, so as to minimise damage caused by damp or vermin (BABAO, 2010).

Traditionally, durable stapled, lidded, acid-free cardboard boxes with acid-free tissue paper have been used to contain disarticulated dry skeletal remains. These need to be of appropriate size and durability to prevent crushing damage to the bones inside but also from bone on bone contact. Several alternatives to the cardboard box have been proposed, including by Bowram (2003) and Cassman *et al.* (2001). These boxes include internal trays and compartments to protect the delicate specimens inside, but also to ease their removal from the box. These boxes have been designed to be easy to handle by one person and fit through doorways. Intricate labels on the outside reduce the need to open and handle the remains. An interesting addition would be to use Perspex boxes or boxes with Perspex lids to facilitate searching for a particular specimen. Some facilities use drawers with foam linings with channels and voids cut to house individual specimens safely.

Some equipment is necessary to ensure correct handling and protection of skeletal material. Polystyrene rings or bean bags should be used for supporting delicate skulls, and sand trays for positioning single bones during analysis.

The use of adhesives for repair of damaged bones is not recommended (Cassman *et al.*, 2007). The use of support trays with a passive cavity cut in inert plastic foam inside an acid-free cardboard box or tray is a good alternative to adhesive as it allows the fragments to lie in the correct position. Parafilm M laboratory film has also been suggested as an alternative to adhesives, as it is stretchy, inert and clings to irregular surfaces (Cassman *et al.*, 2007).

Student Sensibilities

While most students are very eager to see, handle and experience human skeletal remains, some find dealing with real human skeletons difficult, especially at first. In the author's experience, it is usually when examining the skull and particularly the dentition that students initially express concern, presumably due to the closeness of their appearance to that of a living person. Students can be reassured, and allowed to 'acclimatise' to these activities gradually, but if the sensitivity lasts too long or the student finds it too harrowing after a few days or weeks, it is best to advise alternative study, and possibly a rethink of career. In most students, the initial trepidation evaporates very quickly, especially as the enthusiasm for the subject takes over.

Alternatives to Human Skeletal Material

It is possible to teach high-quality anatomy, osteology and forensic anthropology theory and techniques without consistent access to an exhaustive skeletal reference collection. There are many online resources that can be used *in lieu* of a teaching collection. Many beautifully and accurately detailed three-dimensional images and interactive resources are available on the internet, as software, and available to download. Some incur a charge, but there are sites that offer free demonstration versions of software or are entirely free to access.

The use of digitised anatomy teaching aids, computer visualisation software and apps is discussed in depth in chapter 10. There are various free 'virtual' skeleton visualisation tools available, such as The Virtual Skeleton (www.uwyo.edu/reallearning/virtskel.html), which allows the interactive manipulation and rotation of high-resolution photographs of skeletal elements, as well as images of pathological specimens and specimens exhibiting ballistic trauma. The Online Virtual Human Body (www.intelicus.com/the-online-virtual-human-body), and the Virtual Human Skeleton (http://ivl.imnh.isu.edu/VHS.htm) are other examples of interactive reference skeletons that can be used by students to revise anatomy, or by teachers to design quizzes or activities without needing access to real cadavers. One of the most comprehensive for human and primate osteology is e-skeletons, from the University of Texas (http://www.eskeletons.org/index.html), which offers glossy, high resolution, life size and bigger photographs of disarticulated bones and articulated groups of bones, viewable from all aspects. This is an invaluable aid for students without hands-on access to skeletons, but with access to the internet.

The Digitised Diseases project (www.digitiseddiseases.org) allows free access for educational institutions to an archive of interactive photo-realistic images of approximately 1600 skeletal specimens exhibiting a wide range of pathological conditions. It contains high-resolution images that can be viewed, downloaded and manipulated on screen, tablet or even smart phone. The archive includes images of a wide range of pathological conditions including endocrine, metabolic, infectious, neoplastic, immunological and developmental diseases, as well as degenerative and traumatic conditions, and even some post-mortem modifications for comparison purposes. Digital images have been created through the combination of computerised tomography (CT), 3D topographical, radiographic data and realistic surface rendering, producing rotatable 3D images of specimens that can be downloaded or viewed on screen at all angles. These images could be accessed *en masse* in the lecture theatre, or by groups of students or individuals working independently. Assessments or exercises could set to examine or describe different conditions, or to compare symptoms with physical manifestations of different diseases.

It is possible to facilitate and improve students' learning experiences in the absence of real human remains through the use of interactive digital media such as the Anatomage™ table, specifically designed for teaching anatomy, pathology and medicine. It is a life-size interactive 'dissecting' table made of two plasma touch screens at gurney height. It allows instant manipulation of 3D volumetric images that have been constructed from CT scans, radiographic images, topographical data and surface rendering. It allows visualisation of the different anatomical systems of the body in isolation or combination with each other – instigating an appreciation of how the skeletal system interacts with the musculature or circulatory systems, for example. Its regular use would not replace the use of real cadavers or skeletal material for forensic anthropology teaching, but may allow more HEIs to provide quality teaching without access to mortuaries and extensive skeletal collections. Also, digital storage of the data may be advantageous for HEIs without dedicated human remains storage facilities. The pedagogical uses of the Anatomage™ table are described in more detail in Chapter 10.

Although hands-on experience of real human skeletal remains is obviously preferable, it is possible to teach Human Skeletal Anatomy with plastic casts of skeletal elements. These are readily available on the internet, through companies such as Bone Clones™, France Casting and Ossafreelance. For undergraduate and postgraduate forensic anthropology teaching, it is important to buy the best quality replicas the department can afford. There are many medical grade models and replicas available to suit most budgets, with articulated reference skeletons starting at about $250 (accurate at time of printing) and skull models around the $75 mark. Of course, the more detail that is required, the greater the cost.

The rapidly reducing cost of high-resolution and high-fidelity topographical scanning and 3D printing and the increasing availability of 3D printing facilities in most universities raises the possibility of using this technique for the quick production of resin replicas of bones for teaching purposes. CT scans of individual elements of specific skeletal remains can be taken and clones of the particular elements produced at relatively low cost. This is an excellent way of making multiple copies of unique specimens exhibiting unusual conditions. It also means that the robust resin replicas can be manhandled by students, thus protecting the fragile and precious real remains. From a pedagogical perspective, it can allow students to examine identical skeletons, which could mean that assignment marks more closely reflect true ability rather than the differential state of preservation or completeness of the skeletal remains.

Teaching Forensic Anthropology Theory

Although forensic anthropology is an extremely practical subject, heavily rooted in experimentation and empirical experience, there is a significant theoretical aspect to the discipline. For most masters'-level courses and many undergraduate courses, the primary aim of focussing on forensic anthropology theory is to create graduates cognisant of concepts, possibilities, conflicting theories and viewpoints, and to instil in them a critical awareness of the limitations of the techniques used. Clever teaching of the theoretical background of the subject generates mindful, discerning professionals who do not stray out of their area of expertise and who are conscious of their limits.

Imparting first-hand experience of the failings of age or sex estimation techniques (for example) may be difficult to achieve, and could even be counter-productive if the student is penalised for an incorrect or vague answer. Assessments (discussed later) can be centred around – and reward the student for – recognition of limitations and critique of research methods. This method of teaching can be incorporated into courses through the review of journal articles for presentation to the rest of the class. Several universities in the United Kingdom and United States either do this currently or have done in the recent past. Students are asked to select a recent research article from a forensic science or osteology-based journal and to present a critique of the paper's aims, hypotheses, methods, results and discussion to the class in an exciting and lively manner. The aim of this teaching method is to: allow the students to pursue research into an aspect of forensic anthropology that particularly interests them; practice vital presentation skills; effectively multiply the exposure of the class to current research techniques and recent advancements in the discipline; and encourage critical appreciation of research. Other ways to encourage critical thinking include debating the value of a particular technique or identification method, with one group arguing pro-use and another attempting to discredit its use. This can be applied to everything from ageing adults using cranial suture closure to iris recognition or identification from ear-prints. Exercises that make students think about potential pitfalls of techniques are useful too – laminated cards can be made for each biological anthropology technique covered (e.g. Suchey-Brooks age estimation from the pubic symphysis; or Phenice's techniques for sex determination (Buikstra and Ubelaker, 1994)). The students can then be asked to write possible limitations on sticky notes, and discuss in groups which sticky notes can be stuck/attributed to which technique.

Forensic Cases as Training

Most universities or HEIs offer 'mock' cases to their students as a way of simulating the situations that they might be exposed to in professional life and recreating the challenges they might face, whilst maintaining a safe, controllable environment in which students can learn and make mistakes. There is some debate as to whether students should be allowed to participate in 'live' forensic cases as a training tool or learning exercise. Although the American Board of Forensic Anthropologists (ABFA) and the British Association of Forensic Anthropologists (BAFA) both openly support the active training of undergraduate and postgraduate students in all aspects of forensic anthropology, there is clear need for caution to be applied, and consideration for the potential pitfalls of involving students. In her chapter *Ethical Concerns in Forensic Anthropolog* (Walsh-Haney and Lieberman, 2004), Heather Walsh-Haney describes her own experience as an intern at the C.A. Pound Identification Laboratory in Florida, where she, accompanied by both undergraduate and postgraduate students, recovered and examined hundreds of forensic cases under mentorship of Dr William Maples. Despite encouraging this practice, Maples had expressed concern that student involvement could prove a 'legal Achilles' heel' to the forensic anthropologist when questioned in court. He suggested that barristers from both sides can use the fact that students have had access to evidence as a potential source of damage, compromise or contamination, and as such, a reason to disallow evidence or expert witness testimony, which could ultimately discredit an expert witness and potentially affect the outcome of a trial (Walsh-Haney and Lieberman, 2004). However, Walsh-Haney and many other forensic anthropologists involved in teaching (including the author) would defend student participation in forensic cases, with the obvious caveat that the student is properly trained and supervised (Walsh-Haney and Lieberman, 2004). Access to, and involvement in, real cases is an extremely valuable teaching tool. It is not only useful for learning about the particular circumstances of the case, and specific identification issues or techniques, but it also gives students experience of dealing with forensic science and law enforcement professionals, death industry and medical personnel, potentially with families and the public, and (hopefully) furnishes them with the skills to act professionally and to represent their professional bodies and members of their chosen career appropriately.

Assessment Methods

There are several assessment methods that are commonly used in undergraduate and postgraduate forensic anthropology courses in the United Kingdom, United States and elsewhere. Whilst each course will be slightly different, and have diverse learning objectives catered for by a range of assessment methods, there are some elements of coursework and tests that are almost ubiquitous on biological or forensic anthropology courses.

Spotter Tests

Forensic anthropology 'spotter' tests are a common assessment tool found in most undergraduate and postgraduate forensic anthropology (or physical/biological anthropology) courses in the United Kingdom and the United States. They have gained a legendary, almost mythical, reputation for being gruelling and demanding. Each course facilitator runs them in his/her own way, but the main characteristics of a spotter exam remain the same: the students work their way through 'stations', where they are presented with one or more skeletal elements. They are given a question paper that requires them to identify and 'side' the element(s) within a strict time limit. Once the time limit is up, each student moves on to the next station for the next skeletal element(s) and the next question(s). In most variations of the spotter exam, the students are not allowed to refer to any reference books or lecture notes. In some, conditions are made more difficult as the skeletal elements can be placed inside boxes so the students have to identify them by touch alone. The aim of the spotter exam is to increase competence at identification and 'siding' of bones, and to replicate the circumstances of a real forensic case, where graduates might be presented with a single bone or several bones, which they need to be able to identify quickly, easily and accurately, without referring to a textbook. It aims to encourage deep learning of anatomical features, which will prepare the students well for future professional practice. The skills fostered by a spotter exam regime are ultimately transferrable to osteoarchaeology, human anatomy, archaeological excavation and orthopaedics.

Management of a 'spotter' exam will vary from institution to institution, according to rooms, staff and time available. Ideally, there should be a room big enough to accommodate all students and specimen stations at once, so that the examination does not have to be split and conducted twice. The number of specimen stations should be equal to or greater than the number of students. The stations should be clearly marked and their number and order obvious, to make transition and progression through the stations easy and intuitive. The amount of time given to each station is flexible, according to the number of students and specimens, their experience level and the complexity of the question. As a general rule of thumb, 30 seconds should be enough to identify a bone and side it, but 1 minute can be given for ease. One minute should be more than enough for undergraduates, and 30 seconds plenty for masters' students.

Marking schemes for spotter tests vary considerably between establishments and even individual teachers. A clear marking scheme should be created at the time of the choosing the specimens that make up the spotter exam, and in doing so, a consensus should be reached about the range of answers that could be awarded a mark. Some take a particularly dim view of incorrect spelling of osteological terms, and some can be more lenient. In some instances, negative marking is used to discourage guessing. Spotter exams are useful tools, as they tend to be difficult for a student to pre-empt or 'question spot', and for a student to get consistently correct answers without genuinely knowing the material.

Laboratory Reports

Another tried and tested method of assessment in aorensic anthropology courses is the laboratory report. This can take the form of: an academic, reference-laden scientific article; a concise, recipe-like account of methodology and results; or an expert witness statement aimed at the court. Each engenders different learning outcomes and satisfies different criteria, so should be chosen according to the focus of the course. Expert witness reports are useful for giving students experience of formatting the observations and conclusions based on their observations in appropriate ways for the police and ultimately court audiences.

The layout of an expert witness report can be prescribed by the assessor, usually via a template, or be part of the assessment and can be left to the students to research. In general, it should at least include the following headings:

- Statement of Qualifications and Experience
- Description of the Assemblage

- Assessment of Minimum Number of Individuals
- Estimation of Biological Sex
- Estimation of Chronological Age/Age at Death
- Estimation of Stature
- Estimation of Ancestry/Ethnicity
- Description of Trauma
- Description of Pathological Conditions
- Summary of Conclusions Drawn

Depending on the level of the students and the aim of the assessment, marking schemes can incorporate awards for critique and recognition of the limitations of the techniques described, as well as correct referencing, illustrations and inclusion of contemporaneous notes.

Other assessment methods can include: written examinations involving essay-type questions or multiple choice questions related to forensic anthropology scenarios; the examination a real or mock case and preparation of a full report on the human remains; defence of an expert witness statement under cross examination in a court room; defence of an osteological report in a *viva voce* situation; reconstruction of a series of events leading to death in a mock crime scene with human remains; or presentation of a critical review of current scientific literature related to a particular aspect of forensic anthropology. The choice of assessment methods of course depends on the experience level of the students, the intended learning outcomes of the course and the time available for the assessment period.

Post-Mortem Examinations

One of the most valuable learning experiences for a forensic anthropology student – whether undergraduate or postgraduate – is the opportunity to view a post-mortem examination. This is of direct benefit to the students as it is a chance to see first-hand how cause of death is determined by pathologists, and allows students to put the post-mortem examination in its forensic, social and ethical context. It also reiterates the distinction between forensic pathology and forensic anthropology, which is often lost in modern portrayals of the subjects in popular culture, thereby directly adjusting student expectations.

Indirectly, however, there are more profound and arguably more important benefits, which make it a significant, even essential, component to any forensic science or forensic anthropology course. In many cases, students have not been exposed to concepts of death, dying and after-death care other than in an academic context in their lives by the time they enrol on the course. Fortunately, only a few will have experienced the death of a friend or relative. A scheduled, organised visit to a hospital or Medico-Legal Centre to see a routine or forensic post-mortem examination is an appropriate way of introducing students to a vocational career that is likely to involve working with cadavers. It gives students the opportunity to determine for themselves whether they are physically, mentally and emotionally able to cope with confronting death and dead bodies. It aids a decision of whether they are suited to career in forensic science or forensic anthropology, and allows them to make an informed decision about the extent of involvement with fresh or decomposing cadavers that they might wish to pursue in the future. It also allows the students to become familiar with the sights, smells and sounds associated with a post-mortem examination.

Visiting a mortuary and meeting the mortuary staff, pathologists, funeral directors and anatomy pathology technologists is a useful learning experience for making contacts, understanding etiquette and gaining an appreciation of the mechanics of the 'death industry'. Students would also have a chance to see the parts of the mortuary dedicated to the reception and treatment of the bereaved, which is a fundamental aspect of a forensic student's holistic education about death.

The visit should include a tour around the mortuary facilities, short presentations from the staff about their diverse roles, a tour of the viewing room(s) and bereaved reception area(s), culminating in the viewing of one or more post-mortem examinations from start to finish. It is invaluable to watch the pathologist's examination of the internal organs and his/her diagnosis of the cause of death. The level of access and interaction with staff and the deceased afforded to the students is dependent on the amenability of the Her Majesty's Coroner, Procurator Fiscal, National Health Service (NHS) Trust, private hospital, Ministry of Defence (MOD) pathologist or the independent Medico-Legal Centre Director approached.

Ethics

Ethics is clearly an issue that needs to be addressed before organising a student visit to the mortuary. If the visits are to be carried out in a teaching hospital, it is unlikely that informed consent from the relatives of the deceased would be necessary to obtain.

Health and Safety Considerations

It is imperative that the appropriate Risk Assessments for a student visit to the mortuary should be carried out, and to abide by the Health and Safety Guidelines of the university/HE/FE institution and of the host institution. It is likely that the mortuary will provide a Health and Safety disclaimer to be signed by all visitors on the occasion of each visit.

Sensible Precautions

It is recommended that at least two members of staff or responsible doctoral students accompany every group of undergraduate or postgraduate students. This provides support should something go wrong, such as a student fainting, or one staff member being delayed.

It is likely that the post-mortem examinations will happen in the early morning, and therefore attendees should be cautioned not to skip breakfast, but to eat a filling but bland breakfast (cereal or porridge, for example), to prevent fainting. All attendees should bring a bottle of water with them, although all food and beverages should remain outside the post-mortem examination rooms.

Immunisations

It is important to ensure that all students attending the mortuary visit are appropriately vaccinated and immunised. In the United Kingdom, the minimum requirement for a mortuary visit where the student is not expected to touch the cadavers is to have valid, in-date vaccinations against polio, diptheria and tetanus and BCG against tuberculosis. In addition, a hepatitis B vaccination is recommended for those in medical and forensic professions likely to come into contact with blood on a regular basis. Vaccinations against hepatitis A and C are also useful, but not mandatory. From a practical perspective, it is valuable to inform students of the requirements for these vaccinations well in advance, as overseas students may not have been subject to immunisation programmes similar to that in the United Kingdom, and need to arrange appointments with their general practitioner or travel clinics to have the vaccinations, and sometimes several instalments and boosters to confer immunity, which can take months.

Personal Protective Equipment

The level of personal protective equipment to be worn by visitors to the mortuary is usually dictated by mortuary staff, but is likely to include galoshes or wellies, a plastic apron, gloves and possibly a visor-type face mask. Students should be advised to bring hair clips or bands to tie their hair up with. It is unlikely that students would be given permission to observe a high risk post-mortem, unless from behind a screen or from a viewing room. In these situations, students should be informed of the risk and allowed to opt out if desired.

It is also appropriate to conduct a briefing and debriefing session for all students attending the mortuary visit.

Student Sensibilities

It is vital that the students are given the opportunity to make an informed decision about whether or not they want to attend the mortuary visit. In the author's experience, it is best to make the mortuary visit stand alone, distinct from the assessed part of the course, and make attendance optional, as some may not want to, and should not feel pressurised into attending.

Briefing Session

A system of psychological briefing and debriefing for the students before and after their mortuary visit can be very effective, and is advised. The briefing session should take place at least a couple of days before the mortuary visit, in order to allow the students to assimilate the information provided and make an informed decision about whether or not they want to attend.

The briefing session should be conducted by the member(s) of staff who will be escorting the students to the mortuary, and should be compulsory for all those interested in attending the mortuary. Attendance to the mortuary should not be allowed if the student has not attended the briefing session. The session should include practical details about getting to the mortuary, expected times of arrival and departure, directions and parking details, dress code required and advice about breakfast and hydration on the day. It should also provide a run-through of personnel likely to be encountered, correct methods of addressing them, and reminders that the students are representing the university (or HEI) and should act accordingly. Most importantly, the brief should include a detailed, step-by-step account of what they can expect during the post-mortem examination itself, with details about sights, smells and sensations that they might not be expecting. This part is incredibly valuable, as it allows the students to build a mental picture of the location, the room, the body and the process, which serves as mental preparation for the visit.

The briefing session should also be a forum in which students can ask any questions they like about the process, the deceased they might encounter, the examination, the outcome of the examination, and so on. It serves as a learning experience, but also helps to assuage fears about the experience.

During the mortuary visits, it is strongly recommended that a 'buddy system' is employed, whereby each student has a 'buddy' or friend for whom they are responsible during the visit. This ensures that if one person is taken ill, or feels faint, there is a clear role assigned as to whom should take care of him/her and this eliminates panic at the time. It also serves as a distraction from unpleasant sights and smells for each person, as s/he can concentrate on his/her buddy's welfare, providing purpose.

Debriefing Session

After the mortuary visit, it is sensible to hold a debriefing session, either immediately after return to campus, or a day or so afterwards. This provides a forum in which students can describe their individual responses to the sights, sounds and sensations of the visit, recount their worries and fears, or excitement and enthusiasm. They can again ask any questions they like regarding the experience. During this session, students (and staff) should be given advice about the sorts of normal responses that they may experience, immediately or after a delay, and coping mechanisms for these. Experiences such as flashbacks, nightmares, loss of concentration or anxiety are all common and normal responses to such an experience, and students should be encouraged to talk about them and air them in a group of peers. Students should also be provided with contact details of professionals to whom they could talk if they feel it necessary.

The implementation of a briefing and debriefing session has been found to greatly improve the experience for both staff and students, to allay fears beforehand and to ensure that all attending the mortuary are mentally and physically prepared, thereby reducing mishap.

Conclusions

This chapter has aimed to show that high quality forensic anthropology teaching can be achieved in universities and HEIs today without huge budgets and unlimited resources. Quality teaching is about engagement with the students, creativity with resources and 'thinking outside the box' when it comes to student activities. The basic techniques of forensic anthropology can be taught with easily sourced equipment, and although there is no substitute for real human skeletal material, adequate alternatives are available, thanks to modern technologies such as 3D laser scanning, digitisation of remains and public access online, as well as 3D laser printing, which could ultimately mean that vast skeletal collections are reproducible economically.

Successful teaching of forensic anthropology does not just include the comprehensive transfer of anatomical knowledge and competence with the 'standard' techniques. It also requires the installation of critical thinking, the desire for knowledge accumulation, and the means to question accepted thinking. This can be germinated in the minds of students through exposure to valuable experiences, such as: post-mortem examinations; the use of mock courts and case scenarios; inventive practical sessions; and the use of outdoor laboratories, where they can see theory in action. Of course, all this learning needs to be assessed and quantified, by course leaders and lecturers, but also by the students themselves, in order to determine whether goals and learning outcomes have been reached. Assessment is a fertile environment for creativity and innovation, and experimentation with assessment (in a careful, validated way), can lead to exponential leaps in student learning, retention and enjoyment. Some ideas for ways to inject innovation into practical sessions and assessments have been presented here.

The future of forensic anthropology as a discipline depends on universities and HEIs continuing to strive for quality in staff and students, and in teaching practices. Without stringent selection procedures, caps on student numbers to ensure the very best candidates are enrolled, and commitment to evaluating and improving teaching practices, academic and professional quality and standards within the discipline will slip. There is the ever-present balance to be struck between catering for the increased popularity of the subject with courses designed to soak up tuition fees and put 'bums on seats', and the need to create high quality graduates who will maintain and improve the standards currently set by professional organisations, and guide the discipline through the choppy waters of the twenty-first century. Forensic anthropology could well become a victim of its own success, and those on the 'front line', teaching the forensic anthropologists of the future, have a duty to entrench appropriate attitudes in the minds of our students. These include: an appreciation and respect for the deceased individuals who they have the privilege of examining; a healthy criticism of current techniques in forensic anthropology, to encourage them to strive to improve them; an insistence on scientific rigour and academic quality in research; and a recognition of the need for professional competence in forensic anthropology practice.

References

American Association of Physical Anthropologists (2003) *Code of Ethics*. Accessible online at http://physanth.org/association/position-statements/ethics.pdf?searchterm=code+of+ethics (accessed 23 July 2014).

Arriaza, B. and Pfister, L.-A. (2007) Working with the dead: Health concerns, in *Human Remains: Guide for Museums and Academic Institutions* (eds V. Cassman, N. Odegaard, and J. Powell), AltaMira Press, Lanham, MD, pp. 205–221.

BABAO Working Group for Ethics and Practice (2010) *Code of Practice*. British Association of Biological Anthropology and Osteoarchaeology. Available at: http://www.babao.org.uk/about/ethics-and-standards/ (accessed 10 December 2016).

Boud, D. (1986) *Teaching in Laboratories*. SRHE/Open University Press, Buckingham.

Bowram, E. (2003) A new approach to the storage of human skeletal remains. *The Conservator*, **27** (1), 95–106.

Buikstra, J. and Ubelaker, D. (1994) *Standards for Data Collection from Human Skeletal Remains.* Arkansas Archaeological Survey Research Series No. 44.

Cassman, V., Martine, K., Riddle, J. and Underwood, S. (2001) Neglect of an obvious issue: The storage of human remains. Conservation and archaeology: Case sudies in collaboration. *Cultural Resource Management,* **24** (6), 11–13.

Cassman, V., Odegaard, N. and Powell, J. (eds) (2007) *Human Remains: Guide for Museums and Academic Institutions.* AltaMira Press, Lanham, MD.

Cox, M., Flavel, A. Hanson, I. Laver, J. and Wessling, R. (eds) (2008) *The Scientific Investigation of Mass Graves: Towards Protocols and Standard Operating Procedures.* Cambridge University Press, Cambridge.

Human Tissue Authority (2004) Human Tissue Act. Available at: https://www.hta.gov.uk/policies/human-tissue-act-2004 (accessed 10 June 2016).

Idaho Visualisation Laboratory, Idaho State University, *Virtual Human Skeleton.* Available at: http://ivl.imnh.isu.edu/VHS.htm (accessed 28 November 2016).

Intelicus, *The Online Virtual Human Body.* Available at: http://www.ikonet.com/en/health/virtual-human-body/virtualhumanbody.php (accessed 10 December 2016).

Kapit, W. and Elson, L. (2001) *The Anatomy Colouring Book.* Benjamin Cummings, San Francisco.

Kerby, J., Shukur, Z. and Shalhoub, J. (2011) The relationships between learning outcomes and methods of teaching anatomy as perceived by medical students. *Clinical Anatomy,* **24**, 489–497.

Krych, A., March, C., Bryan, R., Peake, B., Pwlina, W. and Carmichael, S. (2005) Reciprocal peer teaching: Students teaching students in the gross anatomy laboratory. *Clinical Anatomy,* **18**, 296–301.

Mann, R. and Berryman, H. (2012) A method for defleshing human remains using household bleach. *Journal of Forensic Sciences,* **57** (2), 440–442.

McGowan-Lowe, J. (2014) *Jake's Bones.* Octopus Publishing, London.

Ministry of Justice (2014) *FAQs Exhuming Human Remains.* Available at: http://www.justice.gov.uk/downloads/burials-and-coroners/exhuming-human-remains-faq.pdf (accessed 28 November 2016).

Morin, A. (1995) *BIODIDAC, A Bank of Digital Resources for Teaching Niology.* University of Ottowa. Available at: http://biodidac.bio.uottawa.ca/index.htm (accessed 11 May 2014).

Overton, T. (2003) Key aspects of teaching and learning in experimental sciences and engineering, in *A Handbook for Teaching & Learning in Higher Education,* 2nd edn (eds H. Fry, S. Ketteridge and S. Marshall), Kogan Page Ltd, London.

University of Texas, College of Liberal Arts, USA. *Eskeletons Digital Resources.* Available at: http://www.eskeletons.org/index.html (accessed 28 November 2016).

University of Wyoming, USA, *The Virtual Skeleton: Human Osteology. Making Learning Real Project,* Available at: http://www.uwyo.edu/reallearning/virtskel.html (accessed 28 November 2016).

Walsh-Haney, H. and Lieberman, L.S. (2004) Ethical concerns in forensic anthropology, in *Biological Anthropology and Ethics: From Repatriation to Genetic Identity* (ed. T. Turner), SUNY Press, Albany, NY.

Working Group on Human Remains (2003) *Report of the Working Group on Human Remains.* Available at: http://www.museumsbund.de/fileadmin/geschaefts/dokumente/Leitfaeden_und_anderes/DCMS_Working_Group_Report_2003.pdf (accessed 28 November 2016).

Further Resources

Biodidac: http://biodidac.bio.uottawa.ca/
Bone Med Leg: http://bonemedleg.host22.com/
Digitised Diseases: www.digitiseddiseases.org
Eskeletons: http://www.eskeletons.org/index.html
France Casting Ltd: www.francecasts.com
The Online Virtual Human Body: http://intelicus.com/the-online-virtual-human-body/
The Virtual Skeleton: Human Osteology: www.uwyo.edu/reallearning/virtskel.html
Virtual Human Skeleton: http://ivl.imnh.isu.edu/VHS.htm

3

Considerations in Using a Crime Scene House Facility for Teaching and Learning

David Rogers

Staffordshire University, Department of Forensic Science and Crime Science, Faculty of Computing, Engineering and Science, Science Centre, Stoke on Trent, UK

In the policing environment, the UK National College of Policing has for many years provided an extensive Forensic Centre training environment at Harperley Hall, Durham. This facility provides a wealth of environments that most, if not all, Higher Education Institutions (HEIs) would aspire to. The issue for HEIs is one of financial cost and a willingness to invest resources in state-of-the-art facilities. HEIs have therefore been obliged to cut their cloth accordingly, and in so doing, adopt and adapt pre-existing structures and environments to suit their particular needs. The Centre at Harperley Hall provides basic and on-going training to police services nationally and internationally. The National Policing Improvement Agency (NPIA) having worked 'closely with the UK Forensic Regulator, Skills for Justice, and Higher Education establishments ensured that the Forensic Centre products are robust, specific and relevant and, most importantly, meet the needs of the operational forensic practitioner.'

In an academic context, it is asserted that some of the undergraduate and postgraduate students undertaking forensic science and allied degree courses will go on to become Crime Scene Investigators (CSI). It is therefore essential that those who choose this career path are provided with a suitable theoretical and practical, yet safe, environment in which the knowledge and skills required to enhance their future employment aspirations can be attained. To that end, HEIs need to provide the student with the basic knowledge and skills through the provision of suitably staffed and equipped facilities, which meet the needs of potential employers.

Within HEIs, a crime scene facility is a safe environment in which undergraduate and postgraduate students can put the theory that they have learnt in the classroom/lecture theatre into practice. The importance of putting theory into practice is underpinned by the learning model that was developed by Kolb (1984), this 'experiential learning' (see Figure 3.1) has a continual cycle of learning that comprises of four parts: concrete experience (where the students are involved in new experiences), reflective observation (the students have time to reflect on their learning), abstract conceptualisation (the students

Forensic Science Education and Training: A Tool-kit for Lecturers and Practitioner Trainers, First Edition.
Edited by Anna Williams, John P. Cassella, and Peter D. Maskell.

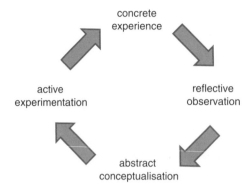

concrete
experience

active
experimentation

reflective
observation

abstract
conceptualisation

Figure 3.1 Kolbs Learning Cycle.

assimilate their new knowledge into current knowledge) and, finally, active experimentation (the students can use new knowledge/understanding to problem solve and make decisions). More detailed discussion of experiential learning and its role in higher education can be found in *A Handbook for Teaching and Learning in Higher Education* (Fry *et al.*, 2014).

The experiential learning model has heavily influenced the teaching of medical professionals, leading to the introduction of problem based learning (Bligh, 1995), which was then utilised by other fields (such as forensic teaching). Problem based learning involves more small group work and self-directed learning, based not around the traditional didactic lecture but a seminar approach, where students encounter a 'problem' and are encouraged to work on the 'problem' themselves with directions from a facilitator (Wood, 2003). This methodology works particularly well with case based scenarios, something that is common in the forensic environment. The use of simulated crime scenes particularly adds to the reality and the learning environment. Evidence from the medical field has shown that an immersive environment can promote learning and consolidation of knowledge (Kleinert and Wahba, 2015), giving more support to the learning that can be achieved with a suitable crime scene facility.

The crime scene facility is commonly referred to as a Crime Scene House, but this is a misnomer. It should not be just one type of environment, a house, but should have the capability and flexibility to encompass a number of different environments. Where possible these should include:

1. any type of building (occupied or unoccupied)
2. any area of land or water
3. any person (whether a suspect, victim or witness)
4. any form of transport
5. any animal

Within the United Kingdom, a number of Universities providing forensic science and allied courses have created these types of environments from pre-existing building stock, furnishing and kitting the facilities out in a variety of ways, including internal furnishings, kitchen equipment, white goods and un-roadworthy vehicles. The scale and variety of facilities vary enormously, and over the years have progressed from mock temporary scenes created in the classroom environment, which can easily be removed and reset as and when required, to dedicated premises that can either be of a commercial or domestic nature, or a combination of both. The recreated scenes not only require skill in setting up by academic staff, but also supervision by the academic staff when the students are processing the scenes as part of the practical aspect of their studies.

The skills required by the staff should come not only from theoretical knowledge, but also from personal experience and training received at establishments such as Harperley Hall. It is not sufficient for a member of the academic staff tasked with setting and supervising the scenes to have read a textbook, as many of the authors of such works have no prior knowledge or practical experience in the area of crime scene preservation, recording, documentation, photography or examination. To highlight this point, one of the basic tenets of contact trace evidence is known as Locard's Principle of Exchange. Many academic authors insist that Edmund Locard's Principle is 'every contact leaves a trace'. Locard should never be maligned in this way. This Principle must never be simplified in such a manner, because in this author's view 'every contact leaves a trace' has no two-way exchange, the phrase does not impart the important aspect of the title of the Principle, that of Exchange. When translated, what Edmond Locard actually stated in his original work of 1920 was:

> on the one hand, the criminal leaves marks at the crime scene of his passage; on the other hand, by inverse action, he takes with him, on his body or on his clothing, evidence of his stay or of his deed. Left or received, these traces are of extremely varied types.'
>
> *Locard, 1920*

The member of academic staff must also understand the issues concerning secondary or tertiary transfer, where contact trace evidence could be inadvertently introduced into the scene by a careless scene setter. Unless those tasked with setting the crime scenes understand Locard's Principle, and that of secondary or tertiary transfer thoroughly, there will be the opportunity for mistakes to be made and students to become confused and misinterpret their findings when it comes to laboratory analysis at a later date.

In real life the CSI is working on behalf of the Senior Investigating Officer (SIO), and it is the CSI's role to ensure that the scene being processed is not contaminated, and that the forensic potential is maximised during the examination and recovery process. To that end, the CSI and the Crime Scene Manager (CSM), along with the SIO, agree the parameters of the examination and designate what scenes will be examined and by whom. In any given real life crime scene there will be a minimum of two scenes: the scene where the offence occurred; and the offender. There may be many more scenes; an example of this might be where an offender abducts a child off the street, takes the child in his motor vehicle, to premises to which he has access, assaults and kills the child, then uses another vehicle to transport the body to a body deposition site. Before the body could be discovered and recovered, animal activity, such as scavenging, may have taken place (Haglund *et al.*, 1989). The body is subsequently discovered by an innocent member of the public who is walking a dog, and the dog indicates to its owner that there is something of interest in the undergrowth, and then the dog and human finder make contact with the clothing being worn by the victim. In this case there are a number of crime scenes, all of which have to be individually examined to avoid cross-contamination:

- the abduction site (land)
- the child (victim)

- the offender (suspect)
- the vehicle 1 (transport)
- the building (occupied or unoccupied)
- the vehicle 2 (transport)
- the body deposition site (land or water)
- the dog walker and finder of the victim (witness)
- the dog (animal)

There may also be other scenes, such as the offender's home address (Figure 3.2) where other evidence may exist. The SIO will be attempting, through the skills of the CSI and the expertise of various forensic scientists to link:

- the offender to the victim through DNA, hairs and fibres, and so on;
- the victim to the vehicles through DNA, hairs, fibres or fingerprints and even toe prints;

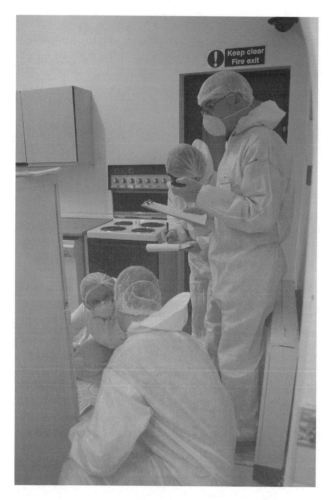

Figure 3.2 Students examining a crime scene in a crime scene house.

- the vehicle to the abduction site through eyewitness evidence, CCTV, or tyre marks or tyre impressions;
- the offender to the vehicle, even though that individual may be the registered owner, through fingerprints, DNA or documentation, which may indicate his movements before or after the abduction (petrol receipts, etc.);
- the victim to the building in which they were held through hairs, fibres, fingerprints or palynology;
- the suspect to the body deposition site through palynology, footwear impressions and tyre impressions;
- the victim to the dog, for elimination purposes, but it may also be that the offender or the victim has a pet, from which either primary transfer of hairs may have taken place as in Locard's Principle, or secondary or tertiary transfer of hairs has taken place.

There are of course many other investigative forensic orientated issues that the SIO will be taking into consideration at the same time:

- suitable pathology provision to maximise the forensic potential from the examination of the victim;
- suitable medical examination of any suspects by suitably trained forensic medical examiners to maximise the recovery of forensic evidence, such as swabs for DNA, forensic odontology for bite marks, clinical examination for injuries, fitness to be detained and fitness for interview;
- technical assistance in the forensic examination of mobile telephones and satellite navigation systems and other IT based equipment.

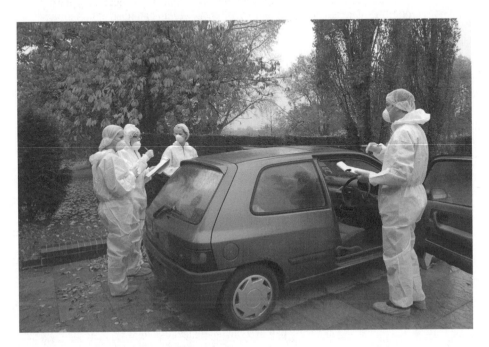

Figure 3.3 Students examining a car based crime scene.

These are complex scenes, with many potential opportunities for contamination and cross-contamination, and the HEI student must be made aware that by starting with just one scene to process, they can build on their knowledge to process a more complex scene in due course.

To that end, the HEI crime scene facility, wherever it is based, must be flexible enough to accommodate most if not all of the scenes described here (Figure 3.3). This will then enhance the student learning experience, and ensure that they have a thorough grounding in the principles of crime scene examination and processing.

References

Bligh, J. (1995) Problem-based learning in medicine: an introduction. *Postgraduate Medical Journal*, **71** (836), 323–326.

Fry, H., Ketteridge, S. and Marshall, S. (2014) *A Handbook for Teaching and Learning in Higher Education: Enhancing Academic Practice*, 4th edn (paperback), Routeledge.

Haglund, W.D., Reay, D.T. and Swindler, D.R. (1989) Canid scavenging/disarticulation sequence of human remains in the Pacific Northwest. *Journal of Forensic Science*, **34** (May, 3), 587–606.

Kleinert, R., Wahba, R., Chang, D.H., *et al.* (2015) 3D immersive patient simulators and their impact on learning success: a thematic review. *Journal of Medical Internet Research*, **17** (4), e91.

Kolb, D.A. (1984) *Experiential Learning: Experience as the Source of Learning and Development*, Prentice Hall, Englewood Cliffs, NJ.

Locard, E. (1920) *L'Enquête criminelle et les Méthodes scientifiques*, Ernest Flammarion.

Wood, D.F. (2003) Problem based learning. *British Medical Journal*, **326**, 328–330.

4

Taphonomy Facilities as Teaching Aids

Peter Cross[1] and Anna Williams[2]

[1] University of Central Lancashire, Preston, UK
[2] University of Huddersfield, School of Applied Sciences, Queensgate, Huddersfield, UK

Introduction

Taphonomy, in its broadest sense, means the study of the events and processes that affect the remains of an organism after it dies (Collins English Dictionary, 2003). It is an integral component of death investigation; understanding of the processes of decay and decomposition of human bodies, as well as materials associated with them, such as hair, clothes and metals, can be very useful for reconstructing death events and estimation of the time elapsed since death. As such, it is a necessary element of a comprehensive education in forensic science, as students need to be aware of the potential contribution that taphonomic analyses can make to the investigation. In order to address that need, the creation and use of purpose-built taphonomic facilities for research and teaching have become more common in UK universities, taking their lead from Higher Education Institutions in the United States.

History of Taphonomic Research in Forensic Science

The field of taphonomy was developed in the 1940s by Ivan Efremov, a Soviet palaeontologist who defined taphonomy as 'study of the transition, in all details, of organics from the biosphere into the lithosphere of the geological record' (Efremov, 1940). Efremov was awarded the State Stalin Prize in 1952 for his work in Taphonomy and Chronological Geology. The word *taphonomy* derives from the Greek words *taphos* (burial) and *nomos* (laws) and was originally only concerned with animal remains. Until the late 1980s, taphonomy was a term used predominantly within vertebrate palaeontology and prehistoric archaeozoology and archaeology. The goals of this 'traditional' field of taphonomy included the reconstruction of palaeo-environments, determining which factors cause differential destruction/attrition/fossilisation of bone, understanding selective transport of skeletal elements and discriminating human from non-human agents of bone

Forensic Science Education and Training: A Tool-kit for Lecturers and Practitioner Trainers, First Edition.
Edited by Anna Williams, John P. Cassella, and Peter D. Maskell.
© 2017 John Wiley & Sons Ltd. Published 2017 by John Wiley & Sons Ltd.

modification. Landmark publications include Weigelt (1927, published in translation in 1989), Behrensmeyer and Hill (1988), which had a significant impact on prehistoric archaeology and archaeozoology, Shipman (1981), Boddington *et al.* (1987) and Lyman (1994) with the publication of *Vertebrate Taphonomy*.

The term 'taphonomy' was not used in the forensic context until the late 1980s and first appeared as a 'keyword' in the *Journal of Forensic Sciences* in 1989 (Haglund *et al.*, 1989). This decade also saw the establishment of the first human taphonomic facility, the Anthropological Research Facility (ARF) at the University of Tennessee in Knoxville, TN, USA. This facility was founded in 1981 by Dr William M. Bass. The establishment of the facility helped drive the interest in human decomposition and boosted the term taphonomy into the forensic science arena. Discussions of human taphonomy began to appear in the forensic literature (Rodriguez and Bass, 1985; Mann *et al.*, 1990) based upon observations made at the University of Tennessee facility. A key publication by Vass *et al.* (1992) introduced the concept of accumulated degree days (ADD) as a measure of temperature and time. However, this work was slow to gain recognition, and was not cited in either volume of Haglund and Sorg's *Forensic Taphonomy* (Haglund and Sorg, 1997; Haglund and Sorg, 2001). A second key publication was Megyesi *et al.* (2005). This work, based on retrospective human case studies, introduced a standardised method of scoring decomposition, the total body score (TBS), and brought together TBS and ADD to allow calculation of post-mortem interval (PMI). Previous publications (Reed, 1958; Payne, 1965; Johnson, 1975; Clark *et al.* 1997; Galloway, 1997) had categorised decomposition into 'stages.' Such studies, whilst valuable, were location specific. Local environment would determine the 'stage' of decomposition a corpse was displaying at a given time, making such studies difficult, if not impossible, to compare. The standardisation of decomposition scoring (Megyesi *et al.*, 2005) and the incorporation of temperature and time into a single measurement (Vass *et al.*, 1992) enabled statistical comparison between geographically disparate studies.

The use of human cadavers is currently exclusive to facilities within the United States, and more recently, Australia and the Netherlands. Forensic taphonomic research within the United Kingdom and Europe has focused on the use of animal models, notably the domestic pig, *Sus scrofa* (Turner and Wiltshire, 1999; Dekeirsschieter *et al.*, 2009; Charabidze *et al.*, 2009; Matuszewski *et al.*, 2008; Özdemir and Sert 2009; Cross and Simmons 2010). Research using animal models provides valuable insights into the processes of decomposition and the factors that influence it. This research also provides important information on local climatic influences and entomological data that are relevant to the conditions found in the United Kingdom (Cross *et al.*, 2009). Whilst studies using human cadavers might be preferable in terms of their direct relevance to forensic cases, animal models facilitate much larger studies of the variables that may influence decomposition, as greater numbers of animals are available for use at one time. In human cadaver studies, numbers of replicates are limited, leading to less robust statistical analysis. Much past and current research on decomposition using human cadavers has produced only anecdotal findings based on single case studies or experiments with low replicate numbers (Rodriguez and Bass, 1983; Mann *et al.*, 1990; Bass, 1997; Schroeder *et al.*, 2002).

Whether human cadavers or animal models are used to study decomposition and factors that influence the process, the goals of modern forensic taphonomy research remain the same. Understanding soft tissue and bone decomposition and distribution, discriminating post- from peri-mortem modification, and more accurate post-mortem interval estimation are the key foci.

Taphonomy Research Facilities

To date, in addition to the University of Tennessee, a growing number of facilities conduct forensic taphonomic research using human cadavers, including: Sam Houston University; Western Carolina University; Texas State University; Southern Illinois University; Colorado Mesa University; Fox Valley Technical College; the University of Technology, Sydney and AMC hospital, Amsterdam, Netherlands. It should be noted that forensic taphonomic research in the United States also involves animal models, as some institutions teaching and researching forensic taphonomy do not possess or have access to facilities that would enable this research to be conducted using humans. Despite the principle of human taphonomic research being already established in the United States, a number of groups have attempted to establish facilities for this but have failed, due to lack of administrative or community support (Melby and Hamilton, 2009).

In the United Kingdom, the first facility dedicated to forensic taphonomic research was established by the University of Central Lancashire. TRACES (Taphonomic Research in Anthropology – Centre for Experimental Study) was opened in 2009 and utilises animal models for its research. TRACES conducts high replicate number experimental projects researching factors that influence the decomposition process and their implications for PMI estimation (Widya *et al.*, 2012; Gruenthal *et al.*, 2012; Cross and Simmons, 2010; Simmons *et al.*, 2010a; Simmons *et al.*, 2010b). Other universities have followed suit, and smaller-scale taphonomy facilities now exist at Cranfield University, University of Huddersfield, Staffordshire University, Gwyndyr University, Keele University and others.

The number of taphonomic research facilities, whether utilising animal or human subjects, is increasing. The research output and resulting publications in forensic taphonomy have also increased dramatically over recent years. Forensic taphonomic research, with its foci on better understanding the process of decomposition and improving accuracy in PMI estimation, has the potential to contribute much valuable science to the discipline and aid death investigation, whether in a criminal or humanitarian context. Forensic taphonomic research is increasingly popular with forensic science students, from a variety of specialities (forensic anthropology, forensic pathology, forensic entomology, forensic DNA), and academic institutions with such facilities are sought after by many students. In addition, those involved in criminal investigation, such as crime scene investigators and search dog handlers, are seeking to learn more about the science behind their work and are undertaking training in forensic taphonomy. They are also increasingly seeking to utilise taphonomic facilities for their own training, such as human remains search and recovery and search dog training, as well as undertaking research collaborations in areas specific to their own requirements.

Currently, no human taphonomic research or teaching facility exists in the United Kingdom, and the reasons for this are unclear. However, a number of institutions do have an interest in the establishment of such a facility, and a single, national centre producing high quality research would be welcomed by many academics, affiliated professionals and members of the public (Witt and Cassella, 2014). There is increased public interest and acceptance of such facilities, and at the established facilities in the United States, there are long waiting lists of people willing to donate their bodies to forensic research (University of Tennessee Knoxville, 2015a; Bellows, 2007).

In addition, there are certain scenarios and conditions that cannot be accurately reproduced using animal models, such as investigations of the effect of particular human diseases or lifestyle choices on the rate of decomposition. Through the use of human taphonomy facilities, it may be possible to determine how diabetes, certain forms of cancer or smoking, for example, may affect decomposition rate and possibly post-mortem interval estimation. In addition, although the use of pigs is considered the best model for human decomposition, there are anatomical differences, for example, limb proportion, which may result in some variation in the decomposition process when compared with humans. This can, for example, necessitate the adjustment of the Megysei *et al.* (2005) total body scoring system when applying it to a pig carcass. Conversely, there are certain factors that may influence decomposition that are better facilitated by animal models. These include the influence of trauma. A variety of traumatic injuries can be inflicted upon a dead animal model and in some cases it may be possible to study the effects of peri-mortem injuries on animal decomposition (Radford *et al.*, 2015), but the peri-mortem injury studies and studies involving inflicting traumatic injuries on donated human cadavers would have severe ethical considerations.

However, despite the increase in the popularity and utilisation of taphonomic research facilities amongst forensic scientists, students, associated professionals and the public, the establishment of such a facility in the United Kingdom has its critics. In additional to financial considerations, the creation of a such a facility might raise a number of legislative, ethical and health and safety issues, and would require extensive consultation with a range of organisations both prior to opening and during its operation. The establishment of a human taphonomic facility may necessitate a change in legislation as, currently, the use of donated human bodies for taphonomy research is not a 'scheduled purpose' licensed by the Human Tissue Authority. There is concern that a donation programme providing cadavers for taphonomic research may negatively impact donation programmes for medical school education. In terms of research, the primary issue for a human taphonomic facility is the likely level of human donation. Taphonomic experimentation, which will provide statistically robust results, requires larger replicate numbers than those provided by the current donation patterns seen in other human taphonomy facilities, and as with all experimental design it is important to carry out an assessment of the number of replicates that will be needed in an experiment by undertaking power analysis (Cohen, 1969). If a taphonomic research facility is using donated human cadavers it is essential that the science produced from such a facility has value and makes a significant contribution to the field.

Teaching Forensic Taphonomy

From a pedagogical perspective, taphonomy facilities are extremely valuable learning and teaching tools. They can be viewed as outdoor laboratories, which allow students to gain precious first-hand experience of all aspects of decomposition. Words or pictures in a book or on a screen cannot fully describe and explain the multitude of processes and factors that influence decomposition, nor can they accurately represent the sensory experience that can be gained from one afternoon monitoring a decomposing carcass. The provision of outdoor facilities enables practical demonstration of the decomposition process in its native environment. It also provides an accurate ecological environment to support the decomposition; it would be practically impossible to observe decomposition complete with correct soil flora and fauna, a full entomological complement of organisms and appropriate weather conditions for different seasons in a laboratory setting.

Such facilities allow students to see, touch, smell and hear decomposition of animal carcasses (or human in the United States and Australia), which is incredibly important for their wider forensic education. It allows them the chance to experience potentially off-putting, unpleasant smells and sights, and decide if this is the career they choose to take. It is obviously better to face these challenges for the first time in a safe, unpressured environment than on a real forensic case. In this way, taphonomy facilities offer an opportunity to 'test the water', and serve much the same purpose as visiting post-mortem examinations (see Chapter 2) on a degree course.

The importance of having accurate decomposition environments that students can observe (or interact with) at close quarters becomes apparent when one considers learning theories, such as the experiential learning cycle proposed by Kolb (1984). This mechanism of learning revolves around reflective observation of experience leading to conceptualisation and active experimentation. A facility where students can observe decomposition in progress as a holistic experience (sights, sounds, smells) and view first-hand the effects of weather, clothing, and so on, on this process, provides a great opportunity for the student to internalise and experience the material to be learned, rather than just try to understand words on a page or pictures in a book.

In addition, the assailment of all the senses in a field decomposition class lends itself well to the active learning enshrined in the VARK (Visual, Aural, Read/write, and Kinesthetic) modalities of learning suggested by Fleming and Mills (1992). In particular, the move away from 'words in a book' to the tangible experience will engage kinaesthetic and visual learners in a unique way. Similarly, the chance for a tutor to explain what students are seeing while it is there in front of them will add depth to the learning experience of multi-modal students. In general, students are enthusiastic about the chance to get out of the classroom and 'see it for themselves'; and this enthusiasm translates into increased engagement and better learning on their part.

A wide variety of forensic science subjects can be explored using animal (or human) carcasses housed in a taphonomy facility. The most obvious is perhaps the identification of the stages of decomposition and subsequent estimation of post-mortem interval. With adequate monitoring of the ambient temperature, this analysis can involve calculation of accumulated degree days. Different scenarios can allow study of the effect of a range of factors on the rate of decomposition, for example, access by insects, submersion in water, ambient temperature, depth of burial, access by scavengers and many other factors. Classes and experiments can be run exploring the use of forensic entomology in estimation of post-mortem interval, extracting DNA from different organs at different times since death, investigations of bone diagenesis and degradation of different materials at varying burial depths or deposition conditions. There is plenty of scope for hands-on exercises, providing students have adequate personal protective equipment and vaccinations. Subjects taught at the Forensic Anthropology Centre at the University of Tennessee Knoxville, for example, include outdoor recovery of scattered and buried remains, human osteology and fire investigation (University of Tennessee Knoxville, 2015b).

Courses and modules can be tailored and timed around the expected decomposition events to be witnessed, and classes can revisit the facility at different intervals during the course. A taphonomy facility also allows for the deliberate creation of a range of decomposition types, in order to expose students to as many decomposition scenarios as possible, for example, hanging, submersion in water, mummification, adipocere formation and burning.

Such first-hand experience is greatly valued by students and prospective students. This is evident as the majority of pedagogical short courses held at existing human taphonomy facilities are consistently oversubscribed. Based on student comments to the authors in the United Kingdom, students have chosen university courses based purely on access to taphonomy facilities.

Establishment of a Taphonomy Facility for Teaching and Research

In order to create a facility for taphonomy research and teaching at a university site, a suitable piece of land has to be acquired. Ideally, the land should not be overlooked by houses or offices, and not have public access across or near it. It is also important to determine if the site is on the flight path of commercial airlines – some of the human taphonomy facilities in the United States are visible from the air and have been photographed by members of the public in aeroplanes or hot air balloons.

The size of the land is relatively unimportant, as a lot can be achieved on a small piece of land, but there is the consideration of the upkeep of the facility, frequency and density of experiments, and the length of time required for research before soil saturation and capacity are reached. The land could be arable, wooded or wasteland and, in an ideal situation, the site would be accessible by road, and there would be electricity and mains water at the site. The site should, however, be assessed to minimise the possible accumulation of decomposition products in water courses and the surrounding environment. In the United Kingdom, The Environment Agency may require a 'groundwater vulnerability' survey to be carried out, after an initial approval based upon known the known geology of the location.

In the United Kingdom, before any animals can be surface deposited or buried, it is necessary to obtain approval from the Department for Environment, Food and Rural Affairs (DEFRA), for the *Use of Animals and Animal By-Products for Research Purposes*. This is a relatively simple process, but can involve visits from DEFRA representatives to the site. Part of the conditions of DEFRA licensing can stipulate that the animal carcasses should be protected from scavengers, such as foxes, badgers, birds and rodents, and so it may be necessary to either erect a suitable rodent-proof fence that extends horizontally underground around the site, in conjunction with overhead netting, or to encase each carcass in suitable netting or a cage. High fencing and possibly a security patrol may also be necessary to keep curious people from trespassing.

The choice of animal species is important, and has implications for equipment, licensing, transport and storage. Ideally, in order perform robust experimentation it is advisable to use pigs (a species that has numerous similarities to humans and are commonly used in taphonomic research (Schoenly *et al.*, 1991; Campobasso *et al.*, 2001; Anderson and VanLaerhoven, 1996). With pigs it is possible to obtain a large number of animals of the same age, size and condition from a local supply of stock that has been bred for human consumption. For teaching purposes it can be cheaper to use animals that have died of 'natural' causes. In the United Kingdom, this means fallen stock (for large domesticates) or even road kill. However, it is important to remember that obtaining animals from fallen stock or road kill for teaching or research purposes comes with an inherent lack of information surrounding the cause of death, time since death and the environmental conditions to which the animal carcasses have been subjected, but this may be necessary if no other animals can be obtained. These can all influence decomposition rate. Irrespective of the nature of supply, whether it be a large number of known carcasses for research or smaller numbers from fallen stock, it is essential to have in place biosecurity protocols to minimise the risk of disease transmission. The biosecurity protocols should be agreed with the DEFRA Veterinary Officer and any additional veterinary advisors. Protocols may involve clinical inspection of animals prior to slaughter and hygiene and disinfection regimes for personnel and vehicles.

Whole domesticated animals intended for food, such as pigs, sheep and cows, with intact intestines, are classified in the United Kingdom by DEFRA as 'Category 2' animals, and DEFRA approval is required to transport and store them. Such animals can usually be obtained direct from farmers, or 'rendering men', sometimes known as 'knacker's yards', for a charge. It is very difficult to stipulate size, sex, breed or postmortem interval when obtaining fallen stock from knacker's yards. University vans and drivers can be registered with DEFRA, and must prove that transportation happens in leak-proof containers. For this purpose, lockable cooler chests or 'game larders' can be purchased.

Carcass disposal after the experimental period is an important consideration for any HEI intending to set up a taphonomy facility. Animal remains should be collected into sealable biohazard or clinical waste bins, which are airtight and waterproof once sealed. These can then be collected by waste management services, for a fee, for complete destruction. Animal remains can also be disposed of as Animal By-Product, collectable by a licensed renderer.

From a practical point of view, there are important health and safety implications to consider. As with any outdoor facility or laboratory, first-aid kits and access to a telephone to summon emergency services to the site are essential. Staff, researchers and students should have a safety induction to familiarise them with safety and evacuation procedures, and the use of full personal protective equipment (scene suits, gloves, face masks, safety goggles) should be encouraged at all times. Attendees to the site should have to provide proof of valid vaccinations, including tetanus (Health Protection Agency, personal communication, 2011). There should be the appropriate number of trained first-aiders available for the number of attendees at any time. Normal, 'common sense' precautions should be taken for working outdoors – drinking water, sunscreen and sun protection in summer months and warm, waterproof clothing and access to shelter and warmth in winter. Steel toe-capped boots and gardening gloves should be worn when digging with spades or using augers. Staff, researcher or students should not attend the site alone.

The Future of Taphonomy Facilities

The future of forensic taphonomy research and, as a consequence, teaching, is uncertain in the United Kingdom. The existence of human taphonomy facilities in the United States and now Australia and the Netherlands means that more and more human decomposition data from a variety of climates and geographic regions is being generated, building a more comprehensive picture of how human decomposition occurs in a multitude of environments. However, none of these are directly applicable to forensic cases in the United Kingdom, which has its own unique combination of climate, fauna, insects and other conditions. Research from the taphonomy facilities in the United Kingdom can supplement this information with data from animal (mainly porcine) analogues. Use of animal carcasses for taphonomy research has important advantages over the use of humans; they can be easily replicated, sample numbers can be high, giving good statistical power to experiments, and variables are easily controlled. Ultimately, however, what we can learn about human decomposition from animals is inherently limited, and it may be necessary for a human taphonomy facility to be created in the UK in the future.

Conclusions

From a teaching standpoint, it is not disputed that taphonomy facilities are extremely valuable pedagogical tools, providing learners with opportunities for hands-on experience of the sights, smells and sensations of decomposition, as well as chances to discover first-hand the influence of different variables on the rate of decomposition. They can be seen as outdoor laboratories from which empirical evidence can be gathered, and they fulfil some of the same pedagogical functions as indoor laboratories, crime scene houses and even post-mortem examination visits. Their use in courses seems to be met with universal enthusiasm from students and learners, and many chose their course based on access to such a facility. Research opportunities are only limited by imagination and resourcefulness, which also makes them very attractive additions to the university repertoire.

References

Anderson, G.S. and VanLaerhoven, S.L. (1996) Initial studies on insect succession on corpse in Southwestern British Columbia. *Journal of Forensic Sciences.* **41**, 617–625.

Bass, W. (1997) Outdoor decomposition rates in Tennessee, in *The Post-mortem Fate of Human* Remains (eds W. Haglund and M. Sorg), CRC Press, Boca Raton.

Bellows, A. (2007) The remains of Doctor Bass. *Damn Interesting.* Available at: http://www.damninteresting.com/the-remains-of-doctor-bass/ (accessed 9 April 2015).

Behrensmeyer, A.K. and Hill, A.P. (1988) *Fossils in the Making: Vertebrate Taphonomy and Paleoecology.* University of Chicago Press, Chicago.

Boddington, A., Garland, A. and Janaway, R. (1987) *Death, Decay and Reconstruction: Approaches to Archaeology and Forensic Science*, Manchester University Press.

Campobasso, C. P., Di Vella, G. and Introna, F. (2001) Factors affecting decomposition and Diptera colonisation. *Forensic Science International*, **2**, 18–27.

Charabidze, D., Bourel, B., Hedouin, V. and Gosset, D. (2009) Repellent effect of some household products on fly attraction to cadavers. *Forensic Science International*, **189** (1-3), 28–33.

Cohen, J. (1969) *Statistical Power Analysis for the Behavioral Sciences*, Academic Press, New York.

Clark, M.A., Worrell, M.B. and Pless, J.E. (1997) Post mortem changes in soft tissues, in *Forensic Taphonomy: The Post-Mortem Fate of Human Remains*, (eds W.D. Haglund and M.H. Sorg), CRC Press, Boca Raton, FL, pp. 151–164.

Collins English Dictionary (2003) *Complete and Unabridged*, HarperCollins Publishers.

Cross, P., Simmons, T., Cunliffe, R. and Chatfield, L. (2009) Establishing a taphonomic research facility in the UK. *Forensic Science Policy & Management: An International Journal*, **1** (4), 187–191.

Cross, P. and Simmons, T. (2010) The influence of penetrative trauma on the rate of decomposition. *Journal of Forensic Sciences*, **55** (2), 295–301.

Dekeirsschieter, J. Verheggen, F., Gohy, M., Hubrecht, F., Bourguignon, L., Lognay, G. and Haubruge, E. (2009) Cadaveric volatile organic compounds released by decaying pig carcasses (*Sus domesticus* L.) in different biotopes. *Forensic Science International*, **189** (1-3), 46–53.

Efremov, I. (1940) Taphonomy: a new branch of paleontology. *Pan-American Geologist*, **74**, 81–93.

Fleming, M.D. and Mills, C. (1992) Not another inventory, rather a catalyst for reflection. *To Improve the Academy*, **11**, 137–155.

Galloway, A. (1997) The process of decomposition: A model from the Arizona-Sonaran Dessert, in *Forensic Taphonomy: the Post-Morten Fate of Human Remains*, (eds W.D. Haglund and M.H. Sorg), CRC Press, Boca Raton, FL, pp. 139–150.

Gruenthal, A., Moffatt, C. and Simmons, T. (2012) Differential decomposition patterns in charred versus un-charred remains. *Journal of Forensic Sciences*, **57** (1), 12–18.

Haglund, W., Reay, D. and Swindler, D. (1989) Canid scavenging/disarticulation sequence of human remains in the Pacific Northwest. *Journal of Forensic Sciences*, **34** (3), 587–606.

Haglund, W. and Sorg, M. (eds) (1997) *The Post-Mortem Fate of Human Remains*, CRC Press, Boca Raton, FL.

Haglund, W. and Sorg, M. (eds) (2001) *Advances in Forensic Taphonomy: Method, Theory, and Archaeological Perspectives*, CRC Press, Boca Raton, FL.

Johnson, M.D. (1975) Seasonal and microseral variations in the insect populations on carrion. *American Midland Naturalist*, **93**, 79–90.

Kolb, D. (1984). *Experiential Learning: Experience as the Source of Learning and Development*, Prentice Hall, Englewood Cliffs, NJ.

Lyman, R. (1994) *Vertebrate Taphonomy*. Cambridge Manuals in Archaeology, Cambridge University Press, Cambridge.

Mann, R.W., Bass, W.M. and Meadows, L. (1990) Time since death and decomposition of the human body: variables and observations in case and experimental filed studies. *Journal of Forensic Sceinces*, **35** (11), 103–111.

Matuszewski, S., Bajerlein, D., Konweski, S. and Szpila, K. (2008) An initial study of insect succession and carrion decomposition in various forest habitats of Central Europe. *Forensic Science International*, **180** (2-3), 61–69.

Megyesi, M., Haskell, N. and Nawrocki, S. (2005) Using accumulated degree-days to estimate the postmortem interval from decomposed human remains. *Journal of Forensic Sciences*, **50** (3), 618–626.

Melby, J., and Hamilton, M.D. (2009) Creating an open-air forensic anthropology human decomposition research facility. Presented at American Academy of Forensic Sciences Meeting, Denver, CO, USA, February, 2009.

Özdemir, S. and Sert, O. (2009) Determination of Coleoptera fauna on carcasses in Ankara province, Turkey. *Forensic Science International*, **183** (1-3), 24–32.

Payne, J.A. (1965) A summer carrion study of the baby pig *Sus scrosfa* Linnaeus. *Ecology*, **46**, 592–602.

Radford, G.E., Taylor, M.C., Kieser, J.A., Waddell, J.N., Walsh, K.A.J., Schofield, J.C., Das, R. and Chakravorty, E. (2015) Simulating back spatter of blood from cranial gunshot wounds using pig models. *International Journal of Legal Medicine*, 10 p. DOI: 10.1007/s00414-015-1219-x.

Reed, H.B. (1958) A study of dog carcass communities in Tennessee, with special reference to the insects. *American Midland Naturalist*, **59**, 213–245.

Rodriguez, W.C. and Bass, W.M. (1983) Insect activity and its relationship to decay rate of human cadavers in east Tennessee. *Journal of Forensic Sciences*, **28**, 423–432.

Rodriguez, W. and Bass, W. (1985) Decomposition of buried bodies and methods that may aid in their location. *Journal of Forensic Sciences*, **30** (3), 836–852.

Schoenly, K., Griest, K. and Rhine, S. (1991) An experimental field protocol for investigating the postmortem interval using multidisciplinary indicators. *Journal of Forensic Sciences*, **36**, 1395–1415.

Schroeder, H., Klotzbach, H., Oesterhelweg, L. and Püschel, K. 2002. Larder beetles (Coleoptera, Dermestidae) as an accelerating factor for decomposition of a human corpse. *Forensic Science International*, **127** (3), 231–236.

Shipman, P. (1981) *Life History of a Fossil: an Introduction to Taphonomy and Paleoecology*, Harvard University Press, Cambridge, MA and London.

Simmons, T., Adlam, R. and Moffatt, C. (2010a) Debugging decomposition data—comparative taphonomic studies and the influence of insects and carcass size on decomposition rate. *Journal of Forensic Sciences*, **55** (1), 8–13.

Simmons, T., Cross, P., Adlam, R. and Moffatt, C. (2010b) The influence of insects of decomposition rate in buried and surface remains. *Journal of Forensic Sciences*, **55** (4), 889–892.

Turner, B. and Wiltshire, P. (1999) Experimental validation of forensic evidence: a study of decomposition of buried pigs in a heavy clay soil. *Forensic Science International*, **101** (2), 113–122.

University of Tennessee Knoxville (2015a) *Forensic Anthropology Center, Donation, Fast Facts*. Available at: http://fac.utk.edu/fastfacts.html (accessed 9 April 2015).

University of Tennessee Knoxville (2015b) *Forensic Anthropology Center*. Available at: http://fac.utk.edu.html (accessed 9 April 2015).

Vass, A., Bass, W., Wolt, J., Foss, J. and Ammons, J. (1992) Time since death determinations of human cadavers using soil solutions. *Journal of Forensic Sciences*, **37** (5), 1236–1253.

Weigelt, J. (1927) (published in translation in 1989) *Recent Carcasses and their Paleobiological Implications*, translated by Judith Schaefer, The University of Chicago Press, London.

Widya, M., Moffatt, C. and Simmons, T. (2012) The formation of early stage adipocere in submerged remains: A preliminary experimental study. *Journal of Forensic Sciences*, **57** (2), 328–333.

Witt, I. and Cassella, J.P. (2014) The feasibility of a United Kingdom Human Taphonomic Research Facility, 10th FORREST Conference, Newcastle, 2014.

5

Forensic Fire Investigation

Richard D. Price

Faculty of Computing, Engineering and Science, University of South Wales, UK

Introduction

Fire and explosion investigation is a highly specialised branch within forensic science and draws upon the application of several scientific disciplines including chemistry, physics, mathematics, material science, computational simulation, criminalistics and forensic methods of analysis.

Fire and explosion investigation theory is studied through traditional lectures but it is the application of these theoretical studies in laboratory experimentation and in realistic practical contexts that further develop the students' independent critical thinking skills.

A fire investigator must possess an understanding of fire science: comprehending the chemistry of combustion, the ignitions of materials, heat transfer mechanisms, fire development and ultimate extinction. Fire investigators draw upon these insights to develop probable routes of fire progression through a building, being aware of the relationship between building occupancy usage, construction and design to the phenomenon of fire spread.

Ultimately, it is the examination of the burnt and charred remains left at the fire scene, the analysis of *in situ* evidence, fire patterns and the reversal of fire progression that lead to the point of origin and the reconstruction of events such as ignition, combustible source and cause (Almirall and Furton, 2004).

These processes must be fully documented as an investigation report suitable for presentation in a court of law, with the expectation that the author may be called upon as an expert witness to give evidence and present their findings.

The fire investigation process from start to finish thus mirrors Bloom's (1959) hierarchy of educational objectives from initial knowledge and understanding through application and analysis and in to final synthesis and evaluation (Almirall and Furton, 2004). The challenge is, therefore, the integration of simulation experiments alongside theoretical studies to achieve these educational goals.

Forensic Science Education and Training: A Tool-kit for Lecturers and Practitioner Trainers, First Edition.
Edited by Anna Williams, John P. Cassella, and Peter D. Maskell.
© 2017 John Wiley & Sons Ltd. Published 2017 by John Wiley & Sons Ltd.

Fire and Explosion Investigation Module

This section of the chapter gives an example of the practical aspects of a final year 20 credit module structure, based on the one taught to final year BSc (hons) Forensic Science Undergraduates at the University of South Wales. This module has been designed and developed in collaboration with fire investigation and crime scene investigation professionals, professional organisations and, finally, academic staff with expertise of the science of chemistry and explosions.

The module is a mix of theoretical studies, research, critical evaluation and practical experimentation, delivered via lectures, tutorials and practical sessions. The assessment comprises a three hour closed book examination (66%) and continuous assessment (34%) and is comprised of: (1) Fire Dynamics Practical (8.5%); (2) Explosion Practical (8.5%); (3) Fatal Fire Investigation (8.5%); and (4) 45 minute online Multiple Choice Question (MCQ) Assessment (8.5%).

Example Practical Sessions

Practical 1: Fire Dynamics – Investigating Flame Speed using the Variable Gas Burner
In this practical, students use a variable gas burner to investigate the speed of a natural gas–air flame speed. Natural gas can form combustible mixtures over a wide range of concentrations in air. As a flame burns, more fuel and air move into the combustion zone to replace the amount consumed. If the fuel and air do not get to the combustion zone fast enough, then the combustion zone moves back to meet the fuel–air supply. This practical investigates the speed of flame propagation over a fixed distance at various different air/fuel ratios in an enclosed environment. Depending on the air/fuel ratio, the flame will propagate at different speeds; at certain ratios, it will not be possible for combustion to take place beyond the 'lower' and 'upper' flammability limits of the fuel. These flammability limits are investigated, which are to be compared with standard reference source values. Students must produce individual structured reports comprising: Introduction, Results, Discussion, Conclusions and References.

Practical 2: Explosion Investigation – An Investigation into the Mechanism
of Gas Explosions
This practical investigates the physical and chemical mechanisms involved in gas explosions, as detailed on the Royal Society of Chemistry (2016) website (*Controlled Explosion of a Methane–Air Mixture Experiment*). A lidded container (such a catering size coffee tin) is evacuated, filled with mains supply natural gas and stoppered at the bottom and top 10 mm diameter orifices (Figure 5.1). In a safe detonation zone, the stoppers are removed and the emergent natural gas ignited as it leaves via the top orifice. During this experiment, air enters the fuel mixture from the orifice at the bottom. As the mixture burns, the concentration of fuel within the container decreases and the concentration of air increases until eventually the limit of flammability is reached, at which point there is a sustained reaction throughout the mixture in the container and an explosion consequently takes place. The progression of the explosion may be measured with a stopwatch and observations researched and reported. Further details of the experimental setup can be found on the Royal Society of Chemistry (2016) website (*Controlled Explosion of a Methane–Air Mixture*). The practical can further be expanded by investigating

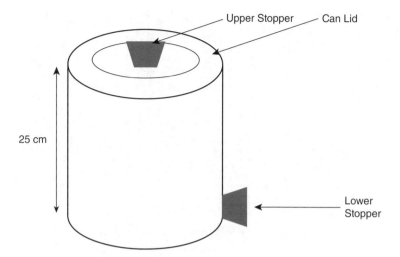

Figure 5.1 Gas explosion experimental setup.

how explosions can be caused by dust of various sorts (e.g. flour, coal) and the concentration of dust in the environment required for combustion by varying the amount of powder in the environment. The experiment is detailed by the Nuffield Foundation (*The cornflower 'bomb'*).

Practical 3: Fire Scene Investigation in a Simulation Fire Scene Scenario
Students conduct a fatal fire investigation within a simulated post-fire scene environment (details on creating a fire scene are discussed later) ensuring that information is gathered in a systematic manner with attention to the relevant details. The detailed fire scene investigation includes descriptions of ceilings, walls, doors and windows alongside smoke, fire, heat patterns and post-fire indicators, in addition to any identifiable points of origin, ignition sources and accelerant. Sketches are to be drawn and to include a key, compass direction, measurements and scale with positions of doors, windows, fixtures, appliances, furniture and relevant items recorded.

Students are expected to consider and evaluate the types of evidence that may be collected from the fatal fire scene, how the evidence is collected, how it is packaged, how it may be analysed and its purpose in ascertaining the cause and spread of the fire and its use as part of the investigation.

This practical is an observational exercise assessing the students' abilities to:

- Appreciate the importance of the use of the correct equipment for investigating a fire scene.
- Identify potential points of origin within the fire scene and predict fire and smoke damage patterns.
- Recognise forensic evidence sources that may be of wider use within a fatal fire investigation.
- Identify the indicators which may be used to distinguish between whether the fatal fire victim died as a result of the fire or otherwise.

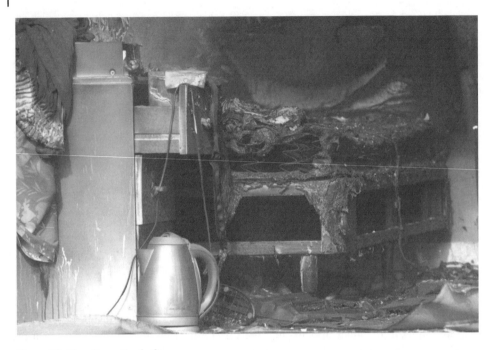

Figure 5.2 The aftermath of a fire.

Working in pairs, the students:

- Select and use equipment (20%)
- Fire scene assessment and sketch (30%)
- Evaluate the forensic evidence (10%)
- Visual examination of the fire victim (20%)
- Photograph the fire scene (Figure 5.2) (10%)
- Fire investigation knowledge (10%)

Practical 4: On-line Multiple Choice Question Test
Multiple choice questions (MCQs) provide a quick and easy formative assessment during the module on several major aspects of fire investigation. These tests allow for students to be presented with visual data in the form of photographs related to fire scenes, undertake their observation and correct identification, for example, stages in the development of a compartmental fire, heat transfer phenomena, flashover (Figure 5.3) and explosion phenomena (Figure 5.4).

Fire Scene Simulation

The study of forensic science provides an opportunity for the application of theoretical knowledge acquired through study to the investigation of simulated crime scenes. This practical approach to forensic investigation education offers the experience through

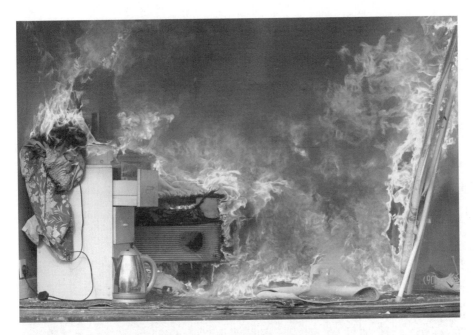

Figure 5.3 Flashover (see colour figure in colour plate section).

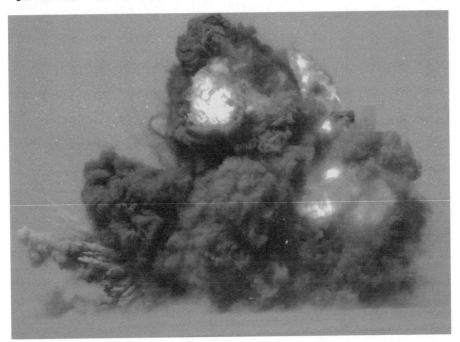

Figure 5.4 EOD teams detonate expired ordinance in Kuwaiti desert. Public Domain Image from Wikimedia Commons. Photographer: Photographer's Mate 2nd Class Aaron Peterson. Source: Peterson https://commons.wikimedia.org/wiki/File:US_Navy_020712-N-5471P-010_EOD_teams_detonate_expired_ordnance_in_the_Kuwaiti_desert.jpg used under CC-BY-SA 3.0 https://commons.wikimedia.org/wiki/Commons:Creative_Commons_Attribution-ShareAlike_3.0_Unported_License (see colour figure in colour plate section).

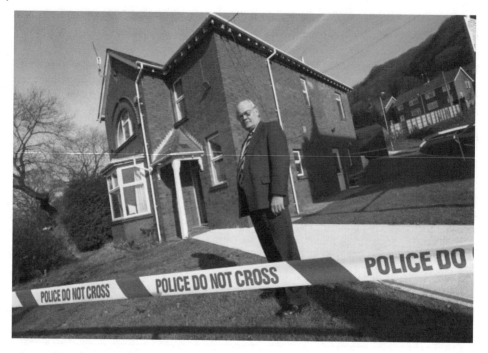

Figure 5.5 Professor Bernard Knight and the Crime Scene House.

which the knowledge and skills involved in the various protocols and procedures can be developed and enhanced into competencies.

The Professor Bernard Knight Crime Scene House at the University of South Wales (Figure 5.5) comprises a ground floor lounge, kitchen and three first floor bedrooms; each room is set up to provide an opportunity to put into practice the skills and knowledge acquired by the student to the investigation of a simulated crime scene in a realistic scenario (Figure 5.6).

It is not usually possible to allow undergraduate students to attend actual fire scenes due to the unsafe nature of the scenes themselves, so in order to allow students to gain experience of fire crime scenes, one of the rooms in the crime scene house has been converted into a simulated post-fire scene. The objective of the reconstruction was to reasonably reproduce the damage and patterns created by a compartment fire involving three separate seats of fire. The most realistic method of producing a fire scene would be to have a controlled fire either by using a blow torch to char specific sections or by having a controlled contained fire within the room to simulate smoke damage. These methods may be suitable in some circumstances, but they do offer an element of risk that may be unacceptable.

The most suitable method is a more cosmetic theatrical approach, still giving the fire effects required without the associated risks of actual fire and smoke.

The walls were painted with black matt emulsion applied using a thick plastic brush to avoid uniform paint coverage and obtain contrasting shades of black colour and a realistic post-fire appearance on the surfaces (Figures 5.7 and 5.8).

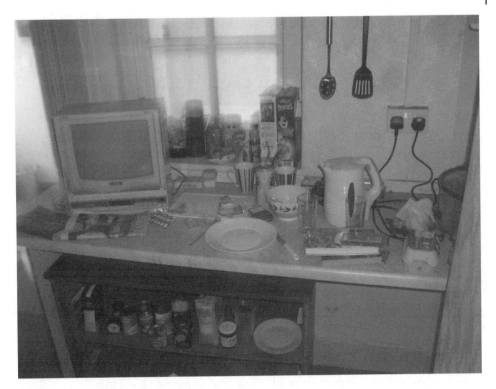

Figure 5.6 Professor Bernard Knight Crime Scene House back room.

Figure 5.7 Fire scene reconstruction – painted walls.

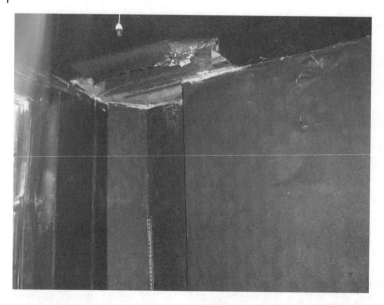

Figure 5.8 Fire scene reconstruction – painted timber (see colour figure in colour plate section).

The doors and glass windows were also painted non-uniformly with the black paint to give the appearance of smoke damage (Figure 5.9).

Surfaces behind wall fixtures were left unpainted to provide areas that were shielded from smoke damage during the fire (Figure 5.10).

Additional smoke hues were added over the black painted surfaces using white and various shades of grey aerosol spray paints (Figure 5.11).

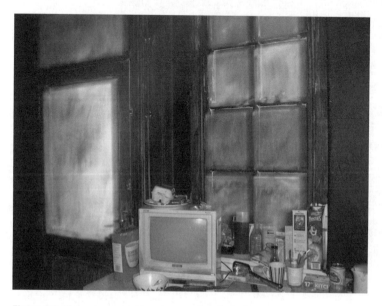

Figure 5.9 Fire scene reconstruction – painted windows.

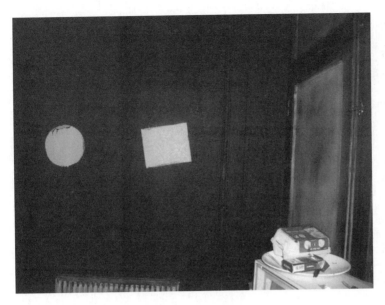

Figure 5.10 Fire scene reconstruction – fixtures.

Areas that were to act as the points of origin of the fire were painted using aerosol spray paints, so as to reflect local damage by fire and heat from the seat of the fire and use of an accelerant (Figure 5.12).

Fixtures and fittings were burned safely away from the room in controlled combustions to add authenticity to the scenario (Figure 5.13).

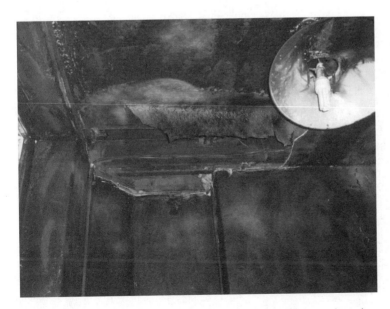

Figure 5.11 Fire scene reconstruction – ceiling (see colour figure in colour plate section).

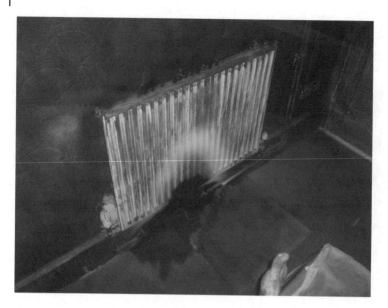

Figure 5.12 Fire scene reconstruction – site of accelerant (see colour figure in colour plate section).

Smoke patterns depicting seats of the fire were added using white and grey aerosol spray paints (Figure 5.14).

Black and grey spray paint was applied as a mist over work surfaces and paraphernalia to create smoke dust appearances (Figure 5.15).

No fatal fire investigation would be complete without an incumbent corpse and a realistic burn victim was purchased from the CSRgroup (http://www.csr-group.co.uk/;

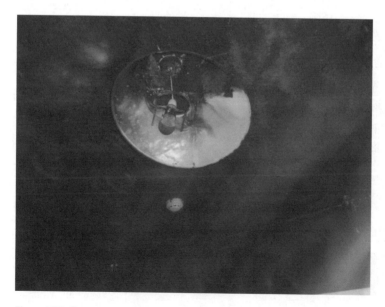

Figure 5.13 Fire scene reconstruction – lamp shade (see colour figure in colour plate section).

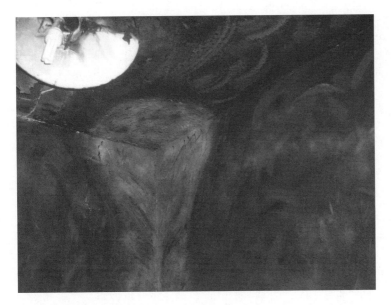

Figure 5.14 Fire scene reconstruction – wastebasket fire.

accessed 26 June 2016), to add reality to the fire scene simulation. These realistic cadavers are hand-made from silicon–latex–urethane and bespoke to requirements.

The white bed sheet upon which the body would lie was masked using the mannequin body and spray painted around to silhouette smoke damage (Figure 5.16).

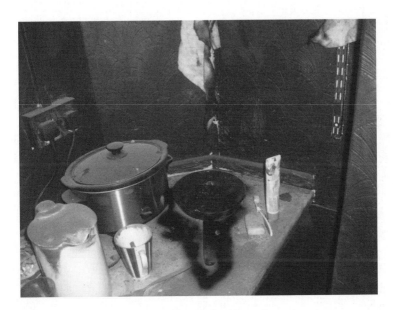

Figure 5.15 Fire scene reconstruction – seat of fire.

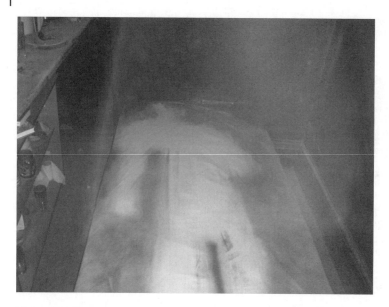

Figure 5.16 Fire scene reconstruction – silhouette on bed linen (see colour figure in colour plate section).

Items of clothing that would be worn by the victim were burned to simulate involvement in a fire (Figure 5.17).

The body was clothed in the burned apparel and placed *in situ*.

Cosmetic touches (moulage) were applied to the mannequin to reconstruct appearance upon death due to the fire (Figure 5.18).

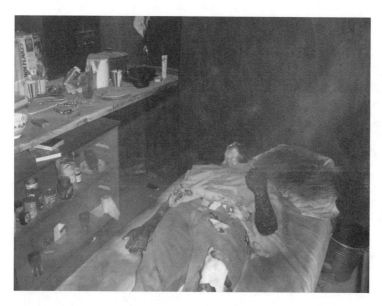

Figure 5.17 Fire scene reconstruction – fire victim.

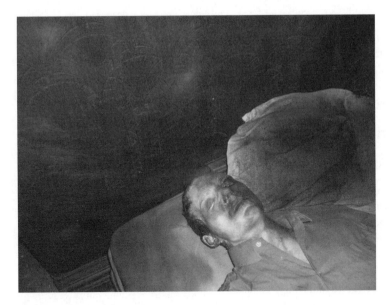

Figure 5.18 Fire scene reconstruction – cosmetic touches (moulage).

Final touches of authenticity to the post-fire scene were added including odours associated with an actual fire scene by using a themed aerosol of woodsmoke (available from DaleAir (http://www.daleair.com/aromas/) sprayed into the room.

The fire scene was thus ready for the student fire investigators to process and record.

Conclusions

The theoretical knowledge acquired by the students through these research studies is consolidated through the practical experimentation described with the student gaining the experience of fire investigation at a post-fire scene.

While only contributing small percentages to the overall assessment of student performance and involving significant effort to create, there is no doubt that practical elements play a very important role in the development of students' knowledge and understanding of subject matter. Experiential learning through undertaking roles discussed theoretically, allows students to actively experience and reflect upon issues and aspects that would otherwise be absent, thus making the process truly worthwhile (Beard and Wilson, 2006).

Future Developments

It is widely recognised that the provision of practical elements greatly enhance the student learning experience (Pearson *et al.*, 2010) and it is the intention to develop an even greater scope of activities available for students to undertake as part of their studies, such as the use and application of field portable devices that may be utilised at the fire scene to assist the fire investigator in the primary detection of accelerants, for example, photoionisation detectors, and also the subsequent laboratory analysis of these fire scene samples for ignitable liquid residues, such as through solid phase micro extraction (SPME) and gas chromatography mass spectrometric (GC-MS) chemical analysis.

Recommended Resources

Introductory Textbooks

Criminalistics, 9th edn (Saferstein, 2007), *Forensic Science*, 3rd edn (Jackson and Jackson, 2011a,b), *Criminal Investigation*, 8th edn (Bennett and Hess, 2006) and *Crime Scene Investigation: Methods and Procedures*, 2nd edn (Pepper, 2010) all provide easily read chapters that are ideal introductions to this aspect of forensic investigation, which orientate the student at the start of their fire investigation studies.

More Detailed Textbooks and Material

More in-depth guidance of fire scene protocols are identified in *The Forensic Science Service Handbook* (2004) and the Cooke and Ide (1993, 2006) series (*A Guide to Fatal Fire Investigations, Principles of Fire Investigation*) remain the stalwart reference sources.

More thorough and comprehensive consolidation of specific in-depth detail related to the full spectrum of fire investigation is achieved through Daeid (2004) (*Fire Investigation*), DeHaan (2002) (*Kirk's Fire Investigation*, 5th edn), Lentini (2006) (*Scientific Protocols for Fire Investigation*) and ultimately the NFPA921 (1994) treatises.

Case Studies

Case studies, such as the Desmond Fennell QC (1988) investigation into The King's Cross Underground Fire, The Tribunal of Inquiry into the Stardust Nightclub, Dublin Fire (Stardust Tribunal, 1981) and The Station Nightclub, New Jersey Fire, provide for reference to actual examples and standard investigative formats.

On-line video materials related to these case studies may be found at http://www .youtube.com/watch?v=1cKTNwnmomk for the King's Cross fire and http://www .youtube.com/watch?v=TdqNtQiVIK4 for The Station Nightclub fire.

References

Almirall, J. and Furton K.G. (2004) *Analysis and Interpretation of Fire Scene Evidence*, CRC Press, Boca Raton, FL.

Beard, C., and Wilson, J.P. (2006) Experiential Learning: A Best Practice Handbook for Educators and Trainers, Kogan Page, Philadelphia, PA.

Bennett, W.W. and Hess, K.M. (2006) Arson, bombs and explosives, in *Criminal Investigation*, 8th edn, Wadsworth Publishing, Belmont, CA, chap. 15, pp. 386–406.

Bloom. B. (1959) *Taxonomy of Educational Objectives. Volume I: Cognitive Domain*, McKay, New York, NY.

Cooke, R.A. and Ide, R.H. (1993) *A Guide to Fatal Fire Investigations*, Institution of Fire Engineers, Leicester.

Cooke, R.A. and Ide, R.H. (2006) *Principles of Fire Investigation*, Institution of Fire Engineers, Leicester.

CSR group, *Authentic Tactical Bodies for Training and Education*. Available at: http://www.csr-group.co.uk/index.php?option=com_content&view=article&id=46:authentic-tactical-bodies-for-training-a-education-&catid=29:products&Itemid=53 (accessed 26 June 2016).

Daeid, N.N. (2004) *Fire Investigation*, CRC Press, Boca Raton, FL.

DaleAir, *Themed Aerosol*. Available at: http://www.daleair.com/woodsmoke-aroma (accessed 28 June 2016).

DeHaan, J.D. (2002) *Kirk's Fire Investigation*, 5th edn, Prentice Hall, Upper Saddle River, NY.

Fennel, D. (1988) *Investigation into the King's Cross Underground Fire*, Her Majesty's Stationery Office, London. Available at: http://www.railwaysarchive.co.uk/docsummary.php?docID=75 (accessed 29 November 2016).

Jackson, R.W. and Jackson, J.M. (2011a) Fires, in *Forensic Science*, 3rd edn, Pearson Prentice Hall, Harlow, chap. 10, pp. 320–351.

Jackson, R.W. and Jackson, J.M. (2011b), Explosions and explosives, in *Forensic Science*, 3rd edn, Pearson Prentice Hall, Harlow, chap. 11, pp. 352–368.

Lentini, J.J. (2006) *Scientific Protocols for Fire Investigation*, Taylor & Francis, Boca Raton, FL.

NFPA921 treatises (1994) *Guide for Fire and Explosion Investigations*. Available at: (http://www.nfpa.org/codes-and-standards/all-codes-and-standards/list-of-codes-and-standards?mode=code&code=921) (accessed 26 June 2016).

Nuffield Foundation. *The cornflower bomb*. Available at: http://nuffieldfoundation.org/practical-chemistry/cornflower-'bomb' (accessed 22 June 2015).

Pearson, D., Moje, E.B. and Greenleaf, C. (2010) Literacy and science: each in the service of the other. *Science*, **328**, 459–463.

Pepper, I.K. (2010) The investigation of a fire scene, in *Crime Scene Investigation: Methods and Procedures*, 2nd edn, Open University Press, Maidenhead, chap. 8, pp. 92–98.

Royal Society of Chemistry (2016) *Controlled Explosion of a Methane-Air mixture*. Available at: http://www.rsc.org/learn-chemistry/wiki/TeacherExpt:Controlled_explosion_of_a_methane-air_mixture (accessed 22 June 2015).

Saferstein, R. (2007) Forensic aspects of arson and explosion investigations, in *Criminalistics*, 9th edn, Prentice Hall, Upper Saddle River, NY, chap. 11, pp. 310–343.

Stardust Tribunal Report (1981) *The Tribunal of Inquiry into the Stardust Nightclub, Dublin Fire*. Available at http://thestory.ie/2012/04/01/stardust-tribunal-report-1981/ (accessed 28 November 2016).

The Forensic Science Service (2004) Fire investigation, in *The Scenes of Crime Handbook*, Forensic Science Service, chap. 10, pp. 65–69.

Further Reading

Barnard, J.A. and Bradley, J.N. (1985) *Flame and Combustion*, Chapman and Hall, New York.

Drydale, D. (1992) *An Introduction to Fire Dynamics*, Wiley-Interscience, New York.
Landrock, A.H. (1983) *Handbook of Plastics Flammability and Combustion Toxicology*, Noyes Publications, Park Ridge, NJ.
Noon, R. (1995) *Engineering Analysis of Fires and Explosions*, CRC Press, Boca Raton, FL.
Quintiere J.G. (1997) *Principles of Fire Behaviour*, Delmar, Albany, NY.
Redsicher, D.R. and Connor, J.J. (1997) *Practical Fire and Arson Investigation*, CRC Press, Boca Raton, FL.

6

Digital Forensics Education

A New Source of Forensic Evidence

Christopher Hargreaves

Cranfield University, College Road, Cranfield, Bedfordshire, UK

Introduction

This chapter discusses a newer area of forensic science education – digital forensics. Digital forensics was defined in the 2001 Digital Forensics Research Workshop (DFRWS) as 'the use of scientifically derived and proven methods toward the preservation, collection, validation, identification, analysis, interpretation, documentation, and presentation of digital evidence derived from digital sources for the purpose of facilitating or furthering the reconstruction of events found to be criminal, or helping to anticipate unauthorized actions shown to be disruptive to planned operations' (DFRWS, 2001), although as will be discussed later, the definition is not as standardised as that for forensic science.

The term 'digital forensics' is used in this section as a concatenation of 'digital forensic science', although there are other terms that are also used, including 'forensic computing', 'computer forensics' and 'cyber forensics'. Digital forensics is used here rather than a term that uses the word 'computer', since the range of digital devices that can be examined has significantly expanded from the traditional beige box stored under a desk to now include smartphones, tablets and wireless routers. This range of devices is continuing to expand into new areas. At time of writing, wearable technology and 'Internet of Things' devices are becoming more commonplace; for example, Wi-Fi weighing scales, personal trackers such as FitBits and Google Glasses.

It is difficult to discuss digital forensics without mentioning that the investigation of computer based evidence in the United Kingdom is steered by the ACPO (Association of Chief Police Officers, now the National Police Chiefs Council) *Good Practice Guide for Digital Evidence* (ACPO, 2012). The document is extensive but summarises four main principles:

1. No action taken by law enforcement agencies, persons employed within those agencies or their agents should change data which may subsequently be relied upon in court.

Forensic Science Education and Training: A Tool-kit for Lecturers and Practitioner Trainers, First Edition.
Edited by Anna Williams, John P. Cassella, and Peter D. Maskell.
© 2017 John Wiley & Sons Ltd. Published 2017 by John Wiley & Sons Ltd.

2. In circumstances where a person finds it necessary to access original data, that person must be competent to do so and be able to give evidence explaining the relevance and the implications of their actions.
3. An audit trail or other record of all processes applied to digital evidence should be created and preserved. An independent third party should be able to examine those processes and achieve the same result.
4. The person in charge of the investigation has overall responsibility for ensuring that the law and these principles are adhered to.

While the definition of forensic science is the 'application of science to law' techniques used for digital forensics can be used more widely than just producing evidence for court. For example, techniques for analysing data on hard disks to extract evidence relating to a crime can also be applied during investigations in corporate environments to determine how a piece of malware got on to a system, whether someone was viewing unsuitable material using work equipment, or whether someone has been sharing proprietary company data with the another organisation.

However, whether digital forensics techniques are used for the purposes of upholding the law, or to come to a conclusion about someone's actions in a corporate environment, there are consequences to the outcome of the investigation and it is therefore vital that the decision reached is the correct one given all the available evidence. Therefore, regardless of the type of investigation being carried out, it is prudent to apply the rigour associated with forensic science.

A Brief History of Digital Forensics Education

Digital forensic science is one of the more recent strands of forensic science to emerge. Yasinsac *et al.* (2003) described the initial development of the field as: 'the child of law enforcement necessity. Computers were being found at crime scenes and investigators were eager to use this new source of information. The investigators sought out people to assist in making this latent form of evidence visible. Often, the few people that were familiar with computers were system administrators of law enforcement systems or other investigators who happened to have either a previous background in information technology or were hobbyists. Early computer forensic practitioners often operated without academic education or formal forensic training. Fewer still had experience working within a structured computer forensics environment.'

To meet this need for training, certainly in the United Kingdom, a small number of short courses (over 1–2 weeks) emerged. Some were at universities and others at police training facilities. These courses were for law enforcement only and had the purpose of training law enforcement to handle computer-based evidence.

Current Digital Forensic Education

The situation regarding education in digital forensic science is now quite different and courses are not aimed solely at law enforcement.

At time of writing, in the United Kingdom there are 41 undergraduate courses with some variation of digital forensics in the title, 21 masters' level courses and many training courses instructing on the use of specific digital forensics software products. It is difficult to comprehend the need for such a large number of specialist courses. However, in reality, some of these courses, particularly at the undergraduate level, are rebranded computer science courses that have been updated to contain a small number of modules that are actually focused on digital forensics.

At MSc level, more courses that are titled with a term such as digital forensics contain a more substantial element of focused content. Nevertheless, there is still a substantial difference in the specific knowledge and skills that students have on completion of a masters' degree. Similar titled courses can have very different focuses; for example, some may have a more substantial computer security element, which better prepares students for incident response work. Some are management focused, which can include the production of security policies. Other courses with a digital investigation focus aim to prepare students for actually performing a digital forensic examination, including substantial technical content on the operation of computer systems, strategies for digital investigation and data recovery, identification of artefacts left from user behaviour and report writing, which includes the presentation of evidence in court.

Such variation in courses offers both advantages and disadvantages for students searching for a course. Choice is obviously a positive thing and students are able to select a course that offers the focus that they want from their education experience and also for their future job prospects. However, the disadvantage is that it is not always obvious what the emphasis of a particular course is. Over time perhaps degree titles will more accurately reflect the particular focus of the course, but this will require substantial collaboration between different parts of the community.

Digital Forensics as a Sub-Discipline?

One reason for the variation in topics taught as part of a 'digital forensics' course is that there is a question over where digital forensics sits in a taxonomy of subjects (Irons *et al.*, 2009). There is debate about whether digital forensics/forensic computing/cyber forensics exists as a sub-discipline of computer science, forensic science, or is a new subject altogether. Irons *et al.* (2009) concluded that digital forensics is a separate subject, but this is not universally accepted. Certainly in most universities, digital forensics courses exist either as part of a computer science department or as part of a forensic science department.

Digital Forensics and Traditional Forensic Science Skill Sets

Compared with traditional forensic science there are certainly some differences in skill sets; for example, digital forensics requires much less emphasis on natural and physical sciences, but deeper understanding and familiarity with computer systems. This involves the use of complex software packages (e.g. advanced hexadecimal editors), understanding the ways in which particular pieces of software store their data (e.g. the internal data structures used in a Microsoft Word document) and the digital artefacts that are created when a user performs a particular action (e.g. the specific digital artefact present that can be used to determine if a web address was typed into the address bar of a browser). Traditional forensic science students also require computer skills but this is focused on the *use* of computer software packages, for example, spreadsheets for data handling or perhaps control software for 3D scanners or other analytical equipment. In addition, while mathematics is important in both forensic science variants, at time of writing there are currently fewer applications for statistical methods and calculus in digital forensics than in traditional forensic science. Conversely, in traditional forensic science it is unlikely that a knowledge is necessary of different number bases, such as binary and hexadecimal, nor an understanding of the different representations of data that are possible, for example, integer and floating point representations, data format representations and text encodings.

Despite these differences in knowledge and skills of traditional forensic science students and those studying digital forensics, both can be considered to be interdisciplinary subjects, and there are commonalities. These include:

- **law** – both digital forensic and traditional forensic science students need an understanding of legal procedures, rules of evidence and courtroom skills;
- **physical crime scene investigation** – it is possible that a digital forensics graduate may be expected to attend a crime scene, for example to assist in the collection of physical items that may contain digital data, or increasingly to conduct a specialised 'live investigation' of a running system, something that requires specialist skills even within the digital forensics field;
- **evidence handling** – both students will need to be able to practically apply evidence handling procedures and maintain chain of custody;
- **scientific method** – both types of student will need to conduct experiments in order to draw conclusions about past events from the state of particular artefacts.

Thus, while traditional forensic science and digital forensics differ in some aspects, they also share a common grounding in law, crime scenes, evidence and the scientific method. There is, therefore, much to be gained from collaboration in both education and research, and sharing of resources (e.g. modules on courses) is likely to be mutually beneficial.

Challenges in Digital Forensics Education

The teaching of digital forensics presents some interesting challenges and this subsection discusses a selection of these.

Different Levels of Study

As discussed in the previous section, digital forensics is an interdisciplinary subject with a need for students to have a thorough grasp of computer science concepts, specific knowledge of operating systems and application behaviour and artefacts, an understanding of the law, forensic science and deep professional ethics (Anderson *et al.*, 2006). Anderson *et al.* (2006) go on to specify that 'due to this large spectrum of skills, graduate level education (at a university degree level) is commonly regarded as the best way to teach computer forensics.' Yasinsac *et al.* (2003) are even more specific, stating that 'computer forensics… is well suited to undergraduate classes,' since there is a 'large body of expertise, techniques, and knowledge that can be presented to undergraduates.'

An earlier section discussed that there are taught courses in digital forensics offered at undergraduate and postgraduate level. There are also a number of doctoral students that are pursuing a PhD in digital forensics. The next section discusses how different aspects of digital forensics map out the Quality Assurance Agency (QAA) for Higher Education degree descriptors offered by different levels of qualifications.

Undergraduate

According to the QAA framework for a bachelor's level degree, students who obtain the qualification should demonstrate 'a systematic understanding of key aspects of their field of study, including acquisition of coherent and detailed knowledge, at least some of which is at, or informed by, the forefront of defined aspects of a discipline' and 'an ability to deploy accurately established techniques of analysis and enquiry within a discipline.'

These points should not be problematic to address, as there is a substantial knowledge base to digital forensics. However, it is clear from the varying syllabuses for undergraduate degrees in forensics, that it is not clearly defined what the 'key aspects' of the digital forensics field are. Since students will usually be starting an undergraduate course after obtaining A-level qualifications, in order to gain knowledge of key aspects of the field, the teaching of a substantial amount of computer science is necessary, including computer architecture, programming, databases, and so on. However, as discussed earlier, digital forensics is a multidisciplinary field and if it is to be considered as an all encompassing digital forensics degree, it must include aspects of law, evidence handling and the scientific method.

Another consideration is that a digital forensics degree is highly specialist at undergraduate level and it is therefore desirable to ensure that students leave with the skills necessary for a wide range of career opportunities in addition to digital forensics. The approach offered by most universities is to provide generic modules on computer science topics, and then offer additional modules that are specific to digital forensics.

Masters' Level

According to the QAA framework for a masters' level degree, students who obtain the qualification should demonstrate 'a systematic understanding of knowledge, and a critical awareness of current problems and/or new insights, much of which is at, or informed by, the forefront of their academic discipline, field of study or area of professional practice' and 'a comprehensive understanding of techniques applicable to their own research or advanced scholarship,' and 'originality in the application of knowledge, together with a practical understanding of how established techniques of research and enquiry are used to create and interpret knowledge in the discipline.'

These masters' level descriptors are more difficult to address than those at undergraduate level. This is in part due to the potential variety of skill sets of students coming into the programme. Since digital forensics is a multidisciplinary field, there are a variety of backgrounds that could be considered acceptable as prior study for entry to a digital forensics masters. Backgrounds could include:

- computer science
- undergraduate digital forensics
- forensic science
- criminology
- law

If it is accepted that some of the material taught on an undergraduate computer science programme forms key aspects of the field of digital forensics, then if students are accepted from backgrounds without that content, the masters' course must include that computer science material for those without the requisite background. This can present a significant challenge since it is then necessary to teach material that for some students is extremely basic, whereas for other students, it is new and challenging. This clearly could be avoided by demanding a computer science background, but experience has shown that some students from non-computing backgrounds are able to comprehend the computing aspect of the course quickly and as a result of their broader background experience perform extremely well in the interdisciplinary field of digital forensics.

Given the speed of change of technology, the requirement for students to have 'a comprehensive understanding of techniques applicable to their own research or advanced scholarship' is extremely important. For example, new versions of web browsers are now released every few months, so assuming that the content taught on the course is cutting edge, the specific artefacts taught at the beginning of the course may be three versions old by the time the students reach the end of their degree. Students will have to realise this as a limitation of teaching in this field, but use this base knowledge as a platform for conducting their own experiments to determine the artefacts left by a newer version of the software. Therefore any digital forensics programme must include not only the scientific method, but also specific digital forensics research techniques, such as virtualisation of test systems for experiments and techniques for monitoring test systems for changes.

Doctoral Level

According to the QAA framework for a doctoral level degree, students who obtain the qualification should demonstrate 'the creation and interpretation of new knowledge', and 'continue to undertake pure and/or applied research and development at an advanced level, contributing substantially to the development of new techniques, ideas or approaches.'

The ideal prerequisite for PhD study of digital forensics is a related masters' degree with a substantial research component, in addition to detailed technical content. It is also worth noting that the study of digital forensics at a doctoral level is likely, at some point, to require programming skills, for example, in the case of researching artefacts left, for substantial evaluation to take place it is necessary to perform some sort of automation.

Education versus Training

Digital forensics is an inherently practical field, with much of the work of a digital forensic practitioner involving the use of specialist pieces of software to acquire, extract and analyse digital evidence. As such, a discussion over digital forensic education and digital forensic training often occurs.

While there are a number of undergraduate and postgraduate courses available in the United Kingdom, there are also many high-quality training courses available on how to use specific software packages that are used in digital forensic investigations, from vendors such as Guidance Software, Access Data and X-Ways.

Yansac *et al.* compared training and education, where: skill equates to knowledge; application to abstraction; using tools to developing tools; applying procedures to establishing procedures; and practice to theory (Yasinsac *et al.*, 2003).

Stevens (2008) discussed this comparison of education and training in the context of the development of an MSc in 'Cybercrime Forensics', and stated that 'Cybercrime Forensics Training is similar in lots of ways to Forensic Computing Education'. This includes: 'practical class student numbers (twenty)', 'the type and specification of the equipment used', 'the variability in student knowledge' and 'the approaches to learning and teaching based on similar theories'. The major differences that were identified included: manpower, the lecture/practical split, the course duration and learning theory interpretation. However, these conclusions come from the development of a single programme and do not necessarily generalise; for example, the differences in course duration (two terms in education and one week in training) do not apply to those education courses that are delivered in 'block mode', for example, over one week full-time, and the lecture/practical split is highly dependent on the way in which the postgraduate education is delivered. Nevertheless, it is difficult to imagine a digital forensics education course that does not include application of theory in *practice, using tools* to investigate a disk image, or *applying existing procedures*. It is likely therefore that the line between digital forensics education and digital forensics training is blurred. The argument is perhaps not that education should only have certain elements, but rather that education courses, in addition to *skills, application, using tools, applying procedures* and *practice*, must **also** contain development of *knowledge, abstraction, developing tools, establishing procedures* and *theory*.

Speed of Technology Change

Another challenge to digital forensic education is the speed of change of technology. This includes big societal changes in technology use, for example, the use of mobile devices such as smartphones and tablets, along with simple version updates of operating systems or applications.

Each new version of an operating system brings new challenges and new opportunities for digital forensic artefact recovery. Fortunately in the Microsoft Windows environment, which is still the dominant operating system, this usually occurs every few years, (Windows XP in 2001, Windows Vista in 2007, Windows 7 in 2009, Windows 8 in 2012, and Windows 10 in 2015). However, some significant applications (e.g. the web browser Mozilla Firefox) now have a very rapid release cycle, meaning that for every new release, research is required to check that the artefacts in the previous release are still present, identify any new artefacts that may have been introduced and check that the user behaviour that can be inferred from the presence of particular artefacts is the same.

Such rapid release cycles have significant impact on teaching digital forensics. Since the field is highly practical, it is not sufficient just to have a lecture discussing the artefacts left; practical exercises and examples are necessary. Therefore, frequent releases of software can quickly make practical exercises out of date. It is possible that data examined during exercises can be student-produced material, but usually in order to make a particular educational point, specific scenarios need to be created in order to produce artefacts with the desired properties. Production of such data is extremely time consuming and rapid application release cycles mean that this needs to be conducted more frequently.

The problem can, however, be mitigated, since despite the rapid release cycles of software, there are often few significant changes. For example, comparing Firefox 7 and 16, there were no changes to the Firefox history databases that affect the reconstruction of websites visited, browser bookmarks or data entered into web forms. Nevertheless, even if the technology in use is extremely similar and the underlying digital forensic principles are the same, using older examples in a fast moving field can create the impression of the material taught being out-of-date. Therefore, ideally, general principles should be taught using up-to-date examples.

Another challenge in providing a comprehensive digital forensic education is that during an investigation, the digital forensic practitioner could encounter any technology, from obsolete floppy disks through to the latest technology. There is therefore a balance that needs to be struck so that a student is provided with an awareness of older technology and enough information to research the topic independently, but making sure that the majority of the teaching time is focused on providing a comprehensive education on modern technologies that are most likely to be encountered. Furthermore, even ignoring obsolete technology, it is not possible to cover the full scope of current technology that may be encountered. This further emphasises the importance of education, abstraction and independent research.

Distance Learning Challenges

Changing student demographics also present a challenge, for example, the need to provide more courses via distance learning. Even when focused on principles, in order to provide a comprehensive and practically useful education in digital forensics, students need exposure to and experience with applications that they will encounter when entering employment in digital forensics. The next section discusses some of the progress that has been made in preparing for delivery of digital forensics education via distance learning.

Software Licensing

One of the challenges with teaching at a distance is access to expensive, proprietary software tools that are central to a modern digital forensics workflow. The tool vendors have made significant progress in making software accessible for teaching in computer laboratories at universities at a reasonable cost, and often include training material. However, students studying remotely may not have access to such labs.

It is possible to provide remote access to laboratories, but such capability usually requires high-level support at the university, as special cases may need to be made to enable such access. It is also possible to utilise some cloud computing technologies, although this is, at time of writing, work in progress. There are also a variety of free open source digital tools available, the usability of which continues to improve. Nevertheless, it is still the case that it is experience of using the commercial packages that is listed in the essential or desirable section of job advertisements.

Size of Disk Images

Even if the problem of access to software is overcome, another challenge is the distribution of course material. If a course includes a practical element that involves the analysis of disk images of a computer, these can be quite large, for example, a compressed version of one of our early assignments is approximately 15 Gigabytes.

This presents challenges for storage online, since this is one of many disk images on a course. It also, sadly, still presents potential bandwidth problems for some parts of the United Kingdom, and indeed other parts of the world that may require access to such distance learning material. It may be the case that broadband speeds mean that the downloading of such material is infeasible.

However, as discussed in the previous section, virtualised environments making use of cloud computing solutions could potentially solve this problem. Since the examination of the data is done through a server hosted virtualised computer system, the data never actually has to be transferred in full from the server to the student, only the current view of the data is transmitted, although some connection speeds may also make this approach infeasible.

Student Support During Practical Exercises

Another challenge to the distance-learning mode of study is how to support students during practical exercises. Typically a practical session has teaching staff that are able to assist a student if they are having trouble with a particular part of a practical. It is not clear if current technology would allow this type of support or if a different model would need to be adopted.

Challenges in Incorporating Law into the Digital Forensics Curriculum

Another challenge to digital forensics education is incorporating law into the curriculum.

Need for Legal Expertise

The first difficulty, and the one that can more easily be overcome, is that a thorough understanding of the law may be outside of the area of expertise of those teaching the 'computing' aspect of digital forensics. However, in large traditional universities, lecturers can be used from the law department in order to assist with these aspects of the course. There are examples of more extensive cross-department collaboration where students studying law are also brought into contact with students from the digital forensics course and cross-examinations of the digital forensics students takes place, which potentially provides benefits for both types of student.

Which Aspects of Law to Teach?

Given that law can be studied full-time for three years, the legal component of a course in digital forensics is necessarily a subset of possible legal issues that could relate to a digital investigation. Assuming that an overview of the legal system is required, and the role of the expert in the legal process will be discussed, a decision will need to be made about which parts of law are of particular interest to the digital forensic scientist. Typically, a digital forensic practitioner will at some point be investigating possession of indecent images of children and therefore sexual offences legislation is often discussed. There are some obvious 'computer crimes,' for example, a computer used to gain unauthorised access to a computer system, and therefore, in the United Kingdom at least, Computer Misuse Act offences are relevant. However, digital evidence from computers or other digital devices could be relevant in any number of offences from fraud to murder. Stalking could involve messages sent via social networking sites, proceeds of stolen goods could be recorded on a smart phone, even a TV recorder may contain digital evidence that provides an alibi for a person's whereabouts. Therefore, a very broad range of legislation could be considered to be within the scope and decisions will need to be made about what is and is not included in the legal component of a digital forensics course.

Which Country's Law to Teach?

Since many crimes could involve digital evidence in some way, the previous section discussed the difficulty in incorporating legislation for all possible crimes into a digital forensics curriculum. In fact, the situation is even more problematic, since laws can be specific to particular localised regions, be that country or state specific legislation. It is commonplace to teach the legislation for the country in which the digital forensics course is hosted, but this potentially causes difficulties for international students without the same contextual knowledge of home students. This may also be particularly problematic if the course is to be offered via distance learning, where students may be geographically scattered and have little knowledge or interest in the legislation of the country in which the course is being delivered. This potentially requires finer granularity in terms of modularisation, and cooperation with universities in other countries. This may allow different legal modules from different institutions to be delivered for students in different countries.

Other Discussions in Digital Forensics Education

Programming for Digital Forensics

As discussed earlier in the chapter, programming is likely to make up some part of undergraduate or postgraduate study in digital forensics. However, there can be challenges to integrating this into a programme.

Lack of Existing Programming Experience

On a bachelor's level digital forensics course, the topics taught are likely to be fairly broad and aiming to provide students with a transferable skill set outside of just digital forensics. It is therefore likely that the amount of programming that is involved on the course is reasonable and that it can be gradually taught over the course of the programme. However, at masters' level, there is much less time available, but it may not be possible to assume any existing programming skills since students may have started the course from a variety of backgrounds. It may be that only a single module is available to teach programming and therefore the choice of language is therefore an important consideration. While there are a number of candidates (Perl, Java, C#, etc.), experience has shown that the use of the Python programming language for a module of this nature is highly effective. Python is commonly used as a teaching language in other areas and certainly has properties that make it useful in digital forensics. Python allows access to file systems, allows raw binary data to be interpreted in a variety of ways, it allows software written in other languages to be called and the output passed to other programs for further processing. There are also modules available for handling a number of different data storage formats, including XML, SQLite and JSON. It is also worth noting that if the decision is made to use Python, it is suggested that version 3 of the language is used, primarily for the different way in which binary data are handled, meaning that explicit conversion between binary and text based data is necessary (using a particular character encoding).

Lab Requirements for Digital Forensics

It has already been discussed that practical exercises and examples are an important part of a digital forensics course. This section discusses some of the requirements for building a digital forensics teaching laboratory.

Hardware

The hardware requirements for a teaching laboratory are not as substantial as a real digital forensic lab. Typically, synthesised scenarios that students will be examining, at time of writing, are unlikely to exceed 40 Gigabytes, which most modern systems will happily process. However, it is worth considering how data will be transferred and high-speed networking and other high-speed connectivity options, such as USB 3 and Thunderbolt, should be seriously considered.

Software

There are a number of different types of software tool that need to be considered for use on a digital forensics course. While the software can be relatively expensive, many vendors will offer substantial discount on the product for use in education environments and may supply training material for the particular tool. One 'type' of forensic software is the large forensic suites that are in use in real-world digital forensic labs, these include EnCase (Guidance Software), FTK (Access Data) and X-Ways Forensics (X-Ways Software Technology). Such tools offer a large range of capabilities, including case management, means to browse disk images, capability to interpret a number of file types that are encountered on a hard disk, searching and indexing, gallery views of images and report generation. There are also specialist packages for recovery of specific artefact types, for example, Internet related artefact recovery using NetAnalysis (Digital Detective) and Internet Evidence Finder (Magnet Forensics). Also, since many entry level positions for digital forensic analysts involve mobile phone data extraction, it may also be desirable to obtain mobile phone specific software, such as XRY (Micro Systemation) or Cellebrite (Cellebrite).

Teaching on a digital forensic course is likely to involve not just the use of tools to recover artefacts, but the knowledge of how these tools actually extract and interpret the data. As a result, the use of a hex editor to view the raw data that makes up the file system or other file type is essential. Typical examples include WinHex (X-Ways Software Technology) and 010 (Sweetscape). Both of these offer the capability to define templates that will interpret a selection of data according to a particular specification. Similarly, other generic data interpretation tools will also be necessary for examining formats such as SQLite, XML and JSON.

All of the software packages discussed are commercial offerings and it would be remiss not to discuss the open source contributions to the digital forensics community. There are a substantial number of open source tools available and it is not possible to discuss all of them in this chapter. A comprehensive catalogue of open source tools is available at http://www2.opensourceforensics.org.

Developing Practical Exercises for Digital Forensics

The need for practical based exercises has been discussed throughout this chapter. This section discusses the development of such exercises.

Lallie (2010) discussed two types of practical exercise in digital forensics, which are 'Skill Specific Case Studies', and 'Holistic Skill Case Studies.'

The first type of case study (skill specific) is designed to improve and/or assess the students' competence in a particular skill in digital forensics. This could be the examination of the partition structure of a disk, a particular aspect of a file system, or perhaps an application level examination, such as recovery of specific information from an Internet browser's SQLite database. Since this exercise is very focused on a particular file or files, construction of test data is usually fairly straightforward. For example, in a simple partitioning exercise it is necessary simply to generate a disk image that contains several partitions so that the students can reconstruct the partition table by interpreting the raw binary data.

The latter type of case study (holistic) requires students to conduct a more thorough investigation, usually of a complete disk image of a 'suspect's' system. In these holistic examinations, a scenario is constructed where some sort of crime has been committed and the disk image needs to be examined. Data generation for this type of exercise usually involves construction of a scenario, a storyboard, and simulating the user's actions over the course of several months. These actions include those that relate to the 'crime' but also normal background activity on the computer system, for example, looking at news pages, shopping, and so on. This type of exercise is much more complex and time consuming to produce. However, in order to create realistic exercises to assess students' ability to perform a digital forensic analysis, it is currently unavoidable.

Summary

In summary, digital forensics is a branch of forensic science associated with the investigation of digital media. Some of the skills required differ from the skill set of those studying for a traditional forensic science degree, with less emphasis on the natural and physical sciences, but with a need for a deep understanding of the workings of computer operating systems and application software. Nevertheless, there are commonalities with traditional forensic science, for example, the need for an understanding of law, crime scene investigation, physical evidence handling and the scientific method.

There are a number of challenges to teaching digital forensics, including balancing education and training on a programme, the speed of change of technology and the time-consuming nature of generating data for exercises and assessment. There are also challenges that are likely to become more prevalent, for example, difficulties in delivering the material via distance learning and how to incorporate law into a course with a diverse, international mix of students. Nevertheless, digital forensics is a new and exciting area of forensic science and the opportunities for research and education increase as technology becomes more integrated into every aspect of our lives.

References

Anderson, P., Dornseif, M., Freiling, F.C., Holz, T., Irons, A., Laing, C. and Mink, M. (2006) A comparative study of teaching forensics at a university degree level. *IT-Incidents Management & IT-Forensics-IMF*, 116–127.

ACPO (2012) *Good Practice Guide for Digital Evidence*. Available at: (https://www.cps.gov.uk/legal/assets/uploads/files/ACPO_guidelines_computer_evidence[1].pdf) (accessed 26 June 2016).

DFRWS (2001) A road map for digital forensic research. *Digital Forensics Research Workshop*, **1**, 1–48. Available at: http://www.dfrws.org/2001/dfrws-rm-final.pdf (accessed 30 November 2016).

Irons, A.D., Stephens, P. and Ferguson, R.I. (2009) Digital investigation as a distinct discipline: A pedagogic perspective. *Digital Investigation*, **6**, 82–90.

Lallie, H.S. (2010) The use of digital forensic case studies for teaching and assessment, in, Presented at the Cybercrime Forensics Education and Training, 1–9.

Stevens, P. (2008) Should Training Be Part Of An Educational Computer Forensics Programme?, 1–20.

Yasinsac, A., Erbacher, R.F., Marks, D.G., Pollitt, M.M. and Sommer, P.M. (2003) Computer forensics education. *IEEE Security and Privacy*, **1** (4), 15–23.

7

A Strategy for Teaching Forensic Investigation with Limited Resources

Crime Scene House: What Crime Scene House?

Janice Kennedy

University of West Scotland, School of Science and Sport, Hamilton Campus, Hamilton, UK

Introduction

In the current teaching reality of increased class sizes and decreased budgets, is it still possible to provide a high-quality learning experience in forensic subjects for our students?

Can we manage, specifically, to instil the critical thinking and evaluation skills that are so vital to forensic science – and indeed to ANY science – graduates?

It is believed that the answer to both of these questions is 'yes,' and in this chapter some ideas will be presented of how that can be achieved with limited resources.

The chapter does not claim to provide a recipe to follow for success, rather it tries to provide a bundle of suggestions that can be dipped into and used – or not – as appropriate.

Historical Background

Analytical skills, both practical and evaluative, are essential transferable skills for science.

In a recent review of skills needed by forensic science graduates, Hanson and Overton (2010) noted that *generic skills* were found by graduates to be of the most use. Of the *forensic science skills*, those most valued by the graduates were the analytical skills.

But what is understood by the phrase 'analytical skills?' Is the definition limited to, for instance, analytical chemistry laboratory skills? In over 20 years of teaching, it has been observed that students certainly favour that definition. As an analytical chemist, that narrow definition has never appeared appropriate: both practical AND evaluative

Forensic Science Education and Training: A Tool-kit for Lecturers and Practitioner Trainers, First Edition.
Edited by Anna Williams, John P. Cassella, and Peter D. Maskell.
© 2017 John Wiley & Sons Ltd. Published 2017 by John Wiley & Sons Ltd.

analytical skills are important. This chapter does not attempt to deal with teaching practical analytical skills, although such skills ARE used as part of the strategy for teaching and assessment discussed later. Rather, this chapter focuses on what is considered to be the most important evaluative skill: critical thinking.

Much of the published work about teaching critical thinking is aimed at psychology. However, the principles appear to translate directly to all sciences, and can certainly apply to the teaching of forensic science. In the past, it has been noted that some confusion about the definition of critical thinking has been an obstacle to teaching and assessing it (Halonen, 1995). For the purposes of this work, critical thinking is taken to involve the three highest categories of the cognitive domain within Bloom's revised taxonomy: analysing, evaluating and creating (Pohl, 2000).

Within critical thinking, consider the set of skills collectively called 'argument analysis skills' (Ennis, 1987; Halpern, 1998): evaluating evidence and drawing appropriate conclusions; distinguishing arguments from non-arguments; identifying assumptions.

These are fundamental critical thinking skills needed by forensic science students to evaluate competing claims in evidence and in interpretation of intelligence.

A review by Abrami *et al.* (2008) suggested that the activities most frequently used when teaching critical thinking skills are not enough *on their own* to produce measurable changes in critical thinking skills.

Such activities might include: using a textbook with specific critical thinking questions or modules; giving lectures critically reviewing evidence and case work; immersing students in challenging course work. Almost all lecturers have probably engaged in the last two activities with students, believing that a good basis for developing critical thinking was being provided.

Indeed, for some students this may be enough. For many, though, more explicit, direct instruction of critical thinking skills may be necessary. Does this mean that academic content must be removed or diluted in order to accommodate this? Absolutely not! Using the 'infusion' method described in Bensley (2010), relevant academic content is used to teach critical thinking rules and concepts along with the subject matter.

Thinking about why something is done, how it is done, what the results obtained mean, how that message can be conveyed and what should or could be done next is the most important transferrable skill set that can be instilled in students. Within this set of skills is subsumed almost all of the generic and forensic science skills sought by employers of science (including forensic science) graduates.

How, then, can this skill set be engendered in students? Savin-Badin and Major (2004), amongst many, have recognised that context or problem-based learning provides a platform for students to view their subject 'for real' and therefore promotes a greater appreciation of relevant underlying theory. As a student-centred approach, it also promotes 'learning by doing,' consistent with the experiential learning theory of Kolb (1984).

In the following section of this chapter, it will be shown how, using Bensley's (2010) seven guidelines for teaching and assessing critical thinking, teaching material and assessment methods were developed for the Forensic Investigation module taken in the third year of a 4-year Scottish system BSc (Hons) in Applied Bioscience with Forensic Investigation. This is a 4-hour per week class taken by 20–30 students.

A change from 12×10-credit modules per year to 6×20-credit modules and the need to have modules-in-common with other programmes, resulted in the number of 'forensic' modules available to students on the BSc (Hons) Applied Bioscience with Forensic Investigation over four years being reduced to 7 (out of 24 in total), followed by a further reduction to 6.5 modules. Previously, an externally sourced scenario called '*The Pale Horse*' by Summerfield, *et al.* (2002) was used in a year 2 module, Forensic Investigation, with some modification to allow flexibility in practical work and final outcome. '*The Pale Horse*', described as 'a problem-solving case study in analytical chemistry', unsurprisingly focused strongly on analytical chemistry skills – technique selection, results interpretation, and so on. This was used with moderate success for several years. In feedback, students said they enjoyed the module, but the results were never as good as the teaching team would have wished.

As part of a programme re-design, the Forensic Investigation module was moved to year 3, necessitating the production of an alternate assessment to avoid repetition. Although at the time this was both annoying and time-consuming, it offered an opportunity to re-focus the entire module.

The teaching team agreed that the general structure of '*The Pale Horse*' was excellent, but that the range of skills students needed to utilise for such a scenario could, and should, be much broader. At this point, the teaching team evaluated the strengths and weaknesses of student skills and came to the following main conclusions:

1. Students tend to compartmentalise knowledge.
2. Students have limited understanding of critical thinking and limited ability in utilising it.
3. That needs to be remedied!

Based on The Council For Industry and Higher Education (CIHE) (2009) recognition of key competencies valued by employers (cognitive skills; generic competencies; personal competencies; technical ability; practical and professional elements), the teaching team reviewed the content of all modules available to our students and agreed which areas of student performance would be targeted in an attempt to strengthen them. These were chosen as: crime scene management and protocol; physical evidence handling; analysis technique selection and interpretation; and critical evaluation of evidence, intelligence and results. Involved in this would be a strong element of interdisciplinary cooperation and group working, but also the need for students to take responsibility for their individual contributions. This is all consistent with 'Guideline 3: Find opportunities to infuse critical thinking that fit content and skill requirements of your course' of Bensley (2010).

The programme taken by these students covers a wide range of topics, forensic and otherwise, which engendered the belief amongst staff that it should be possible to design an open-ended problem based learning scenario for the third year, which both engaged the students' interest and encouraged them to use ALL of their knowledge, thereby increasing their ability to connect their previous and newly-acquired knowledge. However, this would all have to be done with no crime scene house and limited resources.

Methodology

A scenario, whose basic structure was unashamedly borrowed from '*The Pale Horse*,' was written and implemented for the third year module. The scenario was set around a suspicious death in student residences in the fictional university town of Hamley and focused strongly on issues relevant to students (drink, drugs, sex, the pressures of student life). It was at least partially written in student-friendly language, and in the local vernacular. This was done to engage interest and relation to the module content. In the absence of a crime scene house, 2 hours access to the School of Health's teaching/observation suite was secured. The 2 hours were just enough time to set-up, photograph and clear the scene: it was not practical for third year students to actually have access to that room – because of student numbers it would need to be booked for quite some time, and that was not possible. The suite is a single room laid out and furnished as a lounge, with one door leading off that. In reality the door leads only to a cupboard, but for the purposes of the scenario it is access to an internal hallway leading to the rest of the flat.

No crime scene dummy being available, a colleague's son offered to do duty as our body, and the flat itself was dressed with a selection of detritus indicating some sort of student party had taken place. Photographs were taken of the overall scene, the body and all evidence available. This same photograph (Figure 7.1) and evidence has now been in use for 13 consecutive student cohorts, indicting the flexibility of the scenario design.

The most important thing when designing this scene was to build-in that flexibility: the evidence placed at the scene needed to be such that all outcomes and student skills could be reflected.

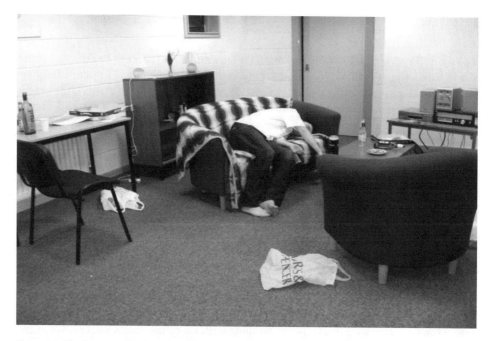

Figure 7.1 The borrowed location and borrowed body.

The teaching team had already decided that it was important that students actually have access to the physical evidence produced from the scene. This meant that we had to have enough duplicates of the evidence available to provide each group with their own collection of evidence.

It should not be obvious from photographs, evidence, or initial analysis whether the death is murder, suicide or accidental death. Students appear to be quite keen to believe it to be murder, so it is good to challenge their assumptions.

The evidence placed at the scene indicated that some serious drinking had occurred (lots of bottles and cans, with or without contents – sourcing duplicates of these was achieved by a connection with one of the staff's bowling club bar, although a student union would be an equally useful source), that drugs may have been taken (pills, powders and cannabis pipe filters – pills can be over the counter (OTC) pharmaceuticals, but having a vet as a friend can produce some very interesting but legal drugs too; powders can be virtually anything; cannabis pipe filters were bought on a trip to Amsterdam) and that food had been ingested (pizza boxes and remains, also receipt for same; pizza boxes came from eBay, remains from the canteen were 'doctored' to match consumption preferred in the scenario, and the receipt was produced to match that). Information about the decedent was also suggested within the evidence: he may have been sick (vomit on the throw over the sofa – the department has access to an artificial stomach, so the contents of the vomit actually match the decedent's stomach contents, but if not available then vegetable soup works quite well); he was on prescription medication (bottle found at bedside – the bottle can be empty and information gained only from the label, or it can contain any prescription drug available; an appeal for leftover prescriptions produced some very interesting drugs indeed) and he was under financial, emotional and academic stress (letters from his bank, ex-girlfriend and the university – easily produced in-house and infinitely adaptable). Further information about the decedent can be gained from transcriptions of interviews with his family, his workmates and those present at the party. Recently 'live' interviews with characters were introduced, which were highly entertaining for the staff playing the roles. Of course, the interviews can be honest and consistent, or otherwise, so students have to evaluate the quality of subjective evidence provided in the same way that they have to evaluate the quality of physical evidence.

The module starts with an introductory week in which a revision session is carried out. In this session, students list, discuss and evaluate as many skills gained from their two and a half years of study as possible. The students subsequently work in groups of (ideally) three, with the groups being allocated by teaching staff to ensure a mix of abilities, personalities and skills, since not all students take exactly the same subjects. The groups are also allocated a strict budget, both financial and in terms of notional man-hours, and are provided with a list giving costs for evidence analysis, as well as a specification of what each test will or will not cover. The costs/hours do not need to be particularly realistic – the intention is to make teams think critically about their requests before wasting notional money or time. This budget/test costs list is given at the end of the chapter as Appendix 7.A and the specifications for each test are given in Appendix 7.B. They are also warned that bankruptcy means losing 5% of their final overall mark. The aims and objectives are explained in critical thinking terms, and students are guided through module descriptor and marking schemes, with critical thinking skills expressly evident within those. This is consistent with Bensley's (2010) guideline 2, 'Clearly state the critical thinking goals and objectives for your class.'

The module then moves into four (possibly five) two-week blocks of activities, depending on the final scenario outcome selected for that year.

In the first week of each two-week block, the students are given written reports (and the scene photograph) associated with the scenario, to evaluate and critique. These are as realistic and believable as possible. As a simple example, the crime number used in the scenario paperwork is in the format used by the local police force. In the critique, students are asked to reflect on and criticise the performance of the 'character' responsible for each report. This helps them to connect their crime scene management and protocol background to the actions, errors and omissions at this scene. It was actually quite difficult to write-in errors and omissions in protocol and performance so that students had enough to critique, and to provide sufficient intelligence within the paperwork for student groups to form multiple theories as to what has happened, without making it TOO obvious what actually has.

At the end of each of the paper exercises, each group must email a request for a limited number of evidence items they wish to receive, with reasons given for why they want them, what they hope to determine from them and how they intend to do that, with the proviso that the group themselves should be able to carry out testing for a specific number of their requests (either one or two – it depends how many laboratory reports are wanted in the final report). They are told that if their reasoning is unsound or techniques chosen are incorrect, they will lose marks. If a suggestion is particularly poorly thought out or expressed, they can easily find themselves bankrupt. Groups do the initial evaluation of the paperwork during class time, with a staff member listening to each group's discussion and reasoning, modelling and scaffolding critical thinking by their responses and interactions with the group. This can be as simple as asking for further explanation of points in the discussion, asking questions to highlight inconsistencies in thinking (the 'What if?' questions), and encouraging students to evaluate the evidentiary strength of their results and conclusions. Bensley's (2010) 'Guideline 4: Use guided practice, explicitly modelling and scaffolding critical thinking' is therefore easily incorporated into the running of this module.

In the second week of each two-week block, students receive the evidence requested (each group has its own evidence locker), and also receive written feedback on each request, except those that they will carry out themselves on that day. If a request is reasonable (appropriate, logical and clear), then their feedback will be the results generated from their request, and students need to interpret them, then consider and reflect on what they learn from them. For some of the requests, in-house results can be produced, while for others information from an open-access site such as the Spectral Database for Organic Compounds (National Institute of Advanced Industrial Science and Technology), can be used. This is particularly useful if you do not have access to a wide range of techniques, or if you have neither the time nor resources to physically run all the student requests. If a request is *not* reasonable (poorly expressed, inappropriate techniques, not enough information provided to actually produce a response, etc.), then their feedback will indicate to the group why they are not receiving the results they had hoped for, and they need to reflect on *that*. One favourite early example was the group who requested receipt of 'all telephone records,' with not so much as a hint of the telephone numbers, or the names of the subscribers. In feedback they were asked as a starting point if they meant records for all telephone numbers in the world? In Europe? In Scotland? Yes, that probably WAS a bit cruel, but the point was made! This strategy corresponds to Bensley's (2010) 'Guideline 1: Motivate your students to think critically' and 'Guideline 6: Provide feedback and encourage students to reflect on it.' Most students *want* to get the best marks possible, so are strongly motivated to think about what they are requesting, and where they went wrong. It has been found that where a group has had a particular problem with the first set of requests, that problem is seldom repeated in subsequent requests.

During the second week of each block, groups also carry out those tests that they CAN carry out themselves. This is another good way of establishing how well a group has thought out the request. For example, a request for 'Presumptive testing for cocaine' applied to a white powder found at the scene, means that students would need to be able to ask the Technician for the correct chemicals and equipment, including those for positive and blank tests. If they arrive at the laboratory without that information, they have to go and research it rather quickly. They would also be asked to consider if presumptive testing for a *single* drug produced the maximum amount of information.

Each two-week block differentiates between the student groups, as each group will request and receive different evidence and feedback, so the information gathered and evaluated will differ for each group. It is possible at this stage to differentiate further, by providing different responses to the same requests, but this can be quite time-consuming. It is also possible, and often desirable, not to pre-determine what feedback will occur for each request, but rather to listen to group discussions and tap into their thinking. It can be quite interesting to cut off an avenue of enquiry upon which a group is set, or to take it in a direction they had not considered.

For each subsequent two-week block the same pattern is followed, and students also need to re-visit information and conclusions from previous weeks in light of new information gained. The whole process is iterative rather than linear: much information provided at the start only becomes relevant later in the process, so students need to keep reviewing, keep analysing and constantly re-evaluating what they think they know.

The first two-week block is all about evidence recovered from the crime scene: students can only request evidence that appears on the evidence list produced by the Scenes of Crime Officer (SOCO) in the scenario.

The second two-week block introduces the samples taken from the body at autopsy: students may request any of those, or may continue with the scene evidence if they feel that would be more useful. (It will not be, but they have that choice.)

Lamb's kidney and liver make suitable substitutes for human ones, and horse or sheep blood and artificial urine (based on lemonade) as well as partially digested stomach contents have been used in the toxicology part of the scenario. All of those are of course pre-treated so that test results match what the scenario demands. This section of work is particularly useful, as students have to consider storage and handling of these samples, as well as sampling protocol and sample preparation. Errors at any of these stages will obviously impact on their results. As an example, occasionally a group will forget to weigh how much of a solid sample is digested prior to analysis, so are unable to achieve any meaningful data from their results. And yes, they are allowed to go through the full process without pointing out their mistakes. It is part of the learning process to reflect on what needs improvement.

The third two-week block may incorporate new evidence being made available to the groups, either from another victim, a suspect or a secondary location. There may be another two-week block with the same criteria, depending on student progress and the complexity of the scenario.

The final block is where students can request other evidence not yet collected, from any character or location in the scenario. The thinking behind their requests must be explained, and they need to know exactly what they want to look for and how they will do it.

After eight or ten weeks, all information has been given, all laboratory work completed and considered and the students then have two weeks to prepare to present their conclusions both orally as part of a group presentation and individually in a final report.

Students are given fairly detailed instructions as to the format of the final report and the evidence of critical thinking required: care has been taken to 'Align assessment with practice of specific CT skills,' according to Bensley's (2010) Guideline 5.

A suggested teaching schedule for this type of module can be found in Appendix 7.C.

Results

The teaching team looked at several ways of evaluating any improvement in student performance.

When considering statistics for these cohorts it should be remembered that the size of the cohort varies from 8 students (year 1) to 28 students (year 7), so small changes in numbers can cause large changes in final statistics.

The first measure of performance, shown in Figure 7.2, was simply the average mark attained at the first attempt at assessment. 'Year 1' was the final year in which the

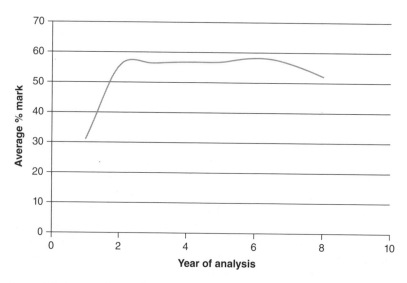

Figure 7.2 Average class mark versus year of data analysis.

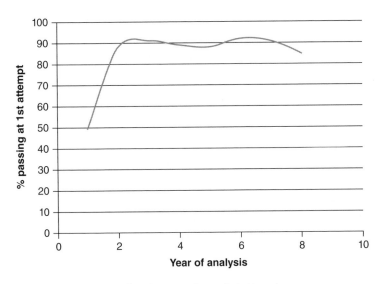

Figure 7.3 Percentage of students passing at first attempt versus year.

previous scenario was carried out, and for which the average mark attained was consistent with previous years.

In year 2 the class average mark increased by over 20%. However, this had to be interpreted with some caution as some of that cohort had already undertaken the previous scenario and so might be expected to have some pre-existing skills in the areas tested. The year 2 cohort also included a group of evening class students and direct entrants who had no previous knowledge of the module. From year 3 to year 6 there was a small percentage increase in average mark each year, but years 7 and 8 showed a small decrease in percentage mark.

The second performance indicator was chosen as percentage passing at the first attempt, shown in Figure 7.3. This was considered to be a good indicator of student engagement with the module.

Again, the large increase between years 1 and 2 was initially viewed with some caution, but that level of attainment has been fairly consistent ever since. Years 5 and 6 were much smaller groups, so their statistics for all measures of achievement were more strongly affected by small changes in results. Years 7 and 8 again showed a small decrease in this measure of attainment.

The final monitor of achievement considered was the percentage of achieving students who attained a grade B1 or better (59.5% or above), shown in Figure 7.4.

Again, the increase between years 1 and 2 was viewed with caution. The percentage of students achieving the two highest grades continued to increase annually until year 7, at which point there was a large dip. Each year's scenario has become increasingly complex, so the initial increase in B1 grades or above was unexpected. It may be that the scenario is now TOO complex, or it may be that the last two years monitored are just weaker overall: each measure of attainment has decreased for these cohorts.

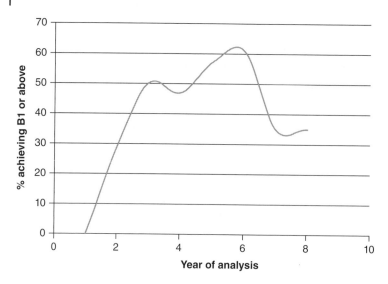

Figure 7.4 Percentage of completing students attaining grade B1 or higher versus year.

Analysis

Many useful lessons have been learned from designing, operating and assessing this module.

- The teaching material and style used has to engage the students. What works best for one individual's students may not work best for another's. Know your students' interests and concerns and scenario content can be designed that they will relate to.
- Learn from the experience each year: reflect on what worked well, what worked less well and why.
- Amend the *module* each year, not just the content. Use what was learned as part of the reflection process, or from student feedback. This is consistent with Bensley's (2010) seventh and final guideline: 'Reflect on feedback and assessment results to improve critical thinking instruction.'
- Engaging the students is just the starting point. Teaching staff also need to engage strongly with the content and with the students. Modelling and scaffolding the students' creative thinking is essential.
- Students must be *fully* aware of what you are asking them to achieve, and *how* you expect them to achieve it.

The main constraint with running a module in this style is time: time to design and plan the scenario and its assessment strategy, time to set up and record the crime scene, time to produce the documentation needed and time to create the feedback sheets necessary for the students. The last of these was initially found to be the biggest issue, consuming several hours every two weeks as open resources to provide feedback were located and incorporated with comments into the feedback sheets. However, although successive scenarios have been different, the team's experience in the first year of delivery means that feedback sheets can now be produced much more quickly, either by adapting already-existing sheets or using information and images from now well-established open sources.

This module incorporates much that is viewed as good practice: alignment of teaching and assessment; motivation; guided practice, modelling and scaffolding; reflective practice; and student-centred learning.

Over the years this module has been running, the main change introduced has been a decrease in the number of experimental reports required for submission. Instead of five reports worth 10 marks each, students in 2012 were asked for only five reports, but each was worth 15 marks. This year (2012) consideration has been given to reducing the number of reports required to 4, but increasing the mark for each to 20 or even 25. For a report worth 'only' 10 marks it was felt that students were not fully utilising their critical thinking skills, something especially evident in the evaluation of results and how they related to the scenario. In 2012, after a thorough briefing on what the change meant, and what was required of them, some improvement was seen for the majority of students.

A non-rigorous evaluation of results in the honours year forensic module linked to this one suggests that student critical thinking skills have been strengthened, as final results for the higher-level module have shown similar improvements to those observed in this module.

Conclusions

Overall, this style of module is a pedagogically-sound, well-tested model, which demonstrably increases student engagement and achievement.

Student feedback is overwhelmingly positive.

Student pass rates and result rates have increased fairly steadily since the module was introduced.

An improvement in critical thinking skills has been observed in the follow-on module in the honours year.

This style of module could be used in almost all academic circumstances: no crime room is needed and no specialised equipment is required: just a good imagination and the willingness to use it.

Acknowledgements

The author would like to thank the following people: Keith Eynon, retired Head of Forensic Support at Strathclyde Police Forensic Laboratory, for support and guidance when our forensic investigation degree was designed; Dr Martin Hall, teaching team member, office mate and sounding board, for patience and his enormous help with the running of this module; all science colleagues at the University of South Wales, who permitted me to use their photographs, or photographs of their nearest and dearest, as part of this module; and the students, for making it such fun despite all the challenges. I hope they feel the same.

Appendix 7.A: Budget Information for Forensic Investigation Scenario

The following types of tests are available to you, but you should consider each of them carefully in terms of financial cost and investigation time. The tests are listed in alphabetical order and no other significance should be attached to their order.

Your budget for this investigation is £5000 and 30 days.

When your money and time has gone, IT HAS GONE. Think first and spend wisely!

Test	Cost/ £	Unit	Time/days
Alcohol analysis (blood or urine)	50	Sample	1
Body fluid or tissue preparation and analysis (chemical/biological)	500	Sample	2
Screening of body fluid or tissue for 'foreign' substances by chemical/biological methods	500	Per test performed	2 days per test performed
Chemical analysis of unknown substance	150	Sample	1
DNA analysis of crime scene stain	500	Sample	5
DNA analysis of reference sample	500	Sample	5
DNA comparison (includes 2 samples)	900	2 Samples	5
Urgent DNA premium charge	600	Sample – cost is additional to analysis costs	2
Drugs identification	125	Sample	2
Drugs screening (blood or urine)	300	Sample	3
Drugs screening (body fluids or tissue)	400	Sample	4
Drugs trace analysis	150	Sample	2
Urgent drugs analysis premium charge	75	Sample – cost is additional to analysis costs	1
Fingerprint examination and evaluation	200	Sample	1
Hair examination (microscopy)	200	Sample	1
Hair preparation and analysis (chemical/biological)	300	Sample	1
Interview with any of the characters in the scenario (15 questions maximum)	100	Interview	1
Presumptive testing for blood	50	Sample	0.5
Presumptive testing for drugs	50	Per test performed	0.5 per test performed
Telephone records request	150	Sample	1
Trace evidence analysis	200	Sample	1
Unlisted test	On request	Sample	On request

Appendix 7.B: Information on Testing Available for Forensic Investigation Scenario

Test	Service provided
Alcohol analysis (blood or urine)	Quantitative analysis of blood and urine for alcohol content
Body fluid or tissue preparation and analysis (chemical/biological)	Analysis for named substance by requested chemical or biological methods
Screening of body fluid or tissue for 'foreign' substances by chemical/biological methods	Screening will be carried out exactly as specified by purchaser: you must state WHAT the substance or type of substance is that you want to screen for
Chemical analysis of an unknown substance	Identification and/or quantification of unknown sample by requested chemical analysis
DNA analysis of crime scene stain	Evidential DNA analysis of crime scene stain including analysis, comparison, interpretation and reporting of case sample, with submission to the National DNA Database where appropriate
DNA analysis of reference sample	As above
DNA comparison (includes 2 samples)	As above
Urgent DNA premium charge	This is a charge made for urgent processing of DNA evidence and is additional to analysis costs
Drugs identification	Identification of common drugs and adulterants by requested method
Drugs screening (blood or urine)	Screening of a blood or urine sample for panel of common drugs (amphetamines, methamphetamines, cannabis, cocaine, and opiates) by requested method
Drugs screening (body fluids or tissue)	Preparation and screening of a body fluid or tissue sample for panel of common drugs as above, by requested method
Drugs trace analysis	Recovery and identification of trace amounts of drugs by requested method
Urgent drugs analysis premium charge	This is a charge made for urgent processing of drugs analysis and is additional to analysis costs
Fingerprint examination and evaluation	Recovery, examination and evaluation of specified mark. Submission to IDENT-1 database for identification
Hair or fibre examination (microscopy)	Examination and results on appearance and condition of hairs or fibres
Hair or fibre preparation and analysis (chemical/biological)	Analysis for named substance by requested chemical or biological methods
Interview with any of the characters in the scenario	YOU must provide the questions you want answered! The interview will deal ONLY with those
Presumptive testing for blood	By Kastle-Meyer
Presumptive testing for drugs	By drug type requested
Telephone records request	Recovery and listing of telephone records for 1 week
Trace evidence analysis	Analysis/comparison of glass, paint etc. samples by requested method
Unlisted test	Purchaser-specified testing

Appendix 7.C: Suggested Schedule for Delivery of This Style of Module

Week	Activity	Content
1	Revision	Discussion/review of current skill set
	Module descriptor	Critical thinking skills explicitly aligned to assessment
	Costing sheets, budgetary constraints	Explanation of consequences of breaking budget
2	Paperwork 1. Read, discuss, evaluate and critique scene documentation	Crime scene report, crime scene manager's report, SOCO's report, evidence list, interview transcripts from family and neighbours
	Requests for evidence from the crime scene	Any six requests, with appropriate level of thought and detail evident
3	Practical work 1	At least two of group's requests should be carried out in the laboratory
	Feedback review. Evaluation of feedback and/or results from evidence requests and practical work	As appropriate to each group
4	Paperwork 2. Read, discuss, evaluate and critique provided documentation	Post-mortem report, Investigating Officer's report, further information about decedent, friends and family
	Requests for evidence from decedent	Any six requests relating to samples recovered at autopsy, with appropriate level of thought and detail evident
5	Practical work 2	At least two of group's requests should be carried out in the laboratory
	Feedback review. Evaluation of feedback and/or results from evidence requests and practical work	As appropriate to each group
6	Paperwork 3	Variable dependent on scenario 'route' chosen. It could include further information on characters involved, on secondary crime scenes or subsequent related events
	Requests for any evidence received thus far	Any four requests relating to any evidence currently available, with appropriate level of thought and detail evident
7	Practical work 3	At least one of group's requests should be carried out in the laboratory
	Feedback review. Evaluation of feedback and/or results from evidence requests and practical work	As appropriate to each group
8[a]	Requests for any evidence received thus far	Any four requests relating to any evidence currently available, with appropriate level of thought and detail evident
9[a]	Practical work 4	At least one of group's requests should be carried out in the laboratory
10	Requests for any evidence from anything associated with the scenario	This is where students can 'tie up' their case
11	Practical work 5	At least one of group's requests should be carried out in the laboratory
12	Group work and final discussions	Group work and final discussions

[a]Optional block.

References

Abrami, P.C. *et al.* (2008) Instructional interventions affecting critical thinking skills and dispositions: A stage 1 meta-analysis. *Review of Educational Research*, **4**, 1102–1134.

Bensley, D.A. (2010) *A Brief Guide for Teaching and Assessing Critical Thinking in Psychology.* Association for Psychological Science. Available at: http://www.psychologicalscience.org/observer/a-brief-guide-for-teaching-and-assessing-critical-thinking-in-psychology#.WEgGILKLTGg (accessed 7 December 2016).

Council for Industry and Higher Education (2009) *Valuing the Views of Employers.* Council for Industry and Higher Education. Available at: http://aces.shu.ac.uk/employability/resources/0802grademployability.pdf (accessed 7 December 2016).

Ennis, R.H. (1987) A taxonomy of critical thinking dispositions and abilities, in *Teaching Thinking Skills: Theory and Practice*, (eds J.B. Baron and R.F. Sternberg), Freeman, New York, pp. 9–26.

Halonen, J.S. (1995) Demystifying critical thinking. *Teaching of Psychology*, **22**, 75–81.

Halpern, D.F. (1998) Teaching critical thinking for transfer across domains: Dispositions, skills, structure training and metacognitive monitoring. *American Psychologist*, **53**, 14–19.

Hanson, S. and Overton, T. (2010) *Skills required by new forensic science graduates and their development in degree programme.* Higher Education Academy, UK Physical Sciences Centre University of Hull. Available at: http://www.rsc.org/learn-chemistry/resources/business-skills-and-commercial-awareness-for-chemists/docs/skillsdoc1.pdf (accessed 7 December 2016).

Kolb, D. (1984) *Experiential Learning as a Source of Learning and Development*, Prentice Hall, Englewood Cliffs, NJ.

National Institute of Advanced Industrial Science and Technology. *Spectral Database for Organic Compounds.* National Institute of Advanced Industrial Science and Technology, Japan. Available at: http://riodb01.ibase.aist.go.jp/sdbs/ (accessed 1 December 2016).

Pohl, M. (2000) *Learning to Think, Thinking to Learn: Models and Strategies to Develop a Classroom Culture of Thinking*, Hawker Brownlow, Cheltenham.

Savin-Baden, M. and Major, C. (2004) *Foundations of Problem-based Learning*, Open University Press/SRHE, Maidenhead.

Summerfield, S., Overton, T. and Belt, S. (2002) *The Pale Horse. A problem-solving Case Study in Analytical Chemistry.* University of Hull. Available at: http://www.rsc.org/learn-chemistry/resource/res00001046/pale-horse-analytical-chem-forensics-c-pbl?cmpid=CMP00001463 (accessed 7 December 2016).

8

Improving the PhD Through Provision of Skills Training for Postgraduate Researchers

Benjamin J. Jones

Abertay University, Dundee, UK

Introduction

Research, and the subsequent peer review and publication of robust scientific studies, is an important way to progress the forefront of knowledge in many fields. This is increasingly true in forensic science, where the UK Home Office Forensic Regulator has highlighted research and peer-reviewed publications as a cornerstone of ensuring both quality and confidence in forensic science (Rennison, 2010). This need to improve and increase research that is of application to forensics is echoed by workers across industry and academic sectors (Jones, 2011).

Research and development requires a high quality skill set, and entry into this world is frequently through completion of a Doctor of Philosophy (PhD or DPhil) degree, a programme of work usually completed over three years with advice and supervision of an established academic, leading to a substantial and original thesis on a specific topic. In addition to research, doctoral level education programmes in some systems include a taught component, although in the United Kingdom the standard route for a doctorate is almost always exclusively research based. However, many PhD graduates will go on to work outside the academic sector, within government or industry, in roles that are not necessarily research-focused (Barnacle and Dal'Alba, 2011; Borrell-Damian *et al.*, 2010; Neumann and Tan, 2011); acquiring and recognising technical and transferable skills, such as management and critical review, can therefore be an important factor for doctoral students.

The desirability of expanding the training element within doctoral programmes is outlined in the Roberts Review (Roberts *et al.*, 2002), which was commissioned by the UK Government to investigate the supply of people with science, technology, engineering and mathematics skills. The Review expresses concern on the suitability of PhD graduates for both academic and industrial employment, and recommends a strengthening of the training element, particularly in non-technical transferable skills. Elements

Forensic Science Education and Training: A Tool-kit for Lecturers and Practitioner Trainers, First Edition.
Edited by Anna Williams, John P. Cassella, and Peter D. Maskell.
© 2017 John Wiley & Sons Ltd. Published 2017 by John Wiley & Sons Ltd.

highlighted include communication and teaching skills, management and commercial awareness (Roberts, 2002). This continued need to extend graduates' training and transferable skills base is echoed in a more recent report from Smith *et al.* (2010). Other works demonstrate the need for training in particular areas such as teaching (Hardre, 2005) and show that the need to develop graduate attributes, both for academic and industrial work, crosses disciplines and international education systems (Foote, 2010; Manathunga and Lant, 2006; Muldoon, 2009). Kehm (2007) investigates European development and global change to doctoral education, outlining the perception that the traditional PhD leaves graduates too narrowly focused, and lacking key professional skills. The Concordat to support the Career Development of Researchers, an agreement between universities and funders, states:

> The importance of researchers' personal and career development, and lifelong learning, is clearly recognised and promoted at all stages of their career.
>
> *Research Concordat, 2010*

Training and development courses conducted during the period of a doctoral programme may assist students to gain skills that benefit their research during their degree, and assist with their future career. This also sets the foundations for an ongoing commitment to Continuing Professional Development (CPD), a recognised industry need and a key competency of many schemes awarding Chartered Status, such as engineering or biology (Engineering Council, 2010; Society of Biology, 2009) or professional accreditation and competency assessment schemes set up in the United Kingdom as the Chartered Society of Forensic Sciences (CSFS) moves from a learned society (The Forensic Science Society) to a professional body (CSFS, 2014).

Many researchers highlight that the PhD course structure is continually evolving in order to cater for future career requirements (Gilbert *et al.*, 2004; Pritchard *et al.*, 2009; Borrell-Damian *et al.*, 2010). Numerous studies (Borrell-Damian *et al.*, 2010; Neumann and Tan, 2011) show that approximately 50% of PhD graduates continue to a position outside the academic sector, Barnacle and Dal'Alba (2011) suggest that only a third of doctoral graduates will be employed in research work. This has contributed to developments in doctoral courses that include both an increase in transferable skills training components and substantial contact with industry. This reflects a change from a PhD focusing on an outcome, a piece of research embodied in a thesis, to an increased focus on the process and training to be a researcher, or developing abilities to utilise acquired skills in a different setting. Professional development is of course not limited to training courses. Pritchard *et al.* (2009) examine training course programmes and show that in some cases these may not be the principal routes to gaining transferable skills; Barnacle and Dal'Alba (2011) highlight that doctoral graduates regularly draw on research knowledge in their current employment, regardless of sector or industry.

The UK's Engineering and Physical Sciences Research Council (EPSRC) planned an increase in user-led skills training within doctoral programmes (EPSRC, 2009) and a number of recent initiatives have incorporated training courses into a doctoral level postgraduate qualification. These include cohort-based study at one of an increasing number of EPSRC Centres for Doctoral Training (CDT) across the UK (EPSRC, 2014), which each concentrate on a particular engineering or physical sciences sector, such as Micro and Nano Materials and Technology at the University of Surrey, Formulation

Engineering (Birmingham) or Photonic Integration for Advanced Data Storage (Queens University Belfast). The outputs from these centres may be applied to forensic science, one centre addresses the subject directly, CDT in Security Science (University College London). A similar scheme across broader disciplines, The NewRoutePhD, was launched in 2001 by a consortium of UK universities, and is available across a range of subjects in different centres. The NewRoutePhD and the EPSRC Centres for Doctoral Training extend the traditional three-year, research-only doctorate to four years, and in addition to research, include advanced technical taught courses and professional transferable skills training (NR PhD, 2014; EPSRC, 2014). This is sometimes reflected in the use of a Master of Research or Postgraduate Diploma as an intermediate or additional award recognising both research and training in research methodology.

Cohort based doctoral training centres increasingly involve industry input, and this is also indicated by the provision of professional or practice-based doctorates, such as the Doctor of Public Health, DrPH, and the four-year Engineering Doctorate, EngD (EPSRC, 2010b), which includes up to 25% training. Such schemes can focus on a primarily industrially based research component, improve links with industry and make graduates better prepared for non-academic employment. However, concerns have been raised on issues such as intellectual property, exploitation of developing ideas, communication and conflicts between professional development of students and the needs of employers (Borrell-Damian *et al.*, 2010; Jones, 2010; Servage, 2009).

With direct relevance to the model of postgraduate provision of forensic science within universities, this chapter investigates research students' assessment of skills gained by attendance on non-mandatory courses throughout postgraduate research degree programmes, and their attitudes concerning course usefulness, structure and integration.

Study of Student Perception of Training Needs

Postgraduate research students responded to a web-based questionnaire, advertised via university web pages, social networking sites and via direct emails through school and departmental contacts. A total of 49 respondents primarily from 'research intensive' or 'research led' UK universities completed the questionnaire; students' research areas were split between life sciences (43%), physical sciences (29%) and humanities (29%). Respondents were also asked if they were part-time students (17%), had had more than three years industrial experience prior to their degree (45%) and if they were members of a professional organisation (60%), which could include organisations such as the Royal Society of Chemistry, Institution of Engineering and Technology or Chartered Society of Forensic Sciences.

Respondents were asked to consider questions on attendance, relevance and format relating to courses in four categories:

- **Technical** (e.g. scientific instrument or technique training or technical software such as Matlab[TM] or Labview[TM])
- **Teaching and Management** (and people skills)
- **Non-technical Computing** (e.g. Microsoft Office[TM] or display equipment)
- **Soft Skills** (e.g. presentation skills, thesis writing)

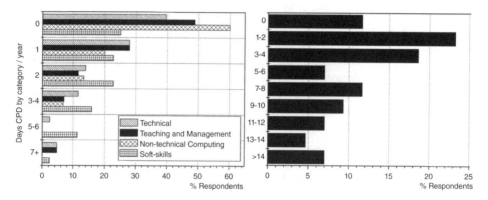

Figure 8.1 Number of days training attended over the past year, by course category (left) and in total (right).

It is worth noting that this classification caused some discussion from respondents on which elements could legitimately be classified as 'professional development.' Some students and supervisors placed emphasis only on technical, subject related courses, rather than what they termed 'vague transferable skills.' However, multiple workers (Roberts, 2002, Smith *et al.*, 2010; Hinchcliffe and Jolly, 2011) emphasise the need for development of attributes in these areas, and categories in this work on *Teaching and Management* and *Soft Skills* reflect these findings.

Training Course Attendance and Usefulness

The number of days of professional development training that students attended over the previous 12 months is shown in Figure 8.1. This is in addition to any requirements for the students' current degree course and is broken down into categories, as collected (Figure 8.1, left) and summed for total days attended by each student (Figure 8.1, right); 53% of students completed four days or fewer over the past year, and 12% conducted no CPD or training over any requirements of their degree programme.

Mean attendance on courses was 5.5 ± 0.7 days over the past year. Breakdown of attendance by course category and students' research topic begins to show some indicative trends. Technical course attendance shows significant variation with students' research subject, with physical science students attending a mean of 2.7 ± 0.9 days, significantly more than humanities or life science students, who attend a mean of 1.4 ± 0.7 or 0.9 ± 0.2 days, respectively. The overall levels of attendance are less than the ten days recommended by EPSRC (2010a) and Roberts (2002).

Nevertheless, students recognise the importance of developing both research and transferable skills; in a survey of approximately 18 000 students conducted for the Higher Education Academy in 2009 (Kulej and Wells, 2009), 89.2% agreed with the importance of developing research skills and 69.6% agreed that opportunities to develop transferable skills were important. However, only 43% agreed they were encouraged to reflect on personal development during their degree. Students were asked to what extent they agree with the statement in Question Box 8.1, to assess their perceptions of the need for training over and above their current degree programme, and aspects of ease of facilitation of this.

Question Box 8.1					
	Strongly Agree	Agree	Neutral	Disagree	Strongly Disagree
Qn1. All my training needs are covered by my degree course (%)	4.4	28.9	20.0	37.8	8.9

From this it can be seen that only 33% students agree that all training needs are covered by their degree. This demonstrates the importance of training courses external to the degree structure of the current UK format, and suggests that students recognise the need to source additional training from their university's graduate school or other providers.

Attending dedicated training courses is one route to acquiring a required or desired skill, and two thirds of respondents indicate they have supervisor support for this. Students who attended courses in the past year were requested to provide an assessment of the usefulness of this training for their current work. Respondents were also asked their opinion on whether attendance on these courses would be useful for their future employment, or in finding future employment. The resultant mean ratings from a scale of 1 (worthless) to 10 (essential) are shown in Table 8.1.

Over this sample set there are no significant differences in scores when results are broken down by course category or student research topic. However, from these data, it can be seen that students find courses useful for their current work, the mean rating for technical courses, for example, is 6.8 ± 0.5. Students also perceive training courses are useful for their future career progression, with similar ratings. Consideration therefore needs to be given to additional factors that may affect student attendance on development courses, or facilitate improved uptake.

The results of this survey suggest that students are attending a low number of courses, relative to their aspirations and recommendations by supervisors and funders (Roberts, 2002; EPSRC, 2010a). Students were asked whether they agreed with further statements reflecting availability and ease of access of courses (Question Box 8.2).

Table 8.1 Mean ratings and standard error for usefulness of courses for current research and future employment.

	Usefulness for current research/10	Usefulness for future career/10
Technical	6.81 ± 0.46	6.45 ± 0.53
Teaching and Management	6.77 ± 0.44	6.70 ± 0.51
Non-technical Computing	6.36 ± 0.53	6.50 ± 0.53
Soft Skills	6.03 ± 0.42	6.44 ± 0.42

Question Box 8.2

	Strongly Agree	Agree	Neutral	Disagree	Strongly Disagree
Qn.2 My supervisor supports my attendance on external CPD courses (%)	21.3	44.7	21.3	8.5	4.3
Qn.3 There are CPD courses in all the areas I need (%)	4.3	26.1	43.5	21.7	4.3
Qn.4 I don't have time to attend all the courses I'd like (%)	12.8	38.3	23.4	25.5	0

Only 30% of students questioned can find courses in all areas they need, and only 26% of students indicate that they have time to attend all courses they wish. Additionally, two-thirds of supervisors indicated that budgetary constraints affect the number of courses that students could attend. Research students were asked if they would like to attend more courses in the next 12 months, compared with their attendance in the previous year. Table 8.2 shows the responses to this question, which are subsequently discussed by category; although this preliminary study has a relatively small sample size, certain correlations can be made with greater than 95% confidence.

Students showed a desire to attend more technical courses; 57% of respondents indicated they wish to attend more technical CPD, with 24% substantially more and only 10% signifying they wished to attend fewer courses (t = test indicated a >99% confidence in positive difference from neutral). This desire for more technical training is correlated with: a perception of an absence of available courses (Pearson $r = 0.43$), the belief of usefulness of courses attended for future career ($r = 0.39$), and, more weakly, with a desire for courses to carry credits for qualifications or chartered status ($r = 0.29$). This is reflected in the Chartered Society of Forensic Sciences' requirement for professional development of 50–75 hours over three years to maintain professional membership (CSFS, 2014). Other professional institutions offer alternative formalising structures for continuing professional development, such as the Society of Biology CPD scheme *Learning for Life* (Society of Biology, 2009) or requirements for Chartered Engineer (Engineering Council, 2010). However, a previous attempt at providing a scheme for structured and evaluated professional development activity, encountered problems with participation. The Professional Formation and Development Scheme, run by the

Table 8.2 Indication of future course attendance.

	Over the next 12 months, would you like to attend more CPD courses (in each category) than over the past year?				
% Respondents	Substantially Fewer	Slightly Fewer	About the Same	Slightly More	Substantially More
Technical	4.1	6.1	32.7	32.7	24.5
Teaching and Management	0.0	8.2	38.8	36.7	16.3
Non-technical Computing	4.1	10.2	40.8	34.7	10.2
Soft Skills	4.1	20.4	32.7	26.5	16.3

Institute of Physics and designed for recent graduates, including those in postgraduate education, was withdrawn due to a lack of participation in reporting of attainment and assessment of competencies (IoP, personal communication, 2002).

However, 53% of respondents state that they wish to attend more Teaching and Managerial CPD courses. In contrast to the technical courses this is not significantly correlated with belief in usefulness for future career, or indeed current work. This notably and worryingly contrasts with the government reviews and other studies. The Roberts Review (2002) and the Smith *et al.* (2010) Government Report on postgraduate education both emphasise the need for development of students' people management skills. Kaplan (2011) highlights that industry sources find that PhD graduates do not necessarily have appropriate business and communication skills. The desire to attend more courses in this category is correlated with the perception of a lack of available courses ($r = 0.42$) and a desire for courses to carry credits for qualifications, chartered status or other recognition ($r = 0.39$). For postgraduate students heading into academia, the recommendation that new academics hold an accredited teaching qualification is in addition to any subject-specific requirements, the review outlines that this training should be available to postgraduate students (Browne *et al.*, 2010). The results of the current survey suggest an increase in the provision of courses in this category, or an increase in advertising or flexibility of provision, is required to meet these needs, and also a shift in mind set of postgraduate students who, in some cases, do not necessarily immediately see the relevance to their future work of what one respondent described as, 'vague transferable skills.'

The non-technical computing course category has the lowest attendance rates, 45% of students wish to attend more courses. However, the profile of responses is not significantly different from a mean neutral response, indicating no significant net desire to attend more courses in the next 12 months. Students' plans for future attendance are correlated with a preference for accredited courses ($r = 0.30$) and for credit carrying courses ($r = 0.43$). This suggests that provision in this category is adequate. Incorporation of a training structure into a more formal scheme may be worth future study.

Desire for additional soft skills courses is negatively correlated with the number of days of soft skill training attended over the past year ($r = -0.33$). This is also correlated with a desire for accredited courses ($r = 0.30$) and courses that contribute towards additional qualifications or other status ($r = 0.43$). This is the only category of courses where there is a significant negative correlation between days attended this year and desire to attend more in the next 12 months. This, and the absence of a correlation with course availability, suggests that there are satisfactory levels of provision in this area, or that students find that a short course is not suitable for growing this type of skill. This may be a reflection of progress since the Roberts Review in 2002, in an increased provision of courses in transferable skills that are geared for specific stages in the PhD (Gilbert *et al.*, 2004; Brunel University, 2010; Pritchard, 2009). This provision well addresses some of the concerns of the Roberts Review (2002), though management and teaching courses are also identified by the review as requiring improvement.

Training Course Delivery

Research teams have reflected that although skills training programmes have become more widespread within PhD studies, questions remain on the more desirable and

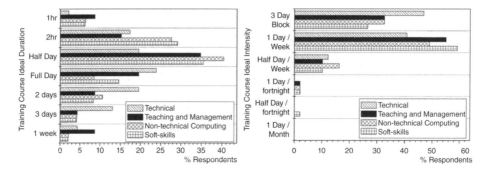

Figure 8.2 Students' preferences on course duration and intensity of training.

effective forms of such programmes (Gilbert *et al.*, 2004; Pritchard *et al.*, 2009). Addressing issues on delivery format, students were questioned on appropriate course duration, assessment of learning and external course recognition or accreditation.

Two questions assessed students' preferences on course duration. The responses are shown in Figure 8.2. Students were first asked their views on the most appropriate course duration, with no further information on content. Modal response is a full day for technical courses, and half day in other categories (Figure 8.2, left). Secondly, a teaching time requirement of three days was specified, and students were asked to express a preference for block teaching, or for the course to be spread over a longer period (up to one day a month). Results are shown in Figure 8.2 (right). For technical courses the mode response was a preference for a three-day block course, for all other categories mode preference was for a course spread over three weeks, with one day of training per week. For all categories, less than 20% indicated a preference for courses running at a lower intensity. This block teaching approach has also been indicated as preferential for industry delegates and would improve flexibility of education provision benefiting both graduates and employers.

Figure 8.3 shows students' preferences on a compulsory assessed component of training courses. Although the principal mode was neutral, a substantial number of respondents were totally opposed to assessment. Students' comments on this question pointed out that attendance does not equate to understanding, a number were concerned with making the test compulsory, or the appropriateness of an assessment on each course. Other researchers have suggested the assessment of a threshold level of competence, particularly for practical work such as veterinary studies or teaching (Cockram *et al.*, 2007; Browne *et al.*, 2010).

Students were asked if they preferred courses to be accredited or otherwise endorsed by an external organisation. A further question asked if there was a preference for courses to carry credits towards additional qualifications, chartered status or other recognition, Table 8.3 details these results. There is a significant proportion in favour for both questions. For example, for technical courses 78% favour accredited courses and 80% prefer courses carrying credits towards additional qualification or chartered status. Respondents highlighted a danger faced by offering recognised qualifications for skills training achievements, that the certificate becomes 'more valuable than the knowledge it is supposed to represent.' Nevertheless, accreditation ensures a benchmark of quality, both to employers and delegates. Particularly for courses taken as general CPD

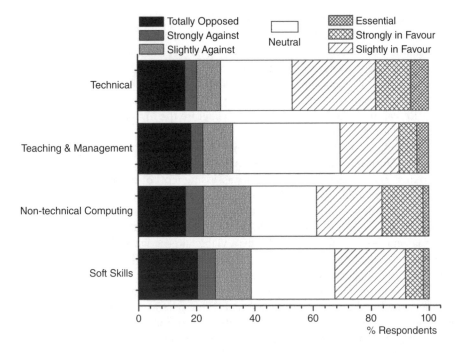

Figure 8.3 Students' preferences on compulsory assessment of training.

rather than for immediate application, additional qualifications enable students to distinguish themselves from their peers by advertising their additional skills set, particularly important given criticisms of the traditional PhD structure (Kehm, 2007; Roberts, 2002). Such qualifications, with inherent portability, may also enable increased freedom of movement in the employment market, which would not necessarily be achieved with

Table 8.3 Students' stated preferences for accreditation and recognition of training courses (values binned from degrees of preference).

Preference for courses to be accredited, endorsed or recognised by an external organisation			
% Respondents	Against	Neutral	In Favour
Technical	2.0	20.4	77.6
Teaching and Management	8.2	24.5	67.3
Non-technical Computing	6.1	32.7	61.2
Soft Skills	8.2	28.6	63.3

Preference for courses to carry credits as part of a scheme leading to additional qualifications, chartered status, or other recognition			
% Respondents	Against	Neutral	In Favour
Technical	4.1	16.3	79.6
Teaching and Management	10.2	14.3	75.5
Non-technical Computing	8.2	24.5	67.3
Soft Skills	12.2	22.4	65.3

uncertificated training. Browne, for example, in the recent review of higher education in England (Browne *et al.*, 2010) specifies not only teaching skills for academics, but accredited qualifications, as an indicator of teaching quality. An approach for postgraduate certificate or diploma courses (MSc level qualifications but one third or two-thirds the content, respectively) has been trialled in particular industry sectors by a number of universities to address particular needs (Tallantyre *et al.*, 2010; University of Nottingham, 2011). Research councils such as BBSRC recognise the importance of training at the masters' level for skills development for industry.

However, it may be counterproductive to introduce further qualifications that may not achieve recognition from employers, and which may necessarily contrast with the responses in this survey suggesting compulsory assessment of courses may reduce attendance. Completion of an additional qualification concurrently with the PhD may also distract from or devalue the doctorate. A structured but flexible route, enabling attendance of CPD courses on a stand-alone basis, but with potential of accrual of credit towards a masters' level qualification may be a viable alternative and enable development of a skill set reflecting the needs of the student; a number of providers offer such qualifications through short courses (University of Oxford, 2011; University of Surrey, 2011). A different approach to provide recognition for training and development would be to promote the link between training and achieving personal accreditation such as chartered status or accredited forensic practitioner. Institutions offering routes to chartered status emphasise the link between commitment to continuing professional development and attainment of status (Engineering Council, 2010; Society of Biology, 2009). The Chartered Society of Forensic Sciences and Institute of Physics offer recognition of CPD courses from a range of academic or commercial providers; however, not all professional organisations offer endorsement of external courses as part of this scheme, indeed, the Institution of Engineering and Technology closed this programme at the end of 2009 (IET, 2010). The use of such a route to improve training uptake would require promotion of recognition of chartered or accredited status as a goal amongst postgraduate students, and emphasis on the link between commitment to CPD and professional status, as well as ensuring a wide ranging set of courses from which postgraduate students can accrue CPD credits in such schemes, all requiring support from universities, training suppliers and professional institutions.

Training courses discussed so far are conducted in addition to the requirements of the students' degree programme. The survey suggests that postgraduate research students wish to have more formal training, and students were further asked if they wished to have more courses as part of their research degree (Question Box 8.3).

Question Box 8.3					
	Strongly Agree	Agree	Neutral	Disagree	Strongly Disagree
Qn5. I would like more courses to be incorporated into my degree (%)	21.7	39.1	23.9	15.2	0

The survey indicates that 61% would like more courses incorporated within their degree. This is correlated with a perception of lack of available courses in relevant areas ($r = 0.42$)

and the desire to attend more courses in technical ($r = 0.31$), teaching and management ($r = 0.36$) and non-technical computing ($r = 0.31$) categories, though there is no significant correlation with additional soft skills courses. Introducing a mandatory training requirement prior to completion of a PhD or transfer from probationary status is an alternative method for providing the needed skills training that has been highlighted by Government reviews and funding bodies (EPSRC, 2010a; Research Concordat, 2010; Roberts, 2002; Smith *et al.*, 2010). However, casting a note of warning, Barnacle and Dall'Alba ask:

> If we are seeking graduates with the ability to work creatively and contribute to innovation, are generic skills really what are required?
>
> *Barnacle and Dall'Alba, 2011, p. 467*

This query on appropriateness of training packages, together with the individual nature of research programmes and projects, as well as variation in student experience and background and subsequent employment route, mean that a rigid compulsory training structure could be counterproductive. Schemes that offer the provision of formal structured training as a component of research degree programmes, such as professional doctorates, EPSRC Centres for Doctoral Training or the NewRoutePhD scheme therefore require a certain element of flexibility and lead to further debate concerning the role of doctorates in education and skills training.

Conclusions

This chapter examines the attitudes of postgraduate research students across disciplines who responded, assessing approaches to development courses in the following categories: technical, teaching and management, non-technical computing and soft skills. Over a period of one year, the students surveyed attended a mean of 5.5 ± 0.7 days non-mandatory training courses across all categories. This is less than the ten days recommended by funding bodies such as the Engineering and Physical Sciences Research Council (EPSRC, 2010a), professional bodies such as the Chartered Society of Forensic Sciences (CSFS, 2014) and Government Review (Roberts, 2002). Students recognise the need to develop their skills by undertaking additional training over and above the PhD structure, as shown in this survey and other works (Kulej and Wells, 2009; Pritchard *et al.*, 2009). This is further reinforced by employers and reviewers (Roberts, 2002; Pritchard *et al.*, 2009; Kaplan, 2011; Hinchcliffe and Jolly, 2011). Rationalising the relatively low attendance, only 30% of students indicate they can find courses in all the areas they need, and only 26% agree they have time to attend all the courses they require. A further survey of supervisors would enable examination of other factors such as budget constraints; however, 66% of students indicate that they have the support of their supervisors to attend external training.

A significant majority of students indicate that they wish to attend more technical and teaching or management courses. This is primarily correlated with the difficulties in finding courses in appropriate areas, and also with a preference for courses to carry credits towards additional qualifications, chartered status or other recognition. Credit carrying courses are significantly favoured; for technical courses 80% indicate this preference. Similarly, courses that are endorsed or accredited by an external organisation such as a professional institute are also favoured. This is reflected in a 2010 review of higher education in England (Browne *et al.*, 2010), which suggests that to ensure quality standards in the sector, new academics require accredited qualifications in teaching, which should be made available to postgraduate students.

These factors may be addressed by increased provision of courses or improved coordination, including wider or more flexible access to existing course provision across the sector. In addition, increased efforts to promote chartered status and emphasis of the link between continued professional development and chartership, may also increase take-up of accredited training courses. Institutions offering routes to chartered status emphasise the link between commitment to continuing professional development and attainment of chartered status (Engineering Council, 2010; Society of Biology, 2009). However, not all offer endorsement of external courses as part of this scheme. Alternatively, to improve uptake and portability, recognition of training or developed attributes could be achieved through a system of credit bearing, masters' level short courses utilised as CPD. This would enable development of skills as required and the accrual of credit over the course of the research degree and potentially during future employment. This would allow students to build training at an accredited, recognised level and to work to the award of a postgraduate qualification over an extended period.

Perhaps suggesting more of a step-change in course provision, and reflecting the increase in Centres for Doctoral Training, 61% of students indicated that they wished for more courses to be incorporated into their research degree programme. This is correlated with the perception of a lack availability of relevant courses, and the desire for more training in categories other than soft skills. The incorporation of a flexible taught component into research degrees merits further investigation. This includes study into the provision of the existing research degree programmes that offer a training component, such as professional doctorates or the NewRoutePhD scheme, or alternatively incorporating training into a PhD programme as a requirement for transition from probationary status. However, PhDs are by nature both novel and individual, which could mean that a rigid compulsory training structure may be counterproductive. Gilbert *et al.* (2004) included comments from supervisors that show an antipathy to establishing a curriculum for PhD study, highlighting a danger that homogenising doctoral students in such a manner will remove the creativity and individualisation, which are essential to science. Barnacle and Dall'Alba (2011) show that doctoral graduates draw on their research work in future employment and question the use of generic skill training as an aid to creative and innovative working. Increased utilisation of centres that offer training in both generic and subject specific skills to the exclusion of other institutions may possibly reduce the effective provision of PhD training, as well as limit choice of supervisor. Flexibility in both provision and requirements for individuals is therefore key to developing the researcher skill set within the PhD framework.

The Roberts review (2002) and a 2010 Government Report into postgraduate education (Smith *et al.*, 2010) have indicated the need for increased training in transferable skills to ensure PhD graduates meet the needs of both industrial and academic employers. The current study indicates a low level of course attendance and a demand for increased management training, which is consistent with these reviews. However, this work also indicates a demand for increased technical training. Principal student concerns are a perceived lack of available courses, time taken out of research for training and recognition of achievement. Some students also fail to recognise the need for training outside their immediate discipline. This suggests improvements are required to the provision, marketing and structure of training for postgraduate research students in order to adequately prepare them for work in academia, government or industry.

References

Barnacle, R. and Dall'Alba, G. (2011) Research degrees as professional education? *Studies in Higher Education*, **36**, 459–470.

Borrell-Damian, L., Brown, T., Dearing, A., Font, J., Hagen, S., Metcalfe, J. and Smith, J. (2010) Collaborative doctoral education: University-industry partnerships for enhancing knowledge exchange. *Higher Education Policy*, **23**, 493–514.

Browne, J., Barber, M., Coyle, D., Eastwood, D., King, J., Naik, R. and Sands, P. (2010) *Securing A Sustainable Future for Higher Education: An Independent Review of Higher Education Funding and Student Finance.* Available at: https://www.gov.uk/government/publications/the-browne-report-higher-education-funding-and-student-finance (accessed 2 December 2016).

Brunel University (2010) *CORE Skills Training Seminars Brunel University Graduate School.* Available at: School http://www.brunel.ac.uk/services/graduate-school/training-development-and-support/research-students/researcher-development-programme (accessed 2 December 2016).

Cockram, M.S., Aitchison, K., Collie, D.D.S., Goodman, G. and Murray, J.-A. (2007) Animal-handling teaching at the Royal (Dick) School of Veterinary Studies, University of Edinburgh. *Journal of Veterinary Medical Education*, **34**, 554–560.

CSFS (2014) *The Chartered Society of Forensic Sciences and Continuing Professional Development (CPD) for Forensic Practitioners.* Available at: http://www.csofs.org/Continuing-Professional-Development-CPD (accessed 2 December 2016]

Engineering Council (2010) *The UK Standard for Professional Engineering Competence.* Engineering Council, London.

EPSRC (2009) *Delivery Plan Scorecard 2008-11*, Engineering and Physical Sciences Research Council, Swindon.

EPSRC (2010a) *Career Development*, Engineering and Physical Sciences Research Council, Swindon. Available at: https://www.epsrc.ac.uk/skills/students/ (accessed 2 December 2016).

EPSRC (2010b) *Industrial Doctorate Centres*, Engineering and Physical Sciences Research Council, Swindon. Available at: https://www.epsrc.ac.uk/skills/students/coll/idc/ (accessed 2 December 2016).

EPSRC (2014) *Centres for Doctoral Training: Current centres*, Engineering and Physical Sciences Research Council, Swindon. Available at: https://www.epsrc.ac.uk/skills/students/centres/ (accessed 2 December 2016).

Foote, K.E. (2010) Creating a community of support for graduate students and early career academics. *Journal of Geography in Higher Education*, **34**, 7–19.

Gilbert, R., Balatti, J., Turner, P. and Whitehouse, H. (2004) The generic skills debate in research higher degrees. *Higher Education Research & Development*, **23**, 375–388.

Hardre, P.L. (2005) Instructional design as a professional development tool-of-choice for graduate teaching assistants. *Innovative Higher Education*, **30**, 163–175.

Hinchliffe, G.W. and Jolly A. (2011) Graduate identity and employability. *British Educational Research Journal*, **37** (4), 563–584.

IET (2010) *Training Provider Endorsement*. The Institution of Engineering and Technology. Available at: http://www.theiet.org/academics/accreditation/index.cfm (accessed 2 December 2016).

Jones, B. (2010) University Challenge: The opportunities for collaboration between industry and academia are now too big to ignore. *Engineering and Technology*, **5** (9), 55–57.

Jones, B.J. (2011) Nano fingerprints: gathering intelligence. *Materials Today*, **14**, 567.

Kaplan, K (2011) Industry-orientated education: the other path. *Nature*, **469**, 569.

Kehm, B.M. (2007) Quo vadis doctoral education? New European approaches in the context of global changes. *European Journal of Education*, **42**, 307–319.

Kulej, G. and Wells P. (2009) *Postgraduate Research Experience Survey*, Higher Education Academy, York.

Manathunga, C. and Lant, P. (2006) How do we ensure good PhD student outcomes? *Education for Chemical Engineers*, **1**, 72–81.

Muldoon, R. (2009) Recognizing the enhancement of graduate attributes and employability through part-time work while at university. *Active Learning in Higher Education*, **10**, 237–252.

Neumann, R. and Tan, K.K. (2011) From PhD to initial employment: the doctorate in a knowledge economy. *Studies in Higher Education* **36**, 601–614.

NR PhD (2014) *NewRoutePhD an Integrated Doctorate*. Available at: https://www.brunel.ac.uk/_data/assets/pdf_file/0019/310528/NewRoute-Programme.pdf (accessed 2 December 2016).

Pritchard, J., MacKenzie, J. and Cusak, M. (2009) The response of Physical Science post-graduates to training courses and the connection to their PhD studies. *International Journal for Researcher Development*, **1**, 29–44.

RCUK (2014) *Training Grant Guide*, Research Councils UK, Swindon. Available at: http://www.rcuk.ac.uk/documents/publications/traininggrantguidance-pdf/ (accessed 2 December 2016).

Rennison, A. (2010) Lund Lecture of the British Academy of Forensic Sciences, London.

Research Concordat (2010) *The Concordat to Support the Career Development of Researchers, Principle 4*. Available at: https://www.vitae.ac.uk/policy/concordat-to-support-the-career-development-of-researchers (accessed 2 December 2016).

Roberts, G. (2002) *SET for Success: The Supply of People with Science, Technology, Engineering and Mathematics Skills*. HM Treasury, London, ch. 4.

Servage, L. (2009) Alternative and professional doctoral programs: what is driving the demand? *Studies in Higher Education*, **34**, 765–779.

Smith, A., Bradshaw, T., Burnett, K., Docherty, D., Purcell, W. and Worthington, S. (2010) *One Step Beyond: Making the Most of Postgraduate Education*. HM Government Department for Business, Information and Skills, London.

Society of Biology (2009) *Continuing Professional Development, Learning for Life*, Society of Biology, London.

Tallantyre, F., Kettle, J., and Smith, J. (2010) *Demonstrator Projects*, Higher Education Academy, York.

University of Nottingham (2011) *Rehabilitation Certificate (PGCert).* Available at: https://www.nottingham.ac.uk/pgstudy/courses/nursing-midwifery-and-physiotherapy/physiotherapy-(neurorehabilitation)-pgcert.aspx (accessed 2 December 2016).

University of Oxford (2011) *Professional Development: Short Courses in Nanotechnology.* https://www.conted.ox.ac.uk/about/nanotechnology-and-nanomedicine (accessed 2 December 2016).

University of Surrey (2011) *Electronic Engineering – Professional Development.* http://www.surrey.ac.uk/eee/study/pd/ (accessed 2 December 2016).

9

Educational Forensic E-gaming as Effective Learning Environments for Higher Education Students

Jamie K. Pringle, Luke Bracegirdle, and Jackie A. Potter

School of Physical Sciences and Geography, Keele University, Keele, Staffordshire, UK

Introduction

Common causes of concern for Higher Education (HE) science lecturers is *students' effective engagement* with topic and the students' ability to learn, understand and apply knowledge in a different situation, or indeed, in a problem-based, real-world scenario. This transfer of knowledge issue may, in part, be due to the structured nature of traditional lecture and associated laboratory practical teaching environments that predominate in the science disciplines. This teaching and learning approach may not prove effective, particularly when compared with accepted experiential student learning models of concrete experience, observation and reflection, subsequent formation of new concepts, and finally, new concept testing (Kolb and Fry, 1975). Other researchers have shown that having an effective teaching and learning environment can result in higher quality student work (Kember and Leung, 2006).

There are also indications from geoscience commercial employers that 'graduates, whilst bright and having the appropriate theoretical knowledge may have difficulty applying the appropriate technique, or more usually, a multi-disciplinary technique combination to solve "real-world" problems in the commercial environment' (Cassidy and Pringle, 2010). Students also 'have the tendency to have difficulties grasping the realities of the real-world world, undertaking commercial projects, keeping to project budgets and tight timescales' (Pringle *et al.*, 2010). The transfer of knowledge has been traditionally hard to replicate in academia although focused fieldwork work-based 'commercial scenarios' for final year students has been shown to partially address this, leading to higher level thinking and learning (see Pringle *et al.*, 2010).

Current HE students are Generation 'Y' generally defined as 1982–2001 birth years (Knight, 2009). Generation Y students are 'fundamentally different in outlook and ambition from any group of kids in the past 50 or 60 years… it is clear that they already know they don't want to live or work the way we do' (Hill, 2002). Generation Y students

Forensic Science Education and Training: A Tool-kit for Lecturers and Practitioner Trainers, First Edition.
Edited by Anna Williams, John P. Cassella, and Peter D. Maskell.
© 2017 John Wiley & Sons Ltd. Published 2017 by John Wiley & Sons Ltd.

have been suggested to be 'mostly "digital natives" connected 24/7, bored by routine and goal-orientated' (Knight, 2009), and as such, may respond positively to technology-based complementary learning environments as much or if not more so than more traditional HE learning environments. However, this is a generalisation as there will be students with different technological abilities, interests and cultural backgrounds and thus the student cohort will be much more diverse and heterogeneous, as pointed out by Sternberg (2012). In addition, the student cohort will also include more mature students, as well as those who may be visually or auditory impaired, so this may affect educational e-gaming teaching and learning.

Educational e-gaming may therefore be a solution for effective learning in HE (see Squire, 2008). This chapter details an action research project undertaken at Keele University. Action research is a pedagogic research tool, which encourages an active researcher–participant intervention approach (for background see Elliott, 2001). There is no set method but the aim of this project was to determine if 'immersive e-gaming could provide an effective complementary learning environment for HE physical science Generation Y students.'

Background

A review of both generic (Harper and Quaye, 2008) and subject-specific educational literature (Olitsky, 2007) has shown student engagement is a high priority, with the Higher Education Academy (HEA) and Quality Assurance Agency (QAA) for the HEA having specific strategies in place to address this issue (UKES, 2016; QAA, 2016). Tallantyre (2008) describes government strategy as 'HE needing to take on board more student engagement', with the HEA 'putting its main emphasis on innovation and developing student engagement skills.' HE engagement takes various forms but commonly reflects students' interest, enthusiasm and participation in a specific topic, with the subsequent benefit of an improved student experience and understanding. However, student engagement with scientific topics is often complex and multi-disciplinary (Thomas, 2008).

Geoscience is characterised by *fieldwork*, which does not have a pre-determined outcome; 'open-ended questions foster greater student motivation, encourages acceptance of uncertainty and serves to enhance transferable skills to graduates' (Williams, 2006). This has been developed pedagogically at Keele University, where Masters-level residential field exercises were evaluated to show how important student-led, group problem-solving, field exercises can be to aid student understanding and engagement (Pringle *et al.*, 2010). However, current university funding, timetable restraints and limited commercial placements mean that there are currently few opportunities for undergraduates to experience a wide variety of learning environments that develop 'interpreting, analysing, evaluating, synthesising and solving complex problems' (Falloon, 2009).

Over 88% of current HE students are Generation Y (Health Education and Statistics Agency, HESA, 2016), who, although having limited computer access in their formative years, by secondary and high school would have been using, and possibly taught by, computer technologies. Nimon (2007) states that these students have general traits of optimism and success, rating participation over achievement; however, they often struggle outside their comfort zone and with not being successful (Hill, 2002). They also have short attention spans. Sheahan (2005) warns employers 'if you can't keep Generation Y entertained, you can't keep them.' A study of 17 000 HE UK post-graduate research students outcomes were 'sophisticated information-seekers and users of complex information sources… not dazzled by technology… highly competent and ubiquitous users of IT' (Joint Information Systems Committee, JISC, 2012).

HE virtual learning through on-line, interactive resources have proved popular with students, Mountney (2009) evidences how computer-generated simulations and video-based animations can improve understanding of how landscapes change over time, which had been difficult to demonstrate prior to the use of computer technologies and digital media. Video podcasts have also aided students' understanding of field equipment before they actually enter the field (see Jarvis and Dickie, 2009). Virtual field trips can also provide 'direct learning opportunities and indeed bridge formal and informal learning,' without the associated logistical challenges and risks involved in running field trips (Stainfield *et al.*, 2000). Warburton (2009) showed that online Second Life™ multi-player immersive online environments could be used as academic learning tools, but required all students to be logged in, undertaking a virtual discussion, which would be variable in content. Chapter 12 discusses these points in further detail.

Educational e-gaming shows great potential, as users become immersed in the online learning environment, providing a 'shift from what a person knows or can store in the head… towards what the person can do, with serious gamers pointing to a future paradigm for e-learning' (Squire, 2008). The sheer variety of game genres (e.g. action, adventure, fighting, role-playing, simulations, sports and strategy game types) 'provide complex learning in which skills and attitudes play important roles' (Gros, 2007). Medical students have been shown to better understand bone fracture morphology, procedure accuracy and operation times have been reduced through the use of Virtual Reality or VR (Citak *et al.*, 2008) technologies. The ability of engineering students to visualise turbine generator assemblages was improved through VR compared with non-participating students (De Sousa *et al.*, 2012). In forensic science, it has been shown that three-dimensional VR can 'accurately reconstruct crime scenes, demonstrates activities at various points in time and allows students to become experienced in crime scene investigations without physically attending a lot of crime scenes themselves' (Ma *et al.*, 2010).

There is clearly scope for science educational e-gaming, although little has been published on this to-date. Leeds University have developed an online geological prospection e-game (see www.see.leeds.ac.uk/misc/miner/), allowing users to become virtual exploration geologists and manage a company, although pedagogic research on its effectiveness has not been published to-date. A pilot geoscience educational e-game to locate a coal mineshaft was generated and shown to be an effective learning tool by Geology, Geoscience and Environmental Science BSc degree students (see Pringle, 2013). Non-educational science-based games have been created for public entertainment, for example, the US-based Crime Scene Investigation (CSI) TV series have had online e-games developed, allowing the user to go through various scenarios to become a criminal detective. Whilst potentially useful and engaging, the primary focus of science educational e-games should be to encourage student understanding and learning.

Methodology

After the initial successful geoscience e-game pilot (Pringle, 2013), two HEA small-project grants funded the development of a forensic science e-game, based on a published real-world case study to locate a clandestine burial of a murder victim in the United Kingdom (Pringle and Jervis, 2010). This case study had always been well received by Keele University BSc Science degree students and thus was considered to be a good basis for an educational e-game. Background resources were needed to provide data for the e-game (Table 9.1), which was developed and iteratively refined through non-project volunteer participant testing. Dedicated computer programmers used commercial computer game generation software and graphical animators to give the game realism and a smooth gaming experience. The game was formalised into the four stages of a forensic terrestrial search (see Pringle *et al.*, 2012 for forensic search best practice), that is: (1) background desk study (Figure 9.1); staged fieldwork including (2) reconnaissance (Figure 9.2) and (3) full surveys (Figures 9.3 and 9.4); and finally (4) excavation of prioritised suspected burial position (Figure 9.5).

An *Action Research (AR) approach* was used (see Elliott, 2001 for AR background) by active participation of 2011–2012 HE Keele University undergraduate taught student volunteers as they studied for Forensic Science (final year) and Geoscience/Geology (second year) BSc degrees ($n = 41$); it would be very difficult if not impossible to evaluate the effectiveness of e-gaming without the students themselves being involved in the process. A smaller cohort of postgraduate research (PGR) Forensic Science/Geoscience/Geology PhD students of varying ages and 50/50 male/female genders ($n = 20$) were also involved to test its effectiveness for students with increased experience. The e-game was directly degree-relevant to the undergraduate cohorts and potentially useful to PGR students. A *sequential mixed methods AR approach* was utilised to provide a 'platform for a variety of intended and un-intended outcomes' (Foddy, 1994) of:

1. Pre-game questionnaire to gain quantitative and qualitative data (as suggested by Gray, 2004) on participating student gaming experience and current usage, preferred learning environment(s), thoughts on their university learning experience to-date, self-rating their forensic search knowledge as well as anything else deemed relevant.
2. Participants undertake the e-game. Simultaneous semi-structured, chronological observations were also made during the exercise, in order to collect 'live data' that may contain insights likely to be missed in a more formal environment, as described by Cohen *et al.* (2005). The exercises were also auditory recorded for later transcribing and comments were grouped into themes (termed coding) to provide qualitative data (see Elliott, 2001).
3. Two post-intervention focus group interviews with undergraduates to discuss (again auditory taped, subsequently transcribed and coded) the learning experience of the e-game for them, its beneficial elements (or otherwise) and any other relevant project thoughts as Wilkinson (2003) suggests.
4. An end-project questionnaire to ask participants to self-rate their search knowledge, determine the e-game student learning experience and learn any un-intended project outcomes.

Table 9.1 List of e-game resources required and sources (see Glossary for detail), intended learning outcomes and time needed to create.

Stage and resource	Teaching and learning tool	Intended learning outcomes	Source	Time to create (h)
(1) *Desk study:* Digital map view data	1 aerial photograph and map	User(s) can visualises the priority search field and surrounding areas	EDINA Digimap download	1
	7 historical and 1 artificial ground maps	User(s) can determine past land use to assist data interpretation		0.5 per map
	1 geology and one soil map	User(s) can determine bedrock/soil type that may assist determine optimum search technique(s)		1 per map
	1 Infra-red (IR) map	User(s) can visualise the search field to detect suspect areas. Red areas indicate mature vegetation and white indicate new vegetation ground	Digitally created by super-imposing areas onto aerial map	8
(2) *Recon-naissance:* User(s) choose resources (limited to 100%)	Search dogs (20%), metal detector (50%), geo-morphology (10%), botany (10%), entomology (30%), thermal camera (50%), methane probe (50%), trial digging (5%) and simulated burial (5%)	User(s) can pick a few of these to simulate realistic restricted budget proportions (%). Some should give indications of suspected burial position(s)	E-game team choose % breakdown and suspect burial position based on case and search knowledge	5
(3) *Full Survey:* User(s) free to roam and choose search equipment	Digital Elevation Model (DEM)	Digital land surface created of search area and surrounding areas	EDINA Digimap download	20
	Site photographs	Programmers used to refine land surface and fill textures	Site visit	4
	VR environment	User(s) can freely roam digital search field surface	Programmers	70
	VR geophysical equipment	User(s) use them to target suspect positions and become 'experienced'	Programmers create from videos	35

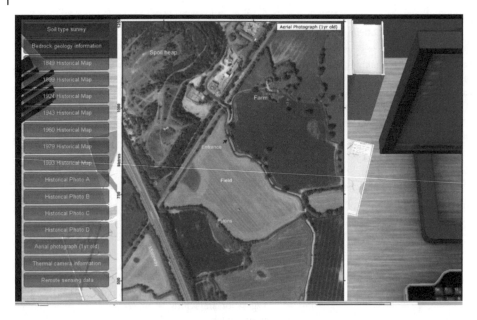

Figure 9.1 E-game screen-shot showing (stage 1) initial desk study data (icons on left) and site image with suspect field marked.

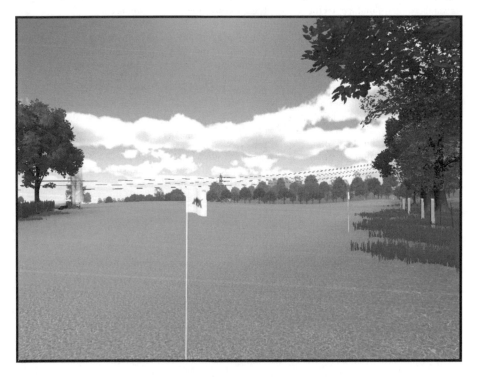

Figure 9.2 E-game screen-shot showing initial reconnaissance (stage 2) suspected flag positions and research van with 'teleport' position (background).

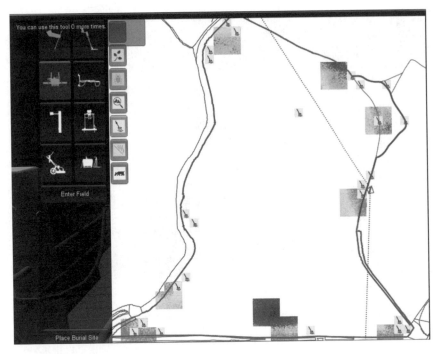

Figure 9.3 E-game screen-shot at (stage 3) with the user in the survey van viewing bulk ground conductivity data (coloured squares) and metal detector results (icons) in the main screen. Bar on left allows user to choose next equipment to be trialled.

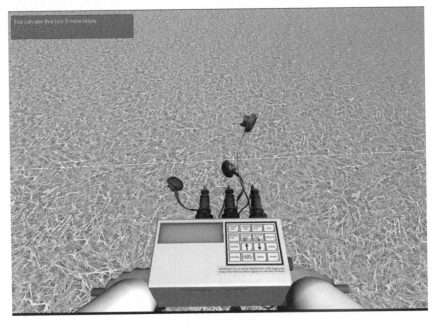

Figure 9.4 E-game screen-shot during (stage 3) collecting electrical resistivity data. Note limited equipment uses for search realism.

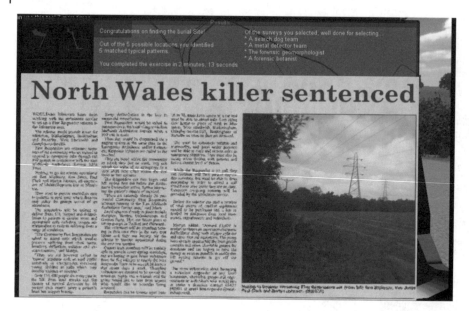

Figure 9.5 E-game screen-shot completion with text and brief user feedback. Alternative finish is 'Killer goes free' newspaper headline.

Results

Analysing the **(1) initial questionnaire**, undergraduate/postgraduate student participants had average ages of 21 and 25, respectively, and were split 61/39 and 70/30 male/female percentages, respectively. All undergraduates and 95% of the PGR students had played computer games before and three quarters of the undergraduates and 40% of the PGR group currently played daily or once a week (Figure 9.6). Almost half of the undergraduates (49%) and over one third of the PGR (35%) students had previously

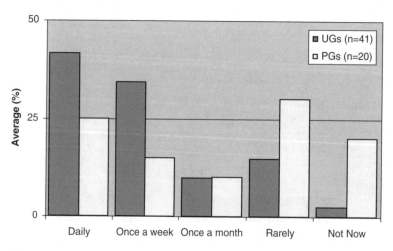

Figure 9.6 Graphical summary of participating HE undergraduate (UGs) and postgraduate research (PGs) students' response to current e-game usage.

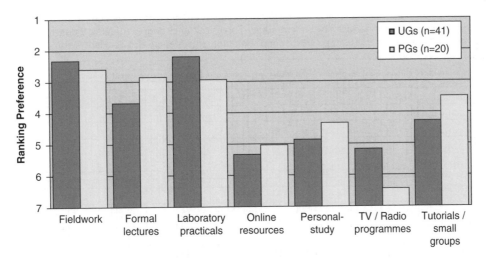

Figure 9.7 Graphical summary of participating HE undergraduate (UGs) and postgraduate research (PGs) students' response to rating (1 = highest) current HE learning environments.

used e-gaming as an educational tool, predominantly in primary school education maths games, and secondary school GCSE revision tools; one commented 'BBC Bitesize made learning key terms fun.' These participants ranked laboratory practicals highest as HE preferred learning environments, followed by fieldwork (2) and formal lectures (3) with other learning environments well behind (Figure 9.7). One fifth of the undergraduates and half of the PGR students had degree-relevant commercial/voluntary work experience, with surprisingly 64% of undergraduates and 60% of postgraduate research students self-rated their search knowledge as either good or average (Figure 9.8).

The **(2) e-game intervention** did not have a user mark for locating the burial as this was not the point of the e-game; however, it was noted that only seven out of 60 were

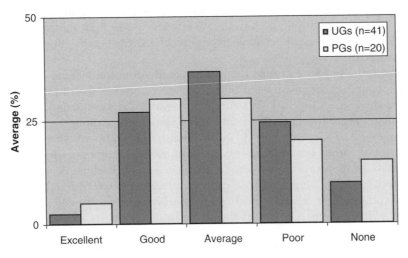

Figure 9.8 Graphical summary of participating HE undergraduate (UGs) and postgraduate research (PGs) students' response to self-rating knowledge to undertake a search investigation.

Table 9.2 Example of chronological 'tick-box' observation record of verbal discussion during the e-game intervention undertaken by undergraduate Forensic Science degree students. It details (A) participant discussions and (B) topics. Expanded contemporary notes are also detailed.

Semi-structured chronological observations and accompanying notes for Forensic Science B.Sc UG students
(A) Participants
Student to student   √   √ √√√√√   √ √ √   √√   √√√ √√   √√ √√   √ √√ √
Student to students √ √√   √   √√√ √   √ √   √√√   √   √   √   √ √
Student to lecturer   √   √√   √√ √   √   √√√
Lecturer to student   √   √√ √   √ √   √   √   √√
Lecturer to students
Student to self   √√   √
(B) Discussion Topic
Task in hand √ √√ √√   √√   √√ √√√√√√√√√√ √√√√√√√√√√√√√√√√√√√√√√ √√√ √√√√√√   √
Relevant documentation
Independent relevant search
Non-Task   √√√√√√√ √√ √   √√   √ √   √√ √√√√√√
Observation Notes (includes initial reflections, points of clarification, etc.)	Initial teething issues with download. Around 1/2 of students looking at other websites (facebook (6), autotrader (2) or indeed gaming(3)) whilst loading. Most students worked through well, read everything and walked around. Others more 'lazy' gamers, wanting to teleport/run everywhere. Most learnt as much by talking to fellow students as playing the game. Some did it 2 or 3 times. Only 2 found body (out of 18).

successful and these participants self-rated themselves as having average to good search knowledge. Contemporary observations evidenced that participants in the three e-game sessions sequentially worked through the search scenario, were task-focused (Table 9.2) and a non-systematic noting of participants e-game completion time varied between 12 and 60 minutes (average of 30 minutes). Observational data showed the importance of the presence of both a group of students, as a significant amount of learning was learnt by student–student interactions, and the 'instructor,' to answer verbal queries (see Table 9.2), although the necessity for the presence of the latter may be due to a lack of e-game text information, which will be rectified in future e-game refinements. There were also a surprising variety of gaming styles used by participants; some were methodological, exploring the entire game environment, whilst others were 'lazy gamers,' one of whom commented 'lots of short-cut buttons to save my time.' A few PGR students also initially struggled with the e-game technology but completed the e-game after some initial e-game familiarisation.

The (3) **undergraduate focus groups** then subsequently discussed educational e-gaming, other learning environments and other relevant comments. From grouping (termed coding) the themes together (in italics): (A) *e-gaming* in general and this *e-game* in particular was positively received with seven comments wishing it to be an assessed component of a course module; (B) there was also discussions on *other learning environments* with formal taught lectures being given a mixed reception, laboratory practicals judged to be useful and, lastly, some ambivalence on the usefulness of group problem classes; (C) participants judged the e-game positively for *job skills*; and (D) *subject engagement* comments evidenced e-gaming was a positive method of a way to learn (Table 9.3). A combined summary of the key themes and number of responses are listed in Table 9.3.

Both focus groups were also very positive about the e-game combining different techniques and datasets, one student commented: 'remote sensing – I never got that until I

Table 9.3 Summary of key themes and codes discussed during the focus groups, with sub-codes also given where appropriate. Key theme letters (A–D) refer to suggested themes in a discussion list.

Themes	Codes	No. of responses	Sub-code	No. of responses
(A) E-gaming	General gaming	16	Positive	12
			Negative	4
	E-game trialled	34	Positive	13
			Suggested improvements	7
			Wanted it to be assessed	7
			Negative	7
(B) Other learning environments	Lectures	38	Lecturer personality (8+/6−)	14
			Positive	9
			YouTube video summary (6+/1−)	7
			Negative	5
			Highly technical	3
	Research project	8	Lit. review	4
			Positive	4
	Practicals	14	Positive	11
			Negative	5
	Problem classes	18	Positive	9
			Negative	9
(C) Job skills	Relevant to job	9	Positive	8
			Negative	1
(D) Subject engagement	New way to learn	7	Positive	7
	Student lack of	6	Negative	6

played the game.' Another participant stated 'I hated it yeah. I'm a girl. Girls don't like games,' which was balanced out by her female peer who commented she was a 'serious gamer.' An unexpected outcome with both focus groups was the discussion on formal lectures and how the lecturers themselves were often more important for effective learning than the content.

Analysis of the **(4) end-project questionnaire** revealed that 95% of undergraduates and 90% of PGR students enjoyed the e-game, giving it an average (non-parametric) rating of 4.1 for undergraduates and 4.0 for PGR students with 5 being the highest. Undergraduates rated 'level of detail' highest, followed by 'value to your studies,' whilst PGR students rated 'accessibility' then 'level of detail' highest (Figure 9.9). The relatively low 'ability to comprehend content' scores may be due to the lack of e-game instructions that was evidenced by the requests for clarification during the e-game intervention itself (Table 9.2). This will be rectified in later e-game versions.

It appeared that 96% of undergraduates and 64% of PGR students self-rated their search knowledge as either good or average, a +32% and 0% change from before the e-game, respectively (Figures 9.10 and 9.11). The majority of the undergraduates (80%) and, interestingly, 54% of the postgraduate participants stated they had an improved search knowledge after playing the e-game.

A simple statistical paired two-tailed t-test of student participants' search knowledge could also be undertaken because the same question was asked before and after the

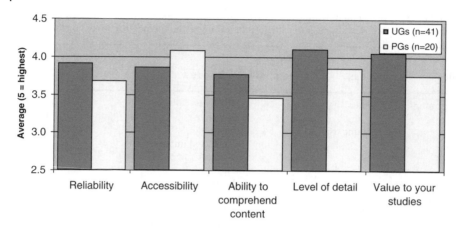

Figure 9.9 Graphical summary of participating HE undergraduate (UGs) and postgraduate research (PGs) students rating the e-game in five areas (5 highest).

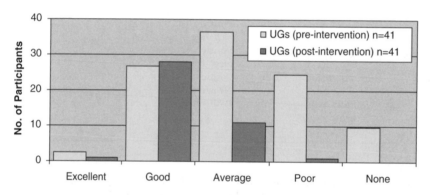

Figure 9.10 Graphical summary of undergraduate participants' (UGs) response to self-rating search knowledge compared both before and after the e-game intervention.

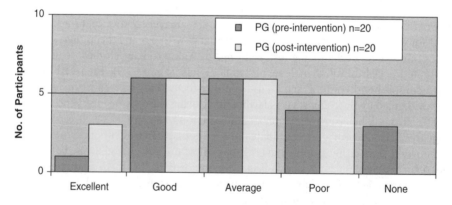

Figure 9.11 Graphical summary of postgraduate research participants' (PGs) response to self-rating search knowledge both before and after the e-game intervention.

e-game intervention. Responses were converted into numerical data (no knowledge = 1, poor = 2, average = 3, good = 4 and 5 = excellent). Results showed that undergraduates showed a statistically significant improvement of search knowledge after the e-game intervention (3.71 post- versus 2.85 pre- with $P = 0$) whilst the PGR search knowledge improvement (3.42 post- versus 2.85 pre- with $P = 0.06$) was not statistically significant (see Till, 1974 for background). Dividing participants by gender showed male search knowledge improvements after the e-game intervention was statistically significant (3.67 post- versus 3.00 pre-) whilst female improvements were not (3.16 post- versus 2.76 pre-), which are consistent with other studies (see Bostock and Lizhi, 2005).

Participants' combined anonymous questionnaire comments showed participants enjoyed the e-game and found it fun (9), that it: aided their understanding (5), showed how searches are conducted (3), was realistic (2), practical (2), good for revision (2) and training (1), although one student commented that it was not as useful as traditional learning environments and another stated that they wanted more detail. Combined suggestions for subsequent e-game improvements included: better avatar movement (41), better instructions (21), more field survey equipment to be available (17), different levels of difficulty (5) and even different scenarios (3). Undergraduate anonymous comments included: 'I think it's a good tool to use, [it] really helped develop my understanding to what sort of results I should expect in the field' and 'useful as get chance to use all equipment in a real-life application, which can be revisited multiple times' although one commented 'just a game, not really representative.' PGR students' anonymous comments included: 'great way to bring together different data sets and synthesize data to reach a conclusion' and 'really good, makes you think about what techniques work best. Much easier when you play again. I used different techniques on the second go.' One PGR student commented that they found it novel that they could select the wrong site, perhaps indicating that current students are used to success or to the complexity of reality that is modelled in the game?

Discussion

This study indicates that, giving current HE students the opportunity to use *complementary learning environments* to traditional lectures and associated laboratory practicals is to be recommended. This is in line with other researchers' findings (e.g. Squire, 2008; Falloon, 2010) who have also used immersive educational e-gaming. Note, however, that all participants rated laboratory practicals, fieldwork and formal lectures highest as their preferred learning environments prior to the e-game. The e-game has both engaged the participating student cohort's learning and teaching experience and has been effective, the latter evidenced by participants improvements in self-rating their forensic search knowledge after the e-game intervention compared with before the intervention. Undergraduate participants' improvements were statistically significant. Interestingly there were gender differences, with male improvements statistically significant whilst female improvements were not. An unintended learning outcome was that some caution should be used when requesting undergraduates to self-rate knowledge – quite a few self-rated they were average or good at search even when they had no search experience. This may be due to the optimistic traits of Generation Y students that others have documented (e.g. Squire, 2008; Falloon, 2010). This contrasted with PGR student participants who may be argued to be more realistic about self-rating their knowledge and who had actual search experience.

It was evidenced when participants were more experienced (i.e. the PGR students), then such educational e-games may prove less effective as an educational tool. These more experienced learners may use educational e-gaming to *hone their search skills* rather than significantly improving them.

Most current HE undergraduate students (at Keele University at least) are Generation Y: half of participants in this study were daily or weekly game users and therefore *e-gaming has great potential* as an as yet relatively untapped educational environment. Over half of the undergraduates had also used educational games before. However, caution should be given to suggestions that e-gaming should be rolled out to all cohorts and formally assessed; a minority of participants were not comfortable with e-gaming, did not enjoy the experience and/or struggled with the technology.

An unintended learning outcome was that it was important to *pilot e-games at an early stage*, in order to ensure alignment with intended learning outcomes. Subsequent iterative game improvements ensured participant engagement and established that the technology could scale to support multiple users simultaneously when using the game. Significant development time was necessary to make the e-game usable but as it has been developed using an established game development framework, its move to a commercial product would not be substantial.

The e-game was almost uniformly appreciated by the participant students as a useful, reliable and informative learning and teaching environment. It was reliable because, unlike some learning environments such as laboratory practicals and fieldwork which may vary between years or even when classes are repeated, e-games give a consistently reliable experience and there is no variation in weather conditions, teaching staff, learner(s) interactions, and so on. It would also be a credible alternative to outdoor fieldwork/laboratory practicals for less physically able students, as others have discussed (see, e.g. Mountney, 2009). Intervention observations showed participants were task focused throughout, showing surprising patience when problems occurred. Undergraduates highly rated the e-game accessibility, level of detail and value to their studies. Participants were also keen to suggest improvements after the intervention. Participants did not seem to mind not being successful at finding the burial position, rather, most enjoyed using their existing knowledge, and information provided in the e-game, to try and locate the burial position.

There were contrasting suggestions and little agreement with having *e-games formally assessed*; some suggested they should to ensure engagement whilst others were worried peers may struggle with the technology and hence would be unfairly penalised if gaining a poor mark. Other suggestions were to run an additional laboratory practical to complement existing teaching module resources.

Clearly *educational e-gaming is a hybrid learning process*, from e-game–participant–participant knowledge transfer, participant decision making, peer group interaction and participant–observer interventions all contributing to the learning experience. Student engagement with the educational e-gaming environment was generally high. However, there needed to be significant time developing and refining appropriate e-game content and related materials for learners to gain the most out of the experience.

Project recommendations show immersive educational e-gaming can be an important complementary learning environment and can be highly effective for current HE Generation Y students, giving a consistent learning experience. However, this study suggests that it should be used in undergraduate, not postgraduate teaching and used to support taught or existing subject knowledge. An unexpected outcome was most participants' requirements to move faster within the e-game virtual environment when in the field, something that was thought better to be realistic rather than replicating commercial games. Upon reflection, this should be a suggestion for future *e-game improvements*. A few students were also keen to have a 'reward' for playing by adding features and abilities available to the player, clues to be included, gold/silver/bronze star rewards or goal-orientated achievements to replicate commercial games, which may be subsequently included.

Conclusions

Educational e-gaming can provide an effective complementary learning environment to more traditional learning methods in Higher Education physical science or potentially humanity studies. E-games can provide a consistent and reliable learning environment, in contrast to field trips and laboratory practicals, especially with the current large cohorts of physical science undergraduates in HE. The e-game developed in this study provided a statistically significant improvement in participant HE undergraduates' knowledge; in this case of forensic search techniques applied to a 'real-world' problem. It also provided a case study for postgraduate HE students to hone their search skills. For others to replicate, it would be necessary to have significant computer programming and design expertise, appropriate scientific input and time spent developing and refining the e-game.

Other Forensic Science degree course staff could make use of this educational e-game for their student cohorts through this book's website. It could also be used before field practicals for fieldwork and/or equipment familiarisation, or for those teaching providers who don't have access to such equipment. It could also be used for in-course assessment to test student search knowledge, although this chapter shows the potential risk for technology-averse students. There is scope to create other educational e-games if experienced software programmers/developers are available, which would require funding. Further e-game developments on mobile device applications or 'apps' could make these fully integrated with current HE student technologies.

Acknowledgements

Karl Reid, Tom Pardoe and David Ledsam are thanked for computer programming and graphical design of the e-game. Keele University participating undergraduates and postgraduate research students are acknowledged for participation in this research project. The Higher Education Academy is thanked for providing two small-project grants to fund the e-game development. Keele University is acknowledged for providing an Innovation in Teaching Award. The Editors and Joanna Wright are thanked for improving this chapter.

Glossary

action research An active pedagogic approach that encourages active researcher–participant interventions.

BBC Bitesize British Broadcast Corporation online examination revision tools/aids.

botany The study of plants.

coal mineshaft Access to below-ground economic coal deposits, usually vertically orientated.

conductivity Geophysical technique used to detect areas with different bulk conductive properties.

CSI Crime Scene Investigation, in this chapter meaning a popular US-based TV entertainment series.

coding Term often used by computer programmers when creating software, but here used in a pedagogical context to group responses into themes and sub-themes to give summarise group discussions.

DEM Digital Elevation Model, digital representation of a land surface.

EDINA Digimap A UK academic-provided resource of digital spatially referenced datasets that can be downloaded, including historical/modern topographic maps, geology, soil and land use maps and DEMs.

electrical resistivity Geophysical technique used to detect areas with different bulk electrical properties.

entomology The study of insects.

GCSE General Certificate in Secondary Education qualifications, usually taken aged 16 in England, Wales and Northern Ireland.

Generation 'X' Students grouped into 1961–1981 birth years.

Generation 'Y' Students grouped into 1982–2001 birth years.

geological prospection The search for economic deposits to extract, generally minerals and/or metals (e.g. gold).

geomorphology The study of land surfaces.

HE Higher education.

HEA Higher Education Academy, UK-based educational institution dedicated to improving teaching and learning.

infra-red map Non-visible wavelength image, used in forensics to detect vegetation maturity, mature vegetation being red and new being white if in colour.

methane probe Specialist equipment used to detect levels of specific gas, normally emitted by organic decay.

QAA Quality Assurance Agency.

teleport In this e-game the ability to instantly transport the user back to a set position beside the equipment vehicle.

thermal camera Specialist equipment used to detect heat sources.

VR Virtual reality.

References

Bostock, S.J. and Lizhi, W. (2005) Gender in student online discussions. *Innovations in Education and Teaching International*, **42** (1), 75–87.

Cassidy, N.J. and Pringle, J.K. (2010) What do students do? Training, research and learning: developing skills for the next generation of near-surface geophysicists. *Near Surface Geophysics*, **8** (6), 445–450.

Citak, M., Gardner, M. J., Kendoff, D., Ségolène, T., Krettek, C. *et al.* (2008) Virtual 3D planning of acetabular fracture reduction. *Journal of Orthopaedic Research*, **26** (4), 547–552.

Cohen, L. Manion, L. and Morrison, K. (2005) *Research Methods in Education*, 5th edn, Routledge Publishers, London, pp. 227–241.

De Sousa, M.P.A., Filho, M.R., Nunes, M.V.A. and Lopes, A. de C. (2012) A 3D learning tool for a hydroelectric unit. *Computer Applications in Engineering Education*, **20** (2), 269–279.

Elliott, J. (2001) *Action Research for Educational Change.* Open University Press, Buckingham.

Falloon, G. (2009) Using avatars and virtual environments in learning: what do they offer? *British Journal of Educational Technology*, **41** (2), 108–122.

Foddy, W. (1994) *Constructing Questions for Interviews and Questionnaires: Theories and Practice in Social Research.* Cambridge University Press, Cambridge, pp. 126–152.

Gray, D.E. (2004) *Doing Research in the Real World*. Sage Publications Ltd, London, pp. 187–212.

Gros, B. (2007) Digital games in education: the design of games-based learning environments. *Journal of Research on Technology in Education*, **40** (1), 23–38.

Harper, S.R. and Quaye, S.J. (2008) *Student Engagement in Higher Education*, Routledge Publishers Ltd, New York.

Higher Education Statistics Agency (HESA) (2016). Available at: from: https://www.hesa.ac.uk/data-and-analysis/students (accessed 7 December 2016).

Hill, R.P. (2002) Managing across generations in the 21st century: important lessons from the ivory trenches. *Journal of Management Inquiry*, **11** (1), 60–66.

Jarvis, C. and Dickie, J. (2009) Acknowledging the 'forgotten' and the 'unknown': the role of video podcasts for supporting field-based learning. *Geography, Earth & Environmental Sciences (GEES) of the Higher Education Academy, Planet*, **22**, 61–63.

Joint Information Systems Committee (JISC) (2012) *Researchers of Tomorrow: the Research Behaviour of Generation Y Doctoral Students.* 85pp. Available at: http://www.jisc.ac.uk/media/documents/publications/reports/2012/researchers-of-tomorrow.pdf (accessed 7 December 2016).

Kember, D. and Young, D.Y.P. (2006) Characterising a teaching and learning environment conducive to making demands on students while not making their workload excessive. *Studies in Higher Education*, **31** (2), 185–198.

Knight, Y. (2009) Talkin' 'bout my generation: a brief introduction to general theory. *Higher Education Academy Planet*, **21**, 13–15.

Kolb, D.A. and Fry, R. (1975) Toward an applied theory of experiential learning, in *Theories of Group Process*, (ed. C. Cooper), John Wiley & Sons, Ltd, Chichester, pp. 33–58.

Ma, M., Zheng, H. and Lallie, H. (2010) Virtual reality and 3D animation in forensic visualization, *Journal of Forensic Sciences*, **55** (5), 1227–1231.

Mountney, N. (2009) Improving student understanding of complex spatial-temporal relationships in earth sciences using computer animation and visualization. *Geography, Earth & Environmental Sciences (GEES) of the Higher Education Academy, Planet*, **22**, 72–77.

Nimon, S. (2007) Generation Y and Higher Education: The other Y2K. *Journal of Institutional Research*, **13** (1), 24–41.

Olitsky, S. (2007) Promoting student engagement in science: interaction rituals and the pursuit of a community in practice. *Journal of Research in Science Teaching*, **44** (1), 33–56.

Pringle, J.K., Ruffell, A., Jervis, J.R. Donnelly, L., Mckinley, J., Hansen, J., Morgan, R., Pirrie, D. and Harrison, M. (2012) The use of geoscience methods for terrestrial forensic searches. *Earth Science Reviews*, **114** (1-2), 108–123.

Pringle, J.K. (2013) Educational environmental geoscience e-gaming to provide stimulating and effective learning. *Higher Education Academy, Planet*, **27**, 21–28.

Pringle, J.K. and Jervis, J.R. (2010) Electrical resistivity survey to search for a recent clandestine burial of a homicide victim, UK. *Forensic Science International*, **202** (1), e1–e7.

Pringle, J.K., Cassidy, N.J., Styles, P., Stimpson, I.G. and Toon, S.M. (2010) Training the next generation of near-surface geophysicists: team-based student-led, problem-solving field exercises, Cumbria, UK. *Near Surface Geophysics*, **8** (6), 503–517.

Quality Assurance Agency (QAA) for HE (2016) Available at: http://www.qaa.ac.uk/partners/student-engagement (accessed 7 December 2016).

Sheahan, P. (2005) *Generation Y: Thriving and Surviving with Generation Y at Work*. Hardie Grant Books, Prahran, Victoria, Australia.

Squire, K. (2008) Video game-based learning: an emerging paradigm for instruction. *Performance Improvement Quarterly*, **21** (2), 7–36.

Stainfield, J., Fisher, P., Ford, B. and Solem, M. (2000) International virtual field trips: a new direction? *Journal of Geography in Higher Education*, **24**, 255–262.

Sternberg, J. (2012) 'It's the end of the university as we know it (and I feel fine)': the Generation Y student in HE discourse. *Higher Education Research & Development*, **31** (4), 571–583.

Tallantyre, F. (2008) HEA Academy support for employer engagement. *Geography, Earth & Environmental Sciences (GEES) of The Higher Education Academy, Planet*, **21**, 44–46.

The Uk Engagment Survey (2016). Available at: https://www.heacademy.ac.uk/institutions/surveys/uk-engagement-survey-2016 (accessed 07 December 2016).

Thomas, C. (2008) An employer's perspective on the recruitment & retention of GEES graduates in the Environmental Sector. *Geography, Earth & Environmental Sciences (GEES) of the Higher Education Academy, Planet*, **19**, 44–46.

Till, R. (1974) *Statistical Methods for the Earth Scientist: an Introduction*, Macmillan Press Ltd, Basingstoke.

Warburton, S. (2009) Second life in higher education: assessing the potential for and the barriers to deploying virtual worlds in learning and teaching. *British Journal of Educational Technology*, **40**, 414–426.

Wilkinson, S. (2003) Focus groups, in, *Qualitative Psychology: A Practical Guide to Research Methods*, (ed. J.A. Smith) Sage Publications, London, pp. 184–204.

Williams, I. (2006) Practical and laboratory work in Earth & Environmental Sciences: guide to good practice and helpful resources. *A Geography, Earth & Environmental Sciences (GEES) Higher Education Academy Learning & Teaching Guide*, 62 pp.

Further Resources

Educational e-game is available to use at: www.keelesop.co.uk/csinorthwales/. Note an internet plug-in is required to download to be able to run the e-game.

10

Virtual Anatomy Teaching Aids

Kris Thomson[1] and Anna Williams[2]

[1] Anatomage, San Jose, California, USA
[2] University of Huddersfield, School of Applied Sciences, Queensgate, Huddersfield, UK

Introduction

In recent years, the number of traditional, 'wet' laboratory practical sessions for anatomy and dissection teaching has steadily declined, in part due to increased student numbers in the Biological Sciences, dwindling resources coupled with the high cost of cadaver donation programmes and technological advances that have offered attractive alternatives (Lewis, 2014). In some cases, virtual laboratory tools have even replaced traditional practical classes, as courses have adapted to the changing needs of the student population, and seized the opportunities afforded by computerised virtual exercises and simulators. Virtual tools being used in laboratory situations now include interactive 'real life' scenarios, patient simulators (Cesari *et al.*, 2006), virtual microscopy and virtual dissection tools for animal and human bodies, 'Second Life' scientific worlds (Clark, 2009) and organ simulators (Lewis, 2014). Much of the virtual pathology world is still quite limited to areas such as virtual light microscopy (Fonseca *et al.*, 2015; Ordi *et al.*, 2015).

This chapter will explore the pedagogical advantages and disadvantages of the use of such virtual tools in the anatomy laboratory environment for forensic science education. Teaching pathology and forensic pathology is an essential aspect in the forensic science curriculum and yet it is not widely taught in the United Kingdom. This has resulted in students demonstrating a lack of basic anatomical skills when considering the body as a crime scene within the wider context of the physical crime scene of a disaster victim identification scenario (Cassella, personal communication).

Virtual Anatomy in Healthcare Education

With the emerging presence of IT based technologies in medical education, virtual anatomy has become an integral part of not only medical training but also the broader realm of healthcare. In particular, these virtual anatomy technologies look to address the difficulties associated with cadaver preparation and usage. Companies with virtual anatomy products such as Anatomage (Anatomage Table) and Touch of Life Technologies (VH Dissector) offer detailed, interactive anatomical images to complement textbooks and traditional cadaveric studies. For smaller anatomy programmes with limited cadaver access (e.g. nursing schools, physician assistant training, undergraduate courses) or institutions with costly donor programmes, these same virtual anatomy products seek to raise the standard of health education by supplying new and innovative tools for exploring the human body.

The unique features of virtual anatomy allow users to engage in a variety of clinical and educational studies including: anatomy and pathology identification, case reviews, procedural training, forensic studies and patient consultation. They supplement existing curricula and procedures with such versatility. In the classroom, traditional textbooks may lack interactivity and cadavers can prove to be expensive and limited. Virtual anatomy products provide reusable and accessible resources to students and instructors for viewing and discussing the same detailed structures.

This is not to say that the use of textbooks and cadavers should be eliminated nor replaced. It has been shown that the use of computer models is effective at demonstrating anatomy even when compared with traditional methods such as dissections or textbooks (Lewis, 2014). Codd and Choudhury's 2011 study evaluated the use of 3D virtual reality computer models to teach human forearm musculoskeletal anatomy at the University of Manchester (Codd and Choudhury, 2011). It was concluded that there were no significant differences between the computer model group and the traditional methods group. Moreover, feedback from all users of the electronic resources was positive. From this, it was determined that virtual anatomy learning can be used to complement traditional teaching methods effectively.

Finally, when compared with the costs of preparing donors for dissection, virtual anatomy platforms offer safe and predictable high quality lab experiences. With less demand for procuring and preparing bodies, institutions can lower the costs associated with embalming chemicals and bio-hazard disposal fees.

For programmes looking to offset the need for costly donor programmes and still provide an effective education, the advantages of virtual anatomy are difficult to ignore. Their inherent interactivity, reusability and cost-effectiveness serve as great complements to traditional anatomical teaching models. Techniques known as virtopsy began at the turn of the millennium as multi-disciplinary applied research projects to implement imaging modalities from diagnostic radiology and surveying technology in forensic sciences. The virtopsy approach is emerging as a robust procedure in forensic investigations (http://www.virtopsy.com/wordpress/about-virtopsy).

The benefit of the techniques used in case work is that the database of material is an exceptional resource in teaching and demonstrating, without the need to have the student and cadaver in the same room or even the same country in real time. Academic colleagues can access the materials now being produced as online resources by the Swiss team who developed the virtopsy technique (http://www.virtopsy.com/wordpress/courses).

The technology used in this technique is not new *per se*, but its application in a forensic investigation and its quality management to ISO 9001:2008 for all three domains (clinical, post-mortem and radiological examination), including reporting and written expert opinions, allowing its use in the Courtroom, is what is new and therefore pertinent to the forensic teaching environment.

Thali *et al.* (2003) reported that the concept of 'virtopsy' is promising enough to introduce and evaluate these radiological techniques in forensic medicine. Using post-mortem multi-slice computed tomography (MSCT) and magnetic resonance imaging (MRI), a number of forensic cases were examined and their findings verified by subsequent post-mortem examination. Results were classified as follows: (i) cause of death, (ii) relevant traumatological and pathological findings, (iii) vital reactions, (iv) reconstruction of injuries and (v) visualisation. In these 40 forensic cases, 47% partly combined causes of death were diagnosed at autopsy, and 26 (55%) causes of death were found independently using only radiological image data. Radiology was superior to autopsy in revealing certain cases of cranial, skeletal or tissue trauma. Some forensic vital reactions were diagnosed equally well or better using MSCT/MRI. Radiological imaging techniques are particularly beneficial for reconstruction and visualisation of forensic cases, including the opportunity to use the data for expert witness reports, teaching, quality control and telemedical consultation.

There are now a variety of materials and a number of courses available online that can be used to access virtual pathology and for 'virtopsy.'

Diaz-Perez *et al.* (2014) reported on the use of new informatics tools to improve the learning process and expand access to medical knowledge, with multimedia and information technology rising to dominance in medical education in recent years. Concurrently, there has been the gradual disappearance of traditional medical museums and autopsies, despite the proven utility in medical education.

The current, traditional passive learning limits the opportunity for reflection, interaction, creativity, clinical correlation and generative thinking. A structural change in how medical schools educate students in the subject of pathology is undoubtedly timely and necessary. Without a peer-based learning group, students also have reduced opportunity to develop social skills in an academic setting. Other limitations of the traditional lecture and demonstration format include the lack of opportunity for self-reflection and social awareness. There is very limited individual interaction when one person lectures to hundreds of students in an auditorium, and most communication is purely unidirectional. The opportunity then for the use of technology to tackle some of these issues is clear.

To fully appreciate the relevance of any pathological findings in a forensic context, students must first appreciate the foundations of anatomy and the nature and placement of organs and tissues in their normal context. Just as with virtual pathology teaching, this can now be facilitated *in part* with the technology of equipment such as Anatomage. Lewis (2014) correctly discusses the limitations that virtual laboratory tools are indeed not perfect, but neither is the use of the real thing; both suffer constraints and limitations. However, in their favour is the fact they are readily available and the issues of cost, facilities and indeed ethics of the use of cadaveric material is a clear advantage of the virtual environment. Lewis (2014) also correctly identifies what may seem obvious but is often overlooked in the Higher Education Industry.

Many resources that Lewis reviewed in his report were over ten years old, and used what are now clearly redundant digital technologies and contain limited interactivity (Franklin *et al.*, 2002). Students in today's Higher Education sector are second and third generation high-tech savvy, known as the 'Digital Generation' in which advanced technologies play a large part in their daily lives. They are used to and indeed, as consumers, expect only the highest quality digital resources and games. It is highly likely that these students would be highly dissatisfied with such technologies should they be introduced into their educational environments. The HEI sector requires technologies to be introduced from other areas, as it is unlikely that financial drivers will see them being created in a bespoke manner.

Anatomage's virtual anatomy product, the Anatomage Table, is a virtual dissection table for anatomy education. A combination of hardware and software, the system showcases real-colour cyrosections, which are photographed slices of a frozen, preserved cadaver. The Anatomage Table also features CT/MR imaging data. The 2D frozen section photographs are converted into a volume that users can clip and rotate to assist with 3D anatomical demonstration and understanding. The product's operating table form factor allows for full body anatomy viewing on a life-size scale. Furthermore, users can upload their own CT or MR data and each system comes with preinstalled, clinical examples of real patient scans. These patient scans are similarly converted into interactive 3D volumes to showcase normal and abnormal anatomical structures.

Anatomage Virtual Anatomy as a Teaching Aid

Like other virtual anatomy products, the Anatomage Table provides tools for educational programmes looking to supplement or substitute cadaver usage. By referencing real patient anatomy from either the colourful cryosections or the radiology scan data, the Anatomage Table can demonstrate intricate details captured in the scan data that may be missed in physical models or artist recreations. Moreover, the ability to upload and view any radiology image set (CT, MR) expands the versatility of the Anatomage Table both inside and outside the classroom.

Anatomy Labs

Full body volume data of male and female virtual anatomy, with minute detailing and surface models of the ligaments, tendons, blood vessels, nerves and the like, serve as a supplement to the existing cadaver curriculum. The Anatomage Table allows for life-size viewing of a scanned cadaver or any patient scan. Medical students can review material with instructors before or after traditional dissection lab sessions. The Table's tools also allow for self-review of labelled anatomical structures and the generation of images for research and presentations.

Users can customise anatomy visualisations by slicing, layering and segmenting through skeleton, muscle, organs and other soft tissue. They can selectively turn on and off independent volume structures or enhance specific features. Users can alternate between the original radiology images and the corresponding 3D images to better link clinical diagnostic images with gross anatomy education.

Medical educators help delineate the high values of virtual anatomy. At Stanford University, the Anatomage Table is becoming a core component of the anatomy courses for both medical and undergraduate studies.

Forensic and Virtual Autopsy Imaging

Virtual anatomy serves as a wonderful tool for autopsy procedures. Software that can support user CT, MRI or ultrasound scans can be used by forensic analysts to scan the body and view data on the software to look for abnormalities as they scroll through the inside of the body. It is difficult to miss important evidence when the analyst can use both the traditional autopsy procedure and the virtual anatomy together. Additionally, as a demonstration tool, displaying the CT or MR images in both 2D and 3D may be more easily understood by the general public especially in courtroom or public presentations.

Moreover, with the use of such technology, archaeology becomes more interesting. Archaeologists are no longer forced into a position where they have no choice but to 'open up' valuable historical material to review its content. They can simply scan their research findings with CT technology and upload it onto the software. Virtual autopsy imaging software such as the Anatomage Table serve as extremely valuable tools for archaeological research as they enable field researchers to study the interior details of their findings while also helping to preserve the original form of the underpinnings of human history.

Advanced Clinical and Procedural Training

In addition to general gross anatomy application, users can utilise virtual anatomy for advanced clinical or procedural training. Specific medical cases, if uploaded in CT, MRI or ultrasound, can be studied in full detail along with general anatomy. As users can review the pathology of the subject, whether it be from a regional standpoint or a systemic one, they can better project progression of a patient's disease. Users can fuse digital models of medical equipment to real scans for simulations or upload scans with surgically placed devices, which greatly enhance their experience in medical education. They can also load their own cases from their radiology department for procedural or clinical teaching. Virtual anatomy with 1:1 life-size image is accommodating to the needs of surgeons, helping visualise medical device and surgical instrument usage on the now-virtual patient. The life-size 3D rendering is perfect for complete medical team case reviews as a collaborative tool. Within the realm of surgery, the patient data can be used as a 3D framework for procedural discussion between radiologists and surgeons.

Visual communication with patients is extremely effective with virtual anatomy. Illustrating a patient's own scan interactively and in 3D is a much more efficient and technologically impressive approach to delivering medical opinion than conventional presentation methods. Three-dimensional presentations may also contribute to enhanced patient understanding of their own illness.

Software such as the one installed on the Anatomage Table that can incorporate user-uploaded CT and MR scans proves invaluable for demonstrating the immense variety of anatomy. Users can even view and interact with animal scans. The technology serves as an ideal instrument for veterinary professions to not only look into the animal's body but also to compare and contrast systematic parts of different species and families for research and teaching. If cryosections of animal data are available, similar reconstruction can be applied and interactive animal volumes can be generated. For forensic anthropology, experts are often called on to investigate remains and exclude human from animal bones, or better, determine key attributes that could identify sex, stature, age, ethnicity and so on. With virtual anatomy technologies such as the Anatomage Table, this knowledge and skill can be introduced to students in a classroom before they are ever called into the field.

Wilco, from the David Geffen School of Medicine at the University of California, Los Angeles (UCLA), showed that virtual 3D models with text and voice-over to delineate anatomy and physiology in detail helped medical students comprehend anatomical rationale much more effectively. As with a cadaver, it is not sufficient to present anatomical structures or variations without context from an expert. For both academia and forensic applications, virtual anatomy content creation software serves to emphasise and highlight key landmarks or features. This can provide more effective understanding from both students and peers alike. When utilising content creation software, users can upload their own medical, dental, archaeological or veterinary scans and manipulate the content to isolate volume, build models, annotate features and create videos. The software allows users to: create high quality medical image visualisations; generate 3D digital models from the MR or CT data directly; or merge existing 3D models to the medical image data.

By creating or merging digital 3D models into the medical images, users can highlight anatomical features or quickly demonstrate medical device functions. The software can be used to create instrumentation simulation. Users can design patient-specific custom fit devices according to the medical images provided. They can fuse 3D device model data into medical images, design verification with medical scans featuring real patient anatomy and adjust and simulate device function within real 3D human anatomy.

Furthermore, these same 3D models may be extracted and used for 3D printing of life-size patient anatomy via stereolithography techniques. Physical samples to demonstrate size, shape, similarities and differences can be prepared for effective presentations.

Virtual anatomy imaging software provides flexibility missing in conventional anatomy studies. For comparative studies, some virtual anatomy products such as the Anatomage Table provide libraries of medically relevant and educationally stimulating 3D images built in. Students can compare the normal and abnormal scans side-by-side. In this way, they can learn to distinguish functional versus dysfunctional and healthy versus unhealthy clinical images.

With the Anatomage software, physicians can compare similar systems for the same or different individuals. Two 3D scans can be superimposed atop one another for immediate 2D and 3D comparisons. The volumetric differences in lung inhalation versus exhalation or the variations in blood vessels in aneurysm cases can be shown to a broader audience. Pre- and post-operative scans can be quickly evaluated together. In addition, depending upon scan availability, these same tools can also be used to track bone remodelling after a fracture or the tumour sizes following treatment sessions.

Outside of the clinical environment, researchers can study comparative anatomy between human and animal skulls or bone structure. Researchers can also easily compare and contrast archaeological data – such as mummified bodies – with modern humans, contributing to research and the understanding of the evolution of the human body. Virtual anatomy content creation software and display platforms, such as those developed by Anatomage and other companies, seek to raise the standard of anatomy education by supplying new and innovative tools for clinicians, instructors and researchers. Relying on real anatomical data from CT or MR scans, these platforms provide the flexibility missing from traditional cadaveric study and make anatomy presentable to a larger audience without sacrificing accuracy or diversity.

Conclusions

In 'Teaching and Learning in a Digital World' (2013), the editor commented upon three themes that permeate the education literature. The first is the need for twenty-first century skills to equip learners with the necessary tools to succeed in the new millennium. As currently articulated, this means knowing how to access content knowledge efficiently and effectively and to acquire inquiry/problem solving skills that are meaningful, adaptable and integrative. The second theme is the importance of developing creative, collaborative, communicative and innovative learners who are culturally sensitive, globally aware and who behave in ethically responsible ways. The final theme is the need for developing digital literacy to keep pace with the exponentially burgeoning digital world that offers vast promise, but at the same time demands a critical stance to ensure that the power of these tools is used responsibly in what Gardner (2012) terms 'good work'.

With this clear three-themed caveat in mind. the use of technology in education is clearly here to stay. How it is used to best effect is the challenge, particularly so when using it to communicate difficult concepts both intellectually and emotionally, so that learners succeed in the themes mentioned here, whilst not losing site of the human aspect that it offers in this artificial medium of Information Technology. This aspect perhaps cannot be developed in the world of Boolean 'ones' and 'zeros' and will require human empathy from the instructors in how best to inculcate the technology. One of the Editors of this text uses a 'mental check-list' to define the correct way to *develop* any such teaching and learning sessions (and indeed assessment) and sessions involving forensic pathology images can be developed with these in mind, see Table 10.1.

Part of the problem in using the new technologies responsibly for TLA is what Fullan refers to as the push–pull dynamic. The push factor is that school is increasingly boring

Table 10.1 Considerations when teaching or demonstrating aspects of Forensic Pathology (in no order of priority).

1. Consider the Learning Outcomes – is the material absolutely necessary?
2. How to present the material – in words or pictures or photographs, video, computer IT and so on.
3. Ensure the class environment is sealed in terms of passers-by, members of the public or colleagues so they cannot see what is on the screen. If necessary, put up a notice on the door preventing entry unless it is an emergency – and they should knock to give you time to *blank* the screen.
4. Build up trust and a rapport with the class, group and so on, so they know they can be honest about what they like, do not like, understand or need reinforcing with further explanation – a quiet group is a group that is not learning.
5. Always use clinical images where possible and show death in the context of a crime scene only when necessary.
6. Show organs and tissues rather than whole body images wherever possible.
7. Consider the audience – if over 18 – clearly define the nature of the lecture, its content and how it will be presented – linked to the Learning Outcomes.
8. Consider how to incorporate real world examples into class.
9. Always show a clear, strong **warning sign** before any images of a disturbing nature and allow students to look away or to leave the room if they feel 'uncomfortable' with the materials – back up the notice-slide with a clear verbal discussion of what to expect.

(*continued*)

Table 10.1 (*Continued*)

10. Be empathetic and sympathetic to peoples' beliefs, cultures, values and expectations – this is as much for the students in the class as it is for the people shown in the material.
11. At the beginning of any session let students know that if they have been affected by any of the four points a–d in the last year, this may be upsetting and they should consider and reflect if they wish to stay and how they wish to engage.
    a. Have you experienced a recent bereavement – within the past 12 months?
    b. Have you previously seen a post-mortem?
    c. Have you witnessed a death – as a relative, carer or bystander?
    d. Is anyone in your family or immediate circle of friends suffering from a life-threatening illness?
12. Remind the class that they must not be judgmental of others – if someone leaves the class, that is the end of it, and there is a clear expectation that no one will mention this outside the class unless it is to offer support to their peer who left.
13. Remind students that they may leave and re-enter the class at any time in case they wish to re-engage with the session.
14. Check to see if anyone in the room is not part of the class – for example, a support note taker and so on – if this is an issue for them then offer to supply appropriate written information so they do not have to stay in that lecture.
15. Know *who and where* your First Aiders are in case anyone feels unhappy or unwell as a result of viewing the images.
16. Watch your class continuously – tell-tale signs of discomfort, unease or possible need to leave the room are fairly obvious – looking down or looking away, whispering continuously to a colleague immediately next to them, perspiration and eye rolling are also signs that have been seen in the past.
17. Be prepared to halt a class to help anyone who may request it – devise a strategy to allow this to happen.
18. Start with images that show a less severe injury to allow students to build up their expectations of what is in the session and how they feel and wish to engage with it.
19. Appropriate gentle humour/banter with students is entirely appropriate to help dissipate stress build-up in the class – this strategy has been well reported in live field situations and has been shown to work over the last decade in mortuary visits.
20. Ensure that images used in examinations or sent to be printed are not viewed by colleagues or administrative colleagues who do not need to see them – this includes External Examiners.
21. Always remind students not to talk about the content of such lectures in an open forum (café, bus, etc.). People do not wish to hear this discussion and may themselves be recently bereaved.
22. BlackBoard PowerPoint will only contain textual information – all of the graphical images and so on are not on BlackBoard.
23. Ask for honest feedback about the nature of what you have taught at the end of each session – allow students to email you or to meet with you privately if they wish to.
24. Accept good advice from wherever it comes about how to teach this subject – it may be that you are too close to the subject and too detached from the graphic nature of the material to appreciate all of the previous points and aspects you may not have considered – be a reflective practitioner.
25. Students attending post-mortems may do so with friendship groups.
26. Students view the facility first so as to familiarise themselves with the environment, noises, smells and so on.
27. A chair (plastic garden chair) was purchased especially so it can be in the post-mortem room when students are there, so they may sit if they feel the need to do so.
28. Students are given an appropriate briefing and can leave the post-mortem room with the attending member of academic staff at any point – the pathologist and two anatomical technical staff are in the room with the remaining students at all times.
29. The pathologist and the technical staff are highly experienced First Aiders.
30. Forensic science students were also given an opportunity for a debriefing session with their peers in a confidential environment.

for students and alienating for teachers. The pull factor is that the exploding and alluring digital world is irresistible, but not necessarily productive in its raw form. This occurs long before students arrive at university and so it will need to be addressed by universities and schools in a unique partnership of development, or by the time they reach tertiary education the problem is deeply entrenched in the educational psyche.

As Fullen identifies (http://www.learninglandscapes.ca/images/documents/ll-no12-vfinal-lr-links.pdf), the digital world of learning and entertainment is exploding, most of it outside (education). The scale of what is becoming available is enormous and it is easy to access. The pull here is incredibly irresistible, but not necessarily productive in the sense that it is largely ungoverned. Given the push–pull tension, we need to avoid either of two extreme reactions. One counterproductive move is to try to rein in students – not a chance against the allure of technology. Another is to marginalise some teachers on the grounds that technology can replace them. This too would be a mistake, as Fullan defines that mere immersion in the land of information does not make one smarter.

Fonseca *et al.* (2015) reported on virtual microscopy as a useful educational methodology, with an excellent compliance of dental students for the transition from conventional to digital microscopy in the teaching of oral pathology. An improvement in the class engagement was reported with questions relating to pathological changes instead of technical problems coming from the class. The simplicity of the software used and the high quality of the virtual slides, requiring a smaller time to identify microscopic structures, were considered important for a better teaching process. Ordi *et al.* (2015) reported similar findings with the use of virtual microscopy in the undergraduate teaching of pathology. Hortsch (2013) discussed the wider aspect of student engagement; this study revealed two important tendencies exhibited by medical students learning histology. In general, most students were reported to prefer to study histology in their own time, and thus scheduled resources, such as lectures and lab sessions, suffered a decreasing attendance as the academic year progressed. A second finding showed a strong and growing preference to use a variety of electronic resources, not only virtual microscopy, but also lecture videos and supplemental histological PowerPoint series. Many traditional learning resources, especially textbooks, were used by only a few students.

The use of technologies such as the Anatomage table is clearly to be applauded but more pedagogical testing will be needed over the coming years to identify the strengths and areas of development for their use in a classroom setting. The technology is indisputably amazing, but it is how it is used and integrated into curriculum that would appear to be the limiting factor at this time. There are some early reports (Fyfe 2013, www.ascilite.org/conferences/sydney13/program/papers/Fyfe.pdf) where students found the Anatomage tables good for ideas of scale and the relationships of organ structures and they liked being able to rotate the images, but were less impressed with the graphics quality and the limitations for group interactions.

References

Cesari, W.A., Caruso, D.M., Zyka, E.L., Schroff, S.T., Evans, C.H., Jr. and Hyatt, J.-P.K. (2006) Study of physiological responses to acute carbon monoxide exposure with a human patient simulator. *Advances in Physiology Education*, **30** (4), 242–247.

Clark, M.A. (2009) Genome island: A virtual science environment in Second Life. *Innovate: Journal of Online Education*, **5** (6), 6.

Codd, A.M. and Choudhury, B. (2011) Virtual reality anatomy: Is it comparable with traditional methods in the teaching of human forearm musculoskeletal anatomy? *Anatomical Sciences Education*, **4** (3),119–125.

Diaz-Perez, J.A., Raju, S. and Echeverri, J.H. (2014) Evaluation of a teaching strategy based on integration of clinical subjects, virtual autopsy, pathology museum, and digital microscopy for medical students *Journal of Pathology Informatics*, **5**, 25.

Fonseca, F.-P., Santos-Silva, A.-R., Lopes, M.-A., Oslei-Paes de Almeida, O.-P. and Vargas, P.-A. (2015) Transition from glass to digital slide microscopy in the teaching of oral pathology in a Brazilian dental school. *Medicina Oral Patologia Oral y Cirugia Bucal*, **20** (1), e17–e22.

Franklin, S., Peat, M. and Lewis, A. (2002) Traditional versus computer-based dissections in enhancing learning in a tertiary setting: A student perspective. *Journal of Biological Education*, **36** (3),124–129.

Gardner, H. (2012) Commentary. Getting at the heart of the creative experience. Creativity: Insights, directions, and possibilities. *Learning Landscapes*, **6** (1), 45–54.

Hortsch, M. (2013) *The FASEB Journal*, **27** (2), 411–413; doi: 10.1096/fj.13-0201ufm.

Lewis, D.I. (2014) The pedagogical benefits and pitfalls of virtual tools for teaching and learning laboratory practices in the Biological Sciences. Higher Education Academy. Available at: https://www.heacademy.ac.uk/sites/default/files/resources/The%20 pedagogical%20benefits%20and%20pitfalls%20of%20virtual%20tools%20for%20teaching %20and%20learning%20laboratory%20practices%20in%20the%20Biological%20Sciences. pdf (accessed 14 April 2015).

Ordi, O., Bombí, J.A, Martínez, A., Ramírez, J., Alòs, L., Saco, A., Ribalta, T, Fernández, P.L., Campo, E. and Ordi, J. (2015) Virtual microscopy in the undergraduate teaching of pathology. *Journal of Pathology Informatics*, **6**, 1.

Thali, M.J, Yen, K., Schweitzer, W., Vock, P., Boesch, C., Ozdoba, C., Schroth, G., Ith, M., Sonnenschein, M., Doernhoefer, T., Scheurer, E., Plattner, T. and Dirnhofer, R. (2003) Virtopsy, a new imaging horizon in forensic pathology: Virtual autopsy by postmortem multislice computed tomography (MSCT) and magnetic resonance imaging (MRI) – a feasibility study. *Journal of Forensic Science*, **48** (2), 386–403.

Teaching and Learning in the Digital World: Possibilities and challenges (2013) *Learning Landscapes*, **6** (2, spring). http://www.learninglandscapes.ca/images/documents/ll-no12-vfinal-lr-links.pdf (accessed February 2016).

11

Online Teaching Aids

Anna-Maria Muller,[1] Luke Taylor,[2] and Anna Williams[3]

[1] Swindon, Wiltshire, UK
[2] University of Kent, Canterbury, UK
[3] University of Huddersfield, School of Applied Sciences, Queensgate, Huddersfield, UK

Introduction

Today's students are members of Generation Y. This is the generation born in the 1980s and 1990s, comprising primarily the children of the baby boomers and typically perceived as increasingly familiar with digital and electronic technology. This generation have grown up holding distinctly different attitudes and characteristics than the generations before them (Tapscott, 2008). Generation Y grew up with the mainstreaming of information technology; they never knew a world without the Internet and regard technology as an essential part of their lives. It is important to characterise this new generation of 'techno-savvy' and open-minded young people in positive terms (Tulgan and Martin, 2001). As these youth grow out of education into the workforce, their mode of engaging with the world and subsequently their world view are challenging the established institutions, businesses and society as a whole.

The high aspirations of Generation Y, and its expectations of immediacy, present organisational challenges to those working with students in an environment that is not yet equipped to present the satisfying answers that they inevitably demand (Prensky, 2001). Generation Y-ers want to have an impact, to make a difference, to improve their world – all of which can be powerful motivators. They thrive on tangible goals, a high degree of flexibility and access in their learning environment.

There are challenges that have to be overcome by educators, who are working in an environment that leaves much to be desired for this particular cohort. The vital lack of financial means and other resources aside, the current systems of Higher Education (in the United Kingdom and elsewhere) are not geared towards motivating this generation to live up to its potential: incentives for Higher Education Institutions (HEIs) to educate an increasing number of students with fewer resources, the alarming consolidated trend of the late twentieth century to evaluate learner achievement and educational success by means of standardised testing, the push towards accreditation within the forensic sector without a consensus on what constitutes a successful and worthy forensic science education or graduate.

Forensic Science Education and Training: A Tool-kit for Lecturers and Practitioner Trainers, First Edition.
Edited by Anna Williams, John P. Cassella, and Peter D. Maskell.

The student body is growing ever more diverse, with HEIs also attempting to recruit more students in programmes of lifelong and distance learning. At the same time educators are left without systematic support mechanisms to help them ensure quality, relevance and success of their efforts to educate the forensic workforce of the early twenty-first century.

For educators, there is the choice to disregard or embrace the attitudes and the ways of engaging that are intuitive to this new generation of students under ever-changing demands and pressures of Higher Education. Meeting the new generation of students 'on their own terms', by being aware of their learning styles, the technologies and forms of interaction students are seeking, will increase effectiveness of study programmes, student retention and goal achievement for students and educators (Slate *et al.*, 2002).

In addition, academics in HE, especially in undergraduate programmes, are conscious of providing students with a broad knowledge base and the necessary cognitive and transferrable skills to cope with uncertain future challenges. This has been customary in higher education systems following the Anglo-Saxon model, which 'provides a broad educational "liberal" base with less emphasis on subject-specific, skills-related content; it is a system with a "loose fit" between higher education and a graduate's subsequent area of work' (Little, 2001). Thus, for UK graduates, 'professional formation is likely to take place after completion of the relatively short first degree, either through further study or through employment (or a mixture of both)' (Lore and Little, 2010).

Students should be empowered to widen their professional expertise, no matter the specific content, later in life and throughout their careers. The strategy to prepare for self-directed learning by developing capabilities that are applicable in any professional context is to be lauded. Too narrowly-defined training courses based, for instance, on the needs of particular service providers, could leave students ill-equipped for other career paths, and may be not as valuable come graduation day, as seen with the closure of the largest forensic service provider in the United Kingdom (Roux *et al.*, 2012). Such 'game-changing' events are outliers and rarely predictable, but when they occur, large numbers of students and graduates are profoundly affected (Taleb, 2010).

This technological revolution coincides with the exponential growth and access to smartphones and mobile devices that allow access to information in real time, at student's fingertips (Taleb and Sohrabi, 2012; Fordham and Goddard, 2013). Allied to this, cheap and free online platforms are being used by teachers and students to create and share knowledge and learning inside and outside of the classroom and at home via virtual learning environments. Plus the new phenomenon of MOOCs (Massive Open Online Courses), such as the EdX, Khan Academy, Udacity and Futurelearn and Mozilla's Open Badges, have started to change the way higher education and indeed learning is accessed, used and accredited. It is in this rapidly changing landscape that Facebook's work (see later section) on the use of its platform as a tool for teaching and learning can be placed.

Employability and Transferrable Skills

The reality is that only a precious few forensic science graduates will find employment in the forensic workforce (Welsh and Hannis, 2011; Hanson and Overton, 2010). However, technological progress, regulatory and public policy developments as well as the general fluidity of demands in the professional sphere have been recognised to be significant long-term trends. The requirement to cope with change is inevitable, for all of them. Whether their career paths lead them into academia, accountancy, legal or the neighbouring scientific professions, these graduates will have to cope with rapid and fundamental social changes in their working lives that are unprecedented and have not been experienced by their parents or grandparents.

The UK labour market in generally is very flexible and employers don't pay premium attention to the disciplines from which their entry level employees come. There is greater flexibility in the UK labour market: only 41% of the senior executives surveyed by CBI and Universities UK cited the degree subject as an important factor to be considered when recruiting graduates. Employability skills (78%) such as, positive attitude (72%) and relevant work experience (54%) ranked higher on the list of consideration for these 581 UK employers (CBI, 2009).

HEIs have an obligation to support students to develop academic, subject-orientated as well as non-cognitive employability skills to cope with these professional demands beyond ticking the boxes on standardised subject-specific quality assessments (Welsh and Hannis, 2011). This is particularly important for forensic science graduates (Hanson and Overton, 2010), as the majority of them will go into a non-forensic science related work environment. According to a CBI-UUK survey (2009) of 880 students, 44% are taking ownership of their development of employability skills, while a third of students (32%) feel that the university should take the responsibility to develop these skills.

With their survey of 147 forensic science graduates, Hanson and Overton (2010) also found a gap in the development of useful employability skills within undergraduate degree programmes in forensic science. Graduates felt skills such as computing, statistics, report writing, oral presentation, time management and organisational skills and managing their own learning were underdeveloped during their programmes of study.

Therefore, moving towards engaging, interactive and tailored curricula cannot be seen as 'pandering to the demands of a generation with entitlement problems and consumer attitudes,' but an acknowledgement of the realities graduates will have to face in the professional world once they leave their *Alma mater*.

Online technologies available to educators today can help you to work with your students, to develop the skills that both employers and students value. These new technologies, strategically employed, can also help you to overcome challenges within the current HEI environment. Last but not least, online media and web-based software will help you to instil values and grounding in the next generation of forensic scientists, that will help to rethink the forensic science community, 'lower the drawbridges' within and create the collegial attitudes that are needed to thrive in the professional world of the twenty-first century.

Science, and in particular forensic educators, have already started to pursue alternative methods to achieve learning goals with their students. Neither trend nor programme, these singular case studies and experiments are found occasionally, as they are attempted by a minority of adventurous and innovative advocates.

The authors argue that online technologies offer a new approach to academia for most forensic educators. It is difficult to imagine a programme of study or class of students who may not benefit from media rich resources, room for debate and exchange as well as learning grounds for professional collaboration.

Online Learning Management Systems

There are a plethora of online and institutional learning tools for universities with such examples as Blackboard and Moodle, and online Learning Management Systems (LMS) designed to bridge the gap between teacher and learner. Virtual Learning Systems have been around for some time now in the varsity space, allowing the boundaries for modern teaching and sharing materials to students to be pushed. Blackboard is constantly adapting to modernisation, and deepening its prowess in the social aspect of the learning environment. There is the facility for lecturers to create courses and upload files, notes and further 'self-learning materials' as well as interacting with students to guide them in the right direction.

The students gain enormously from this. They are able to download course material, further work and guidance on research material and publications instantly, and there are now powerful tools available at the touch of a button to allow self-learning. Students are able to post questions and receive answers from their peers, and interact seamlessly with them about all aspects of work, creating an online student environment. This in turn reduces the amount of time spent by the lecturer, who may previously have had to repeat explanations to individual students. This then enhances the ability for independent thinking and personal structure. With the latest updates, it is now possible for staff or students to link Dropbox accounts to Blackboard to save course content and upload content to specific courses created.

LMS is mentioned briefly here due to the availability of mobile applications for both of these services. There are also apps to convert online LMS into a native app for tablets and pads, facilitating use and creating a portable learning service to students and lecturers without the need for printing materials. A social learning environment is also much easier to create when all students are able to easily interact and exchange ideas and questions on assignments, examinations and research projects with peer-to-peer support.

The days of students walking to lectures with reams of handouts are becoming a thing of the past with the advent of handheld electronic devices such as mobile phones and tablets.

iTunes U

iTunes U is a variant of the Blackboard and Moodle systems designed by Apple Inc. It is a freely available platform through which lecturers and students can interact and share information; and due to its ease of availability, it will be detailed here. There are 20 GB of storage available at no cost, for uploading all types of materials required by the lecturer (videos, images, documents, presentations, etc.) to a central private inbox. This material can then be cherry-picked to place into any number of modules or packages for students.

Timings are also at the control of the course planner. Modules can be activated or sent out at selected times and can be student-specific to restrict access to certain information only to the people who need it.

When iTunes U is opened, the student is greeted with an overview of the course with tabs along the left set by the course instructor (overview, instructor, outline and syllabus, optional apps/books, etc.). Along the bottom of the screen is a set of tabs that allows the student to navigate through: posts added by the Course Leader, notes that have been taken by the student and the materials uploaded by the Course Leader. These create a separated view of the information provided through iTunes U and create a clearer method to process this information.

Within the posts tab, it is possible to add modules or topics in relation to the overall course and release these to the students. Again a list of modules/courses are available along the left tab. Posts appear as a topic header, with a brief explanation of what is within the topic, and a list of links to specific sections of the topic. These can be videos, documents and presentations, links to websites, journals and other reference materials, and are listed in the order in which it is intended for the student to approach the course. Once the student makes a selection, they are able to view within the app (useful for video) or download the file locally.

Note-taking Apps – The Age of Evernote and OneNote

Platforms that remove the need for paper are much appreciated by the student as well as staff. Not only does this reduce overall costs for both the students and the institution, it increases the university's ability to be a 'green source' of learning. The ability to take notes on the fly and edit later with instant synchronisation between devices can be much more useful than the traditional notepad. These apps can reduce the amount of time spent on writing notes, and allow instant searching and sharing of lecture information and resources, giving the student much more time to absorb information from the lecture, rather than having to constantly switch between listening and writing. This listening and writing method can cause a 'Doppler Effect' in which partial amounts of information are recorded, whilst other information is missed.

Two examples of popular note-taking apps are Evernote and OneNote (Microsoft). Both offer a range of features. Evernote offers quick, easy access to notes and capturing thoughts, and the ability to add photographs and diagrams instantly, as well as a verbal dictation function. OneNote is much more complex and can take more time to master, but offers a more comprehensive range of note taking, with the traditional structure of a notepad with tabs and sections for each subject/topic.

Scientific Demonstration Apps

With the continuous development of computer and mobile applications, progression in the educational market is stronger than ever. Mobile devices are currently at the forefront of many sectors, and forensic science is no exception. These technologies (especially within software) are being developed and optimised to aid in education of forensics (King and Gwinnet, 2011) and practitioner use (Tanner and Duncan, 2013). For the purpose of this book, the focus will be on education, and specifically on how mobile technology and applications can vastly improve the ways in which educators provide material, and how students can facilitate and supplement their learning.

A multitude of applications are university oriented, including areas such as medical and biological, chemical and analytical sciences, as well as scientific instructional applications. These vary in price and scope of use, and range from free but relatively limited apps to expensive apps with one off payments and/or subscriptions. Useful applications are not just limited to specifically targeted software for university education. Several 'lite' versions of practitioner-orientated software exist for mobile devices, which are of great use for students, enabling them to reach an understanding of forensic practice as well as providing a strong basis for research.

Such software includes that of 'ForChem' by Griffith University in Australia. ForChem (available on Mac OS X, Microsoft Windows, IOS and Android) allows the student to follow the scientific process of scene investigation from arrival to recovery of evidence and continuity processes in a step by step manner. The student is able to attend a mock crime scene, scan evidence via QR codes and load them into the application. They input the method for collecting specific types of evidence and if incorrectly collected, the application will prompt the student to try again and collect the evidence another time. The application excels with its ability to carry through the entire process, with each student's report being collated and made available to all. The students are then able to write a report based on the information fed back from the evidence collected. This provides constructive feedback to allow the student to learn from their mistakes and to think around why some of their choices may have been incorrect.

Taking skeletal anatomy apps as an example: there are many basic products offering low resolution imagery of bones with limited function. Examples of this are '*The Human Skeletal System HD*' by Erik Haugen Media, and '*Essential Skeleton 2*' by 3D4Medical. Both applications offer a stripped down experience of a 3D model of the skeletal system, showing the bones in anatomical position, but not much more in terms of learning aids. This is where '*Skeletal System Pro III*' by 3D4Medical excels (see Figure 11.1). It is a much more feature-rich app, as it allows the user to fully manipulate the digital human skeleton. It allows the isolation of individual bones with full 3D rotation, sagittal and coronal cross sections of the cranium and colour coding of the complex cranial/pelvic structures. The operator is able to present this application interactively to the class through projection with live annotation and manipulation, whilst students who own the application are able to follow along or direct themselves to suit their individual learning needs.

There are a plethora of more generalised apps for higher education purposes available on multiple platforms.

Within the Forensic Curriculum

Online technologies may enhance your forensic science curriculum, by providing more layers of learning and more opportunities to be inclusive and encourage student participation. The potential for Web 2.0 tools to facilitate and enhance student learning has been described in numerous articles over the past few years (Alexander, 2006; Brainard, 2007; McDonald, 2009; Minocha, 2009; Nachmias, 2002; Oradini and Saunders, 2008; Reuben, 2008; Thompson, 2008; Wesch, 2009).

Specific benefits include:

- Learning-related benefits: facilitation of collaborative learning, development of independent learning skills, problem solving, team work, reflective learning, quick/early feedback from instructors, overcoming isolation of geographical distances, peer-to-peer support/feedback, visibility of students' work, integration of multimedia assets and the creation of informal relations between educators and students.

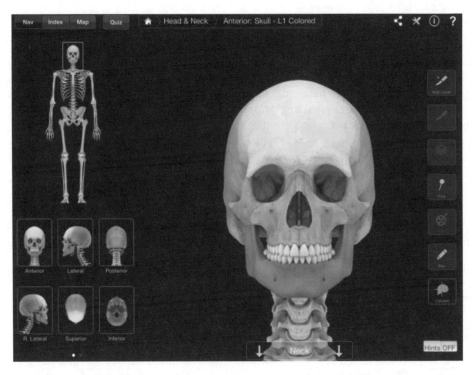

Figure 11.1 Skeletal System Pro III demonstrating colour coded cranium (see colour figure in colour plate section).

- Social benefits for students: increased engagement in course material, development of a sense of community and of transferable skills that enhance student employability, increased sense of achievement, control and ownership of their work.
- Benefits for HEIs: increased cross-institutional collaborations, support and community building outside the course environment, development of communities of practice, increased student enrolment and retention (Foroughi, 2011).

Practical Guidance for Using Online Tools

Being mindful about the advantages and drawbacks of these different tools, how can we introduce them into forensic science curricula to enhance the student experience?

Online, electronic and video games

Pringle was able to enhance attainment and learning experience for his undergraduate students. In addition, his 'CSI North Wales' e-game provided an environment to experience some the realistic constraints of a work environment (see Chapter 9).

Now, creating a realistic, detailed and iteratively evaluated and improved online game is a very involved approach that is not within the reach of every forensic educator. However, a resource that lists existing e-games and applications may be achievable using crowdsourcing amongst our target audience.

Virtual Learning Environments (VLEs)

'Learning platform' is a generic term to describe a broad range of ICT systems that are used to deliver and support learning. A learning platform usually combines several functions, such as organising, mapping and delivering curriculum activities and the facility for learners and teachers to have a dialogue about the activity, all via ICT. So, the term learning platform can be applied to a virtual learning environment (VLE) or to the components of a managed learning environment (MLE). A VLE is a software tool that brings together resources for curriculum mapping, delivery, assessment, tutor support, communication and tracking. A managed learning environment (MLE) refers to the whole range of information systems and processes that support learning and the management of learning within an institution. It includes VLEs or other learning platforms, administrative and other support systems (BECTA, 2006).

Blogs

Blog Web log (blog): an online journal/commentary with simple automated content-creating facilities, links and response mechanisms. Blogs often use RSS (see later) so that readers can subscribe and receive new content as it is published (BECTA, 2006).

Podcast

Podcasts are audio files that can be easily distributed via the web and downloaded to computers and personal audio players. Podcasts are often syndicated so that users can subscribe (usually for free) to a particular service and have new content automatically downloaded. The software required to produce and distribute podcasts is available for free or at little cost, making this form of 'broadcasting' extremely accessible (BECTA, 2006).

RSS

Really simple syndication (RSS): a set of XML-based specifications for syndicating news and other website content and making it machine readable. Users who subscribe to RSS-enabled websites can have new content automatically 'pushed' to them. This content is usually collected by RSS-aware applications called aggregators or news readers. Some web browsers now have these news readers built in (BECTA, 2006).

Wikis

Wikis are collaborative web pages that can be viewed and modified by anyone with a web browser and internet access (BECTA, 2006).

Creative Commons

This is a licensing system developed by Lawrence Lessig and others at Stanford University, CA, USA. Creative Commons (CC) licences allow a content creator to decide how published work may be copied, modified and distributed. UK versions of the licence are now available (BECTA, 2006).

Folksonomy

Derived from folk + taxonomy, a Folksonomy is a way of categorising data on the web using tags generated by users. Folksonomies are used on collaborative, 'social' websites for photo sharing, blogs and social bookmarking. Social bookmarking websites are services that allow users to store their favourite websites online and access them from any internet-connected computer. Users tag their favourite websites with keywords. These are then shared with other users and build into folksonomies of the most popular sites arranged under different categories (BECTA, 2006).

Social Networks and Forums

Twitter

The character restriction of tweets can be used for educational purposes – to encourage the learner to distil and summarise concepts in 140 characters. It allows classes or researchers to communicate the crux of their research in a short, pithy way – useful for those trying to engage the public with their research.

Hashtags can be used effectively too, to signpost thousands of students at once to information. For example, Anna Divinsky of Penn State University, PA, USA, used twitter to allow the 58 000 learners enrolled in her MOOC to share, evaluate and comment on each other's work using the hashtag #artmooc (Fee, 2013). Hashtags can be used to encourage and facilitate discussions around guest speaker contributions to courses, by providing a focal point that allows questions to be put to the speaker in an open forum. Live tweeting during public lectures raises awareness inside and outside the class, and doesn't interrupt the speaker, but allows all the questions to be seen. It can also encourage contributions from those external to the course (Fee, 2013).

Facebook

In the broadest sense Facebook (or for that matter any equivalent networking system) can enable communication, collaboration and network building around areas of common interest in the discipline or specialism being studied. In a more structured way it can be used at course level to build activities to augment face-to-face interaction (Fordham and Goddard, 2013). The use of Facebook for formal learning benefits from students' familiarity with the interface. Most already use it, are comfortable with it and so it is easy to integrate into their routine. The creation of a closed Facebook group is a useful tool for learners on a single module or course, as it facilitates interaction between all members of the group, but no-one else. It effectively extends the classroom and allows contact between group members outside class time.

Facebook can be used successfully for induction, assessment, feedback, time management and resource management. Examples of how Facebook can be used in the classroom include the following (Online College, 2009):

- News gathering – students can use Facebook to search for news and media stories relevant to the topics covered in class.
- Documenting change over time using photographs and commentary – particularly useful for practical sessions on ageing of bloodstains, diagenesis of bone, changes in fingerprint development or all sorts of other forensic investigations.

- Resource curation – students can collect and point each other to valuable resources relevant to the class.
- Exam practice – practice exam questions can be posted, so all students can see them and see each other's answers. There is potential for formative assessment here, and even extra credit for the fastest correct answers posted.
- Students can be asked to post summaries of each lecture after the session to allow formative assessment or reflection on the topics covered.
- Mock forensic scenarios can be created using fictitious profiles for victims, suspects, friends of both, police and so on, to demonstrate different types of evidence.
- Lessons in biometrics, identity theft, online fraud and internet crime can be demonstrated using Facebook as a platform.

More examples can be found on the Online College (2009) website.

Academia.edu or Similar

Websites such as Academia.edu (https://www.academia.edu/) or Researchgate (https://www.researchgate.net/) allow researchers to upload their own authored or co-authored peer-reviewed journal articles or other articles. This allows students to directly access articles to which they may not have institutional access, and even to engage in direct correspondence with the authors of the research relevant to their classes. These websites encourage networking, cross-pollination of ideas and collaborative research.

LinkedIn

LinkedIn works in a similar way to Academia.edu or Researchgate, in allowing students direct access to the experts in their field, access to original sources and opening up networking opportunities. It is also possible to link to professional organisations and practitioner groups, where information about conferences, workshops and courses can be exchanged

Deciding Which Technology to Use

Different tools exist for use in different scenarios and to serve diverse audiences. There are various questions you can ask yourself and criteria to assess in order to find a good approach for your students and teaching environment.

In any case, there is a need to guide students in their use of the technology and set expectations early on about what happens with these resources after projects are assessed and declared 'finished.'

Some criteria to consider when choosing a technology or service for a particular scenario are:

- openness for participation open/semi/closed
- event-based versus topical resources
- infrastructure versus control
- ease of use, media sharing.

Openness for Participation

Another aspect to consider when choosing one of these web services is their ability to control the access to content and discussion groups. Facebook provides invitation based access, giving moderators granular control over who has access to groups and pages and who won't be able to access the resource. Blogs and wikis can be passworded or even user-role restricted, to enable different actions for different user-roles — from merely browsing the site as visitors to contributing as authors and editors. Moderators can be setup to approve user generated content, such as comments or posts.

Open online resources have the potential to invite contributions from the wider online and professional forensic community, whereas closed or invitation-restricted sites offer a safe place for learners to try different modes of public debate and contribution, finding their voice through 'learning-by-doing' and experiencing peer-review first hand.

Resources that are open to the wider online audience, however, have to maintain a certain degree of editorial integrity, observing the rules of fair use, copyright and privacy protection for students. The potential visibility of general access sites means they are less of a safe learning environment and more suitable for student groups who have reached a certain level of ICT literacy as well as familiarity with 'netiquette.' Learners working towards information literacy skills and an understanding of the basic tenets of professional communication online may be better served taking their first steps into online publishing and public debate in the gated confines of more closely monitored Virtual Learning Environments or other controlled-access websites. More guidance about best practices for using social media for education purposes can be found at NASUWT The Teacher's Union (www.nasuwt.org).

Transient Versus Permanent Solutions

Factors to consider when choosing a technological solution:

- Are you creating a temporary support structure or a permanent resource? That is, is your use case event-based, for instance, used during one lecture run per term, a certain period of time during a one-off training, practical or short course? Or, are you trying to build a resource that may be more permanent?
- The burden and responsibility of infrastructure versus the handling your content over to third parties.
- Having your own infrastructure can be a blessing and a curse. Of course, if your HEI already provides the online tools and spaces to explore web-based technologies, you can take advantage of these resources. Over the past decade VLEs, wikis, blogs and even institution-specific social networks have been adopted by a majority of HEIs. The access to these online technologies is often managed by IT departments and IT support staff.

However, there can be a number of reasons to look elsewhere to find a 'digital playground,' for instance:

1. when gaining access to the internal tools is too cumbersome or takes a lot of administrative work to get started and find out if it's for you and your learners;
2. internal services may not offer the features you are looking for in your specific use case;

3. you already have personal or professional experience with a system that is not supported internally, but easy for you to setup and maintain;

4. you may be intimidated by your IT department – there is no shame in admitting this — you are certainly not alone.

Don't underestimate support issues, ranging from technical support for individual students to training your students to use the system.

If you can, work with your IT department to get started: they will be able to spare you the responsibility of maintaining the technical infrastructure of the application you are looking for. In addition, if something is officially approved and sanctioned by the IT department, they will have training resources and documentation at hand, for you and your learners.

If you introduce a system of your personal choice, more likely than not, you will end up producing documentation, guides and deliver the student training for the system yourself. This can add up to a significant workload on your part, which will not benefit the intended learning outcomes you want to achieve — these will merely be the first steps to get you and your learners 'off the ground.'

To date, Delicious, Twitter, Facebook, Tumblr, and so on, provide a free service to their user base. However, these companies are operating under business-objectives, and in a fast-paced environment of 'change policy first, apologise later.'

Twitter currently saves your 3200 most current tweets and makes them available to you. Third party services or software such as ThinkUp, BackupMyTweets and Tweet Nest may assist in archiving your timeline for as long as Twitter allows them to connect to their programmable interfaces. A Facebook page may be a great way to organise and facilitate discussions around an event or a campaign, more structured services such as self-maintained wikis and blogs, or services in the custody of individual HEIs hold stronger long-term appeal as permanent resources.

Free blogs from service providers such as Tumblr, blogger.com, wordpress.com have proved more reliable in terms of archiving content and provide access to individual posts via permanently accessible links — until the account holders decide to delete their own content.

There are considerable advantages of choosing these, not education specific, social services: general ease of use and familiarity; participants will immediately benefit from the 'network effect' of being on a platform with millions of other users, and learners are somewhat likely to have experience using these services or even be registered already. This lowers the adoption barrier noticeably, as students will not experience the learning curve that comes from using a completely new environment. With more and more university services adopting online communication channels, it will also be a relief to all participants not to have to safeguard one more login and password, for example, when Facebook is used as a platform to host discussions and course relevant content.

If you want to evaluate the use of the new tools by your learners, third party services may not allow you insight into certain analytics about user behaviour, popularity of content or access to certain resources over time. These metrics are valuable and certainly instructive, if you want to acquire data on using these tools in order to build them into your regular curricular activities, course work and student assessment. Formalising and standardising a self-reflective online teaching practice will allow you to optimise the use of these tools for you and your students. It will also enable you to share case studies with colleagues and the wider community of forensic educators. Working towards the development of best practices within the forensic community is one pillar upon which the adoption and strategic use of new technologies rests.

Conclusions

Online tools enable self-directed learning and allow you to provide resources that address students with diverse backgrounds, knowledge or skill gaps, previous experience and more advanced learners.

The explosion in the technology available and the software and processes that drive them are far ahead of the knowledge and skills in academia on how to use them. Despite international conferences on e-learning and the tools (e.g. those discussed here) to disseminate the good practice, there is a lag behind.

Multi-media content can direct students to vetted learning materials catering to different preferred learning modes, and facilitates learning for those with non-traditional or particularly visual learning styles. It allows for asynchronous learning – students can pick up their notes when it suits them, enabling learning amidst employment and family life. Online teaching aids allow for multiple engagements with the session or topic – students can return to the topic at their own convenience. It can also foster a habit of collaboration and developing team working skills, which are invaluable when it comes to elusive employment in forensic science.

References

Alexander, B. (2006) Web 2.0. *A New Wave of Innovation for Teaching and Learning*, 32–44.

BECTA (2006) *The BECTA Review 2006: Evidence on the progress of ICT in education*. British Educational Communications and Technology Agency (BECTA), London, UK. Available at: http://dera.ioe.ac.uk/1427/1/becta_2006_bectareview_report.pdf (accessed 25 July 2016).

Brainard, J. (2007) Boston College Case Study. *Socialtext*. Available at: http://www.socialtext.net/cases2/index.cgi?boston_college_case_study (accessed 23 April 2016).

Confederation of British Industry (CBI), with Universities UK (2009) Future fit: Preparing graduates for the world of work. Available at: http://www.voced.edu.au/content/ngv:13894 (accessed 29 July 2016).

Fee, J. (2013) 7 Ways Teachers Use Social Media. MashableUK. Available at: http://mashable.com/2013/08/18/social-media-teachers/#fG19ySR68ZqV (accessed 29 July 2016).

Fordham, I. and Goddard, T. (2013) *Facebook Guide for Educators*. The Education Foundation. Available at: http://www.ednfoundation.org/wp-content/uploads/Facebookguideforeducators.pdf (accessed 12 July 2016).

Foroughi, A. (2011) A research framework for evaluating the effectiveness of implementations of social media in higher education. *Online Journal for Workforce Education and Development*, **5** (1), 5.

Hanson, S. and Overton, T. (2010) *Skills Required by New Forensic Science Graduates and their Development in Degree Programmes.* Higher Education Academy UK Physical Sciences Centre.

King, I. and Gwinnett, C. (2011) The investigation into using e-learning technology as an improved delivery method of forensic science education for the CPD of lawyers. Presented at British & Irish Legal Education and Technology Association Annual Conference, Manchester Metropolitan University, 11–12 April 2011 (unpublished).

Little, B. (2001) Reading between the lines of graduate employment. *Quality in Higher Education*, **7** (2), 121–129.

Lore, A. and Little, B. (2010) The REFLEX study: exploring graduates' views on the relationship between higher education and employment. *Centre for Higher Education Research and Information*, The Open University, London.

McDonald, F. (2009) Five steps to developing a powerful social networking strategy. *University Business: Solutions for Higher Education Management*, May.

Minocha, S. (2009) A study on the effective use of social software by further and higher education in the UK to support student learning and engagement. Report and case studies. Available at: http://www.jisc.ac.uk/whatwedo/projects/socialsoftware08 (accessed 3 September 2015).

Nachmias, R. (2002) A research framework for the study of a campus-wide Web-based academic instruction project. *The Internet and Higher Education*, **5** (3), 213–229.

Online College Staff Writers (2009) 100 ways you should be using Facebook in your classroom – updated. OnlineCollege.org. Available at: http://www.onlinecollege.org/2012/05/21/100-ways-you-should-be-using-facebook-in-your-classroom-updated/ (accessed 21 July 2016).

Oradini, F. and Saunders, G. (2008) The use of social networking by students and staff in higher education. University of Westminster, London, UK. Paper presented at the iLearning Forum, Paris.

Prensky, M. (2001) Digital natives, digital immigrants Part 1. *On the Horizon*, **9** (5), 1–6. Available at: http://www.emeraldinsight.com/doi/abs/10.1108/10748120110424816 (accessed 10 May 2016).

Reuben, R. (2008) The use of social media in higher education for marketing and communications: a guide for professionals in higher education. *eduGuru*, August 19. Available at: http://doteduguru.com/id423-social-media-uses-higher-education-marketingcommunication.html (accessed 14 May 2016).

Roux, C. Crispino, F. and Ribaux, O. (2012) From forensics to forensic science. *Current Issues in Criminal Justice*, **7**.

Slate, J. Manuel, M. and Brinson Jr, K. (2002) The 'Digital Divide': Hispanic college students' views of educational uses of the Internet. *Assessment and Evaluation in Higher Education*, **27** (1), 75–93.

Taleb, H. (2010) Gender and leadership styles in single-sex academic institutions. *International Journal of Educational Management*, **24** (4), 287–302.

Taleb, Z. and Sohrabi, A. (2012) Learning on the move: The use of mobile technology to support learning for university students. *Procedia-Social and Behavioral Sciences*, **69**, 1102–1109.

Tanner, A. and Duncan, S. (2013) On integrating mobile applications into the digital forensic investigative process. *(IJACSA) International Journal of Advanced Computer Science and Applications*, **4** (8), 56–61.

Tapscott, D. (2008) *Grown Up Digital: How the Net Generation is Changing Your World.* McGraw-Hill, New York.

Thompson, J. (2008) Is education 1.0 ready for web.2 students? *Innovate*, **3** (4). Available at: http://www.socialtext.net/cases2/index.cgi?boston_college_case_study_(accessed 20 May 2016).

Tulgan, B. and Martin, C. (2001) *Managing Generation Y: Global Citizens Born in the Late Seventies and Early Eighties.* Human Resource Development, HRD Press, Amherst, MA.

Welsh, C. and Hannis, M. (2011) Are UK undergraduate forensic science degrees fit for purpose? *Science & Justice*, **51** (3), 139–142.

Wesch, M. (2009) From knowledgeable to knowledge-able: Learning in new media environments. *Academic Commons*, 7.

12

Simulation, Immersive Gameplay and Virtual Realities in Forensic Science Education

Karl Harrison[1] and Colleen Morgan[2]

[1] *Cranfield University, Cranfield Forensic Institute, College Road, Cranfield, Bedfordshire, UK*
[2] *University of York, Centre for Digital Heritage Research, King's Manor, York, UK*

Introduction

This chapter considers the nature and use of simulation within the context of forensic science education. It is curious to note that despite the massive growth in popularity of forensic science-based programmes of education, initially in the UK's higher education sector, but increasingly as a vehicle to teach a broad range of applied science in further and schools education as well (Paton, 2009), there has been little formalised discussion of how the resulting education products and processes might best be shaped, let alone what their intended outcomes might be. Forensic science, which encompasses a broad range of scientific principles, investigative processes and contexts of application, is particularly given to education and training practices that include scenario building, simulated activity and role-play within their content. If it is accepted that forensic science education has thus far lacked coordinated direction, then this is particularly so with regard to considerations of where simulations and scenario-based learning might feature, which have thus far escaped detailed consideration.

The purpose of this chapter is to explore the nature of immersive gameplay-based learning within forensic science, something that is common, and has proven to be a success in the medical sciences (McGaghie *et al.*, 2010). To provide context, one must first consider the existing structure of forensic science education and provide a background of virtual education and serious games. We follow this with an elaboration on the application of a full spectrum of immersive gameplay within forensic science education and, finally, conclude with recommendations for best practices in the field. As will be demonstrated, this chapter seeks to suggest that far from being a novel concept, immersive gameplay has been inextricably linked with key elements of professional training in crime scene investigation and forensic science practice since such training was first formalised in the United Kingdom; and that, far from being an educationalist's gimmick or the latest fad, virtual reality and simulation-based learning feed directly from the notions

Forensic Science Education and Training: A Tool-kit for Lecturers and Practitioner Trainers, First Edition.
Edited by Anna Williams, John P. Cassella, and Peter D. Maskell.
© 2017 John Wiley & Sons Ltd. Published 2017 by John Wiley & Sons Ltd.

of dynamism and complexity that underpin (or undermine) concepts of science as they are understood within forensics (Marsh *et al.*, 2005).

Terms of Reference

The debate that centres on the relative places of education and entertainment is one that has become particularly poignant since the penetration of computers into the classroom, but its roots clearly pre-date such developments. The entertainment of children as a part of their education, linked with traditional concepts of game-playing or charismatic teaching styles had been considered a distraction from learning objectives and had been addressed in terms as strong as 'irresponsible' (Swartz, 1974).

More recently this stance has been reconsidered as a misconception; the dictum of *pathein mathein*[1] had been seen as requiring not just an active struggle to acquire knowledge and understanding, but more importantly a painful one in which there is no place for entertainment (Woudhuysen, 2004). Mutual antagonism between the conflicting interests of education and entertainment have been traced to more deep-rooted concepts of the separation between work and leisure in the western world (Greenhalgh, 1989), and this debate has been conducted as much in the field of media communications as it has in pedagogical studies (Singhal *et al.*, 2003). These distinctions have, however, been seen as becoming ever more tenuous as a growing number of people make use of internet-based multi-user platforms for work, social interaction and gameplay.

More recent pedagogical innovations support alternative approaches to education; *Situated Learning*, which encourages a recognition of learning as a 'social phenomenon constituted in the experienced, lived-in world, through legitimate peripheral participation in ongoing social practice' (Lave and Wenger, 1991). Legitimate peripheral participation as a learner involves membership in a community of practice that is a 'two-way bridge between the development of knowledgeable skill and identity' wherein apprentice learners achieve mastery through a 'social process of increasingly centripetal participation which depends on legitimate access to ongoing community practice' (Lave and Wenger, 1991). Although tacit knowledge exchange and production has been utilised and identified in forensic science education (Doak and Assimakopoulos, 2007), the field of forensic science education has an incredible and primarily unrealised potential in actively cultivating situated learning through simulation and immersive gameplay.

Computer-based approaches to situated learning have been cultivated in multiple contexts for nearly two decades. Though there was initial resistance to virtual learning environments as 'true' situated learning through a perception of inauthenticity of experience (Hummel, 1993), further research demonstrated virtual or 'anchoring' contexts as acceptable surrogates (McLellan, 1994). This is further supported by the development of augmented reality and more realistic virtual environments in education. Recent developments in the construction of Collaborative Virtual Environments (CVEs) (DeLucia *et al.*, 2009), Augmented Reality (AR) systems (Di Serio *et al.*, 2012), Virtual Reality Learning Environments (VRLEs) (Huang *et al.*, 2010) and Virtual Situated Learning Environments (VSLEs) (Jones, 2007) have complicated the issue of computer-based immersive education still further, particularly for the non-specialist teacher or

---

1 Παθειν μαθειν, 'to suffer is to learn,' a classical Greek concept best known from Aeschylus's *Agamemnon*.

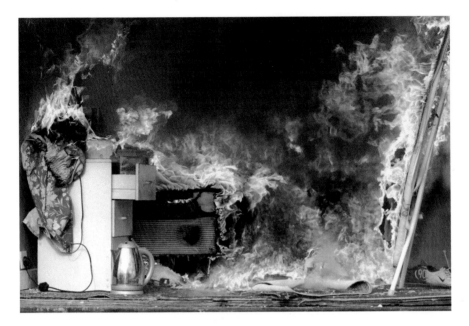

Figure 5.3 Flashover.

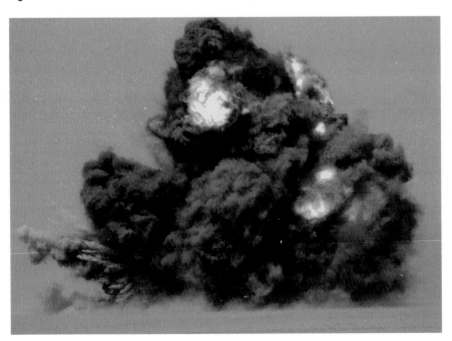

Figure 5.4 EOD teams detonate expired ordinance in Kuwaiti desert. Public Domain Image from Wikimedia Commons. Photographer: Photographer's Mate 2nd Class Aaron Peterson. Source: Peterson https://commons.wikimedia.org/wiki/File:US_Navy_020712-N-5471P-010_EOD_teams_detonate_expired_ordnance_in_the_Kuwaiti_desert.jpg used under CC-BY-SA 3.0 https://commons.wikimedia.org/wiki/Commons:Creative_Commons_Attribution-ShareAlike_3.0_Unported_License.

Forensic Science Education and Training: A Tool-kit for Lecturers and Practitioner Trainers, First Edition.
Edited by Anna Williams, John P. Cassella, and Peter D. Maskell.
© 2017 John Wiley & Sons Ltd. Published 2017 by John Wiley & Sons Ltd.

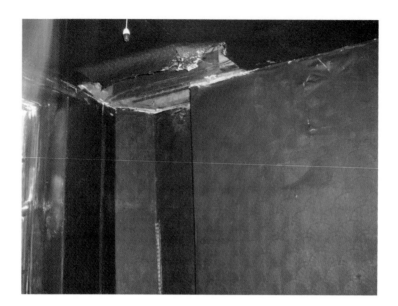

Figure 5.8 Fire scene reconstruction – painted timber.

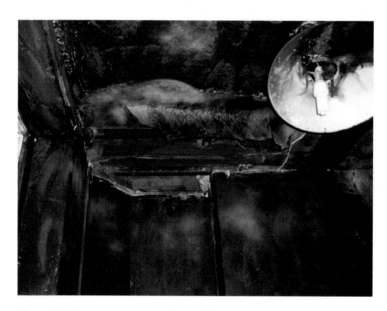

Figure 5.11 Fire scene reconstruction – ceiling.

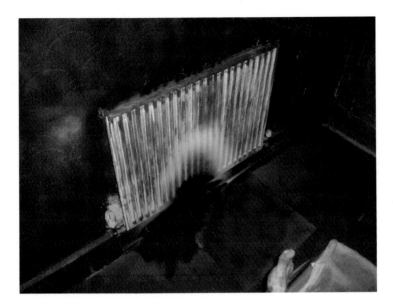

Figure 5.12 Fire scene reconstruction – site of accelerant.

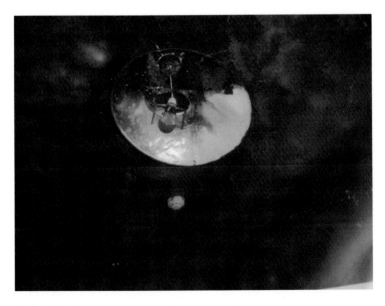

Figure 5.13 Fire scene reconstruction – lamp shade.

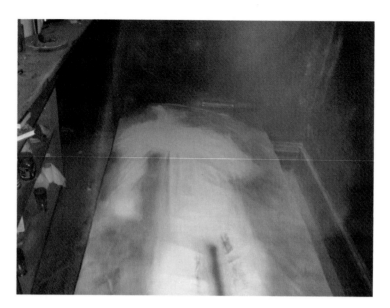

Figure 5.16 Fire scene reconstruction – silhouette on bed linen.

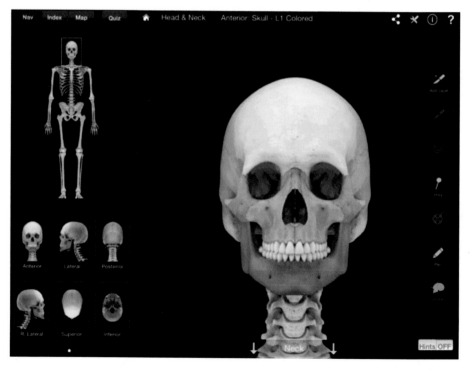

Figure 11.1 Skeletal System Pro III demonstrating colour coded cranium.

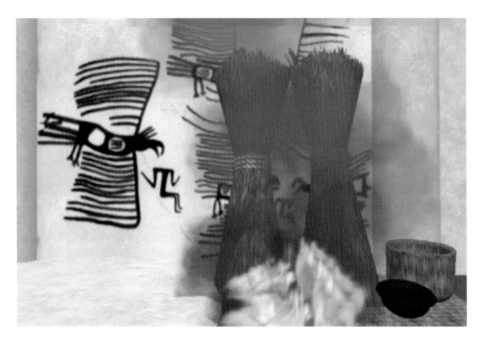

Figure 12.3 Interior view of the burning of Building 77. Recreated within the virtual reconstruction of Çatalhöyük in *Second Life*.

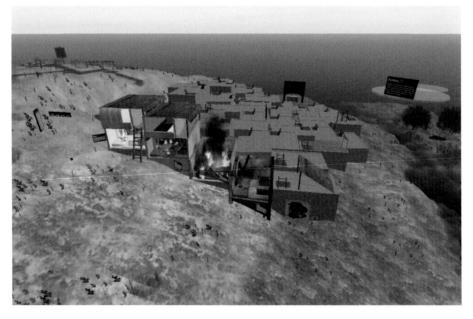

Figure 12.4 Exterior view of the burning of Building 77. Recreated within the virtual reconstruction of Çatalhöyük in *Second Life*.

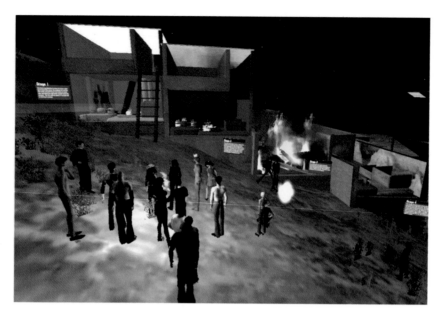

Figure 12.5 Exterior view of the burning of Building 77, showing avatars watching. Recreated within the virtual reconstruction of Çatalhöyük in *Second Life*.

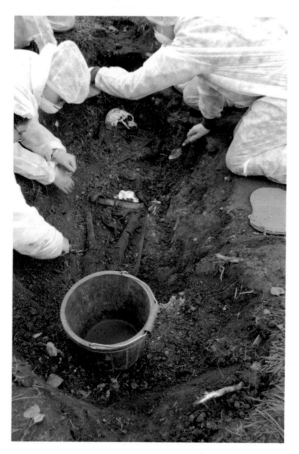

Figure 12.6 Forensic professionals excavating a mock grave; the final exercise in a four-day scenario-based Forensic Ecology training course (Courtesy of Alecto Forensics).

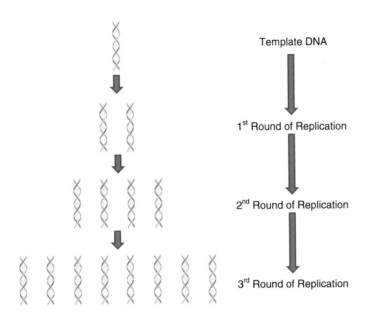

Template DNA

1st Round of Replication

2nd Round of Replication

3rd Round of Replication

Figure 13.1 DNA replication during PCR.

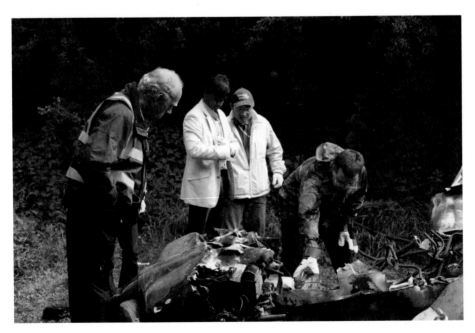

Figure 15.2 A typical light aircraft accident featuring disrupted and burnt metal and manmade material fibres (photo: author's own).

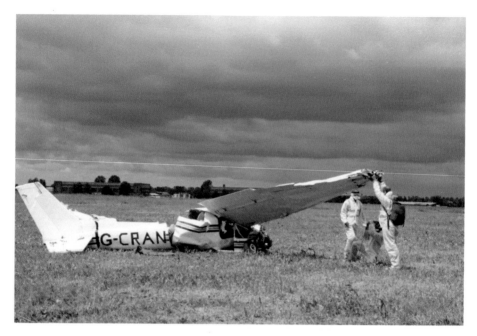

Figure 15.4 A 'real' wrecked aircraft on simulated crash site (photo: author's own).

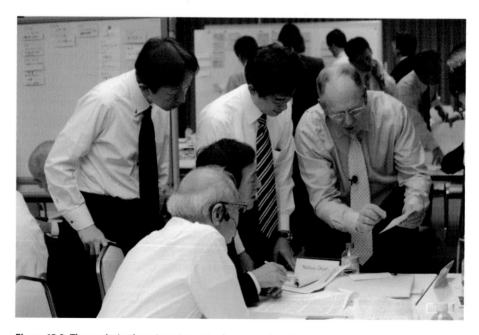

Figure 15.8 The analysis phase is an intensive learning phase (photo: author's own).

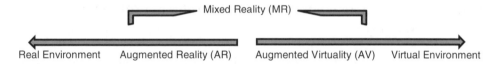

Virtual Continuum (VC)

Figure 12.1 The Virtual Continuum, after Milgram and Kishino (1994). *Source*: Milgram and Kishino 1994. Reproduced with permission of Milgram.

lecturer. All three are recognised as forming part of a 'virtuality continuum' within the overarching concept of Mixed Reality (MR) (Figure 12.1).

While Milgram and Kishino's (Milgram and Kishino, 1994) conceptualisation of mixed reality is old in the terms of published research in computer education, it offers a valuable tool in linking a range of educational methods, from scenario-based simulation in the Real Environment to augmented reality systems; both of which have a proven track record in the delivery of forensic and investigation training. The technologies used for mixed reality approaches to education, for example fully virtual, immersive environments versus augmented reality, have different affordances. While virtual reality allows instructors to fully control all aspects of a scenario, augmented reality brings phenomenological elements of a crime scene into play. Examples of each kind of simulation will be considered with respect to forensic education, following a discussion of Serious Games.

Serious Games

While Johan Huizinga notes the growth of seriousness in game-playing from the nineteenth century (Huizinga, 1949), and Clark Abt recognised game play as a legitimate educational method in the 1970s (Abt, 1970), the concept of serious games is intimately tied to the growth and eventual dominance of computers in education and everyday life in industrialised nations. The oft-cited definition states: 'a serious game is a game in which education (in its various forms) is the primary goal, rather than entertainment' (Michael and Chen, 2005). Serious games have been developed in a wide variety of educational contexts; deep government investment has led to games regarding military and governmental training (Michael and Chen, 2005), yet topics of serious games have become incredibly diverse, representing teaching to different ages and skill levels. Within these extremely diverse contexts there are also a multitude of approaches to the concept of serious games, including framing, identification and assessment of their efficacy (Marsh, 2011).

While serious games have been developed for many purposes, in the field of Forensic Science Education there have been relatively few examples of serious games. These examples run from simulation-based real environment learning that is familiar to forensic scientists, particularly those who work in the field as crime scene investigators, to an example of arson investigation in the highly stylised virtual reality of *Second Life* (www.secondlife.com). By describing these examples in depth, we highlight their usefulness as well as their detriments, and propose to form a more cohesive, rigorous approach to simulated learning in Forensic Science Education.

Simulation-based Real Environment Learning in Professional Forensic Training

Crime Scene Investigators (CSIs) working for UK police forces are now almost entirely a body of civilian specialists operating in a niche role. The shift away from warranted police officers began as early as the late 1960s in some police forces, but this small number greatly expanded following the publication of the recommendations of the Touche Ross Report in 1987 (Tilley and Ford, 1996). A further expansion of civilian specialists followed as a consequence of the growing importance of DNA evidence, as the required level of technical knowledge increased beyond the general forensic awareness of most warrant-holding police officers.

This need for technically proficient specialists brought about the formation of the National Training Centre for Scientific Support to Crime Investigation (NTCSSCI), a training facility based at Harperly Hall, County Durham, UK. The role of the CSI centres on the identification, preservation, recording and recovery of evidence from crime scenes, as laid down in national guidelines communicated to CSIs via a programme of training coordinated by the College of Policing (formerly National Policing Improvement Agency, NPIA).

In the College of Policing (CoP) model (see CoP Training), CSI training is designed to continue over an extended period, beginning with a two-stage initial course, in which each stage consists of a phase of pre-course learning, a formal residential training element and the subsequent completion of a Professional Development Portfolio. Following this initial training, CSIs would complete two years' of work before attending Harperly Hall to complete a two-week 'development course.' Beyond this, further specialist training would be delivered within specific courses (i.e. fire investigation, crime scene management) (see Figure 12.2). CSI training is competency based, with a framework of skills demonstrated in class and their successful use being evidenced on return to operational duty in force. Whilst challenges to police budgets have resulted in some forces adapting this standard training model, it still forms the exemplar on which alternative systems have been based.

Simulation-based Real Environment exercises have formed a fundamental part of the CoP training model from the outset, with mock crime scenes being utilised to develop investigative and evidence gathering skills at every level of delivery. Whilst these would generally feature limited levels of scenario development and immersivity, scenes would be dressed to simulate particular room or space types, an introductory narrative related to the crime committed would be provided, and on occasion an actor playing the role of the crime victim would be on hand to allow the trainee CSI to practice their interview skills (Sawyer, personal communication, 2011). Nick Sawyer, an NTCSSCI trainer, was an early adopter of more immersive scenario-based training exercises at Harperly Hall:

> The training in crime scene management that was put in place was as realistic as could be achieved given that a fictional practical scenario was used to provoke 'real time' reactions to a dynamic and progressive murder scene examination, which included the role play of 'Pathologists' and other scene attending expert scientists.
>
> The focus of the facilitation was on the Crime Scene Manager (CSM) and how they personally managed the dynamics.'
>
> *Sawyer, personal communication, 2011*

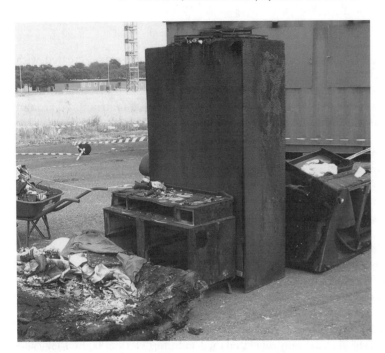

Figure 12.2 Wreckage of a 'suspicious fire' being investigated as part of the NTC Fire Investigation Training Course. Perhaps the most ambitious of dynamic and immersive programmes, the Fire Investigation Course centred on the real-time investigation of simulated fire scenes set out in ISO containers.

Hydra Augmented Reality

Whilst augmented reality systems have yet to make any great inroads into forensic training, they are a well-established means of depicting the multi-faceted nature of police investigation of major crime and associated serious incidents. The Hydra and Minerva systems (Hydra Foundation, www.hydrafoundation.org) utilise video, audio, operational radio traffic, telephone, maps and documentation to build an immersive, but fundamentally non-virtual, 'real' scenario world within which trainee senior detectives would be expected to make decisions and engage in critical thinking throughout an extended exercise (see CoP Training). These systems seek to replace in part traditional means of delivering scenario-based training, which would encompass paper-fed narratives, printed maps and model buildings as vehicles of communicating the problems a given exercise sought to highlight.

Whilst the Hydra system has the benefit of being able to support divergent narrative paths prompted by the decisions reached by participants, it is limited by the number of available places and the associated cost (Mooney *et al.*, 2012). As a consequence, an initial attempt has been made to produce a 'lighter' low-cost model of e-tabletop software, specifically for the purposes of major incident training (Mooney *et al.*, 2012). Such a system might then be appropriate for training lower ranks not requiring the full overview of such a demanding scenario, although thus far the software has been tailored for major incident management, rather than forensic investigation.

Virtual Reality

CSI North Wales is a collaboratively built 'forensic geoscience e-game' created with *Unity*, a flexible game engine used to develop a wide variety of games and virtual simulations (www.unity3d.com). The details of this game can be found in Chapter 9. *CSI North Wales* is an example of a virtual learning environment that is structured around a linear game. The user is represented by a pair of hands that holds on to various forms of equipment in the hopes of finding buried human remains and there is a beginning, middle and an end, marked with either success or failure in solving the crime. *CSI North Wales* employs a limited virtual environment that is specifically tailored as an educational venue.

Another approach is to embed educational material within larger virtual worlds. *Second Life*, a virtual world owned by Linden Labs, encourages users to create avatars and build 3D objects to populate the landscape. *Second Life* debuted in 2003 as a place 'where people could build whatever they liked, and become whoever they wanted' (Guest, 2007). Many educators have taken advantage of this flexibility to build simulations to support their classroom activities. While it is possible to create a game inside *Second Life*, gaining levels and achieving specific outcomes is not inherent to the format.

In 2007, the Open Knowledge and Public Interest research group (OKAPI) at the University of California, Berkeley, digitally recreated the Neolithic (7400–6000 BCE) tell site of Çatalhöyük, located in modern-day Turkey (Morgan, 2009). During the archaeological excavation of Çatalhöyük, several buildings were discovered that had been burned, with visible scorching and burnt artefacts. One of the authors of this chapter investigated Building 77 and Building 80 in 2008 to assess the cause and intensity of these fires, and to help determine if they were accidental burning incidents or arson (Harrison *et al.*, 2013). The preservation of the archaeological remains and Neolithic architecture allowed the identification of the main focus of burning in Building 77, due to heat shadowing and smoke staining (Figure 12.3).

The burning of Building 77 was recreated within the virtual reconstruction of Çatalhöyük in *Second Life* (Figure 12.4). The reconstruction contained an interpretive museum, a guided tour of the tell, a 'sandbox' wherein visitors could build their own objects, a photography and video area, a zone for discussing the site with archaeologists in avatar form and a large area of Neolithic buildings. Using information and images captured during the forensic analysis of Building 77, we built a series of four rooms that demonstrated progressive stages of the fire with accompanying written explanation, video taken onsite and the presence of the archaeologists involved in the re-creation of the houses (Figure 12.5). *Burning Çatalhöyük* was subsequently hosted – an in-world event to attract the attention of educators and *Second Life* users to the site (Morgan, 2009). During this event a tour was held and a lecture explaining the process of building the virtual rooms and burning in prehistory. There were a total of 30 avatars present, and the event was held in conjunction with an undergraduate workshop on virtual worlds at the University of California, Berkeley.

There were a number of advantages to hosting the burning demonstration in an open, online venue such as *Second Life*. While the demonstration was not fully interactive the buildings could be left as they were for many months, providing a point of interest for the larger reconstruction. Avatars could explore and interact with the space and

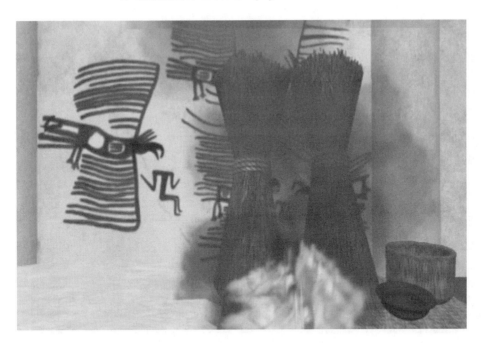

Figure 12.3 Interior view of the burning of Building 77. Recreated within the virtual reconstruction of Çatalhöyük in *Second Life* (see colour figure in colour plate section).

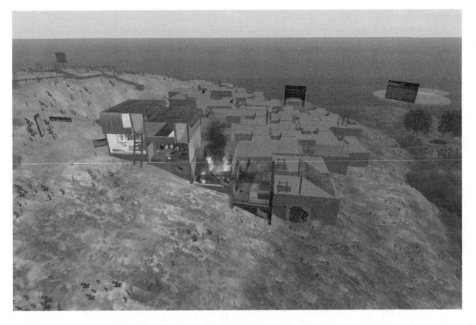

Figure 12.4 Exterior view of the burning of Building 77. Recreated within the virtual reconstruction of Çatalhöyük in *Second Life* (see colour figure in colour plate section).

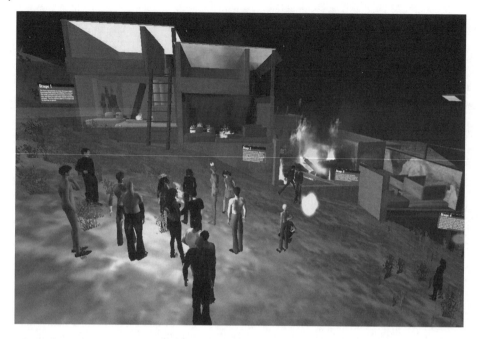

Figure 12.5 Exterior view of the burning of Building 77, showing avatars watching. Recreated within the virtual reconstruction of Çatalhöyük in *Second Life* (see colour figure in colour plate section).

with each other, asking questions about the forensic demonstration as well as regarding archaeology in general. Finally, students who reconstructed burning buildings in a virtual, 3D world were able to more fully appreciate flame overs and their effects on architecture. These students also became experts in building virtual worlds and the difficulties that can arise in reconstructing landscapes, even those that have excellent preservation such as Çatalhöyük. As legitimate peripheral participants they moved through a process of increasingly centralised knowledge production. They were then able to teach each other and provide expert tours of the reconstruction to avatars who came for the *Burning Çatalhöyük* event. *Second Life* is a particularly appropriate environment for situated learning, providing an incentive to learn, 'an idea crucial to understanding the viability of virtual worlds as learning spaces' (Ondrejka, 2008).

Though there was a substantial interest and investment in *Second Life* by educators initially attracted by educational pricing, many educators and projects including OKAPI's Çatalhöyük have left the format after a substantial increase in pricing in 2010. The instability inherent in using private, for-profit resources for education and outreach has encouraged many to seek Open Source and Open Access options. Accordingly, many institutions have turned to *OpenSimulator* (opensimulator.org), an Open Source virtual world generating software that is similar to *Second Life*. The barriers to both accessing and using *OpenSimulator* make it an awkward and under-utilised option, but continued development may increase the suitability of the platform for education.

United Kingdom based CSI training has long recognised the sophisticated response that is elicited from trainees undergoing dynamic, scenario-based exercises. These not only require a flexibility of response and analytical consideration to ensure optimal evidence collection, but also more faithfully reconstruct the nature of the crime scene and require a much broader range of ancillary skills (communication, cooperation, leadership and decision-making) from their subjects.

This model of scenario-based training appears to have become partially embedded in later-developing HEI offerings to university students attending courses in Forensic Science or Forensic Investigation. The interactivity and kinaesthetic learning offered by crime scene houses has become so popular that such a resource is now a *de rigueur* feature of undergraduate Forensic Science programmes; indeed, the University of Central Lancashire (UCLan), who have perhaps invested more than any other UK university in the provision of crime scene houses, describes them as an 'essential facility in which to teach' (UCLan, 2011). In contrast with the physical resources of providing a space for practical exercises, the time and attention to detail required of more immersive scenario-based learning has not been seen to feature so centrally.

Compounding these trends of development away from the realities of crime investigation still further, many undergraduate forensic science courses are housed within the structure of traditional science departments, the senior staff of which seek (understandably) to emphasise the importance of laboratory-based exercises in their curricula.

This overarching structure, plus a defensive reaction to these universities against challenges to the veracity of forensic science degree courses (Forrest, 2004) have resulted in a structure of academic provision and assessment that emphasises individual, task-based analytical exercises over more open-ended, scene-based interpretation and problem solving.

In fact, much of the undergraduate student cohort's exposure to the realities of crime scene investigation constitute some of the more traditional and static provision on forensic science programmes, with former-police officers and CSIs communicating case studies from scene photographs to students. They remain passive recipients of an investigation reconstructed as a meaningful narrative, even when many of the ex-police employees delivering this provision would have had direct personal experience of dynamic scenario-based learning through their own training.

To address these shortcomings in the traditional approaches to forensic science education, further development of simulation-based roleplaying scenarios is suggested. Each position on the virtual continuum has benefits and detractions that must be considered to assess the efficacy of these methods for forensic science education. Accordingly, the following characteristics for the assessment of situated learning for multimedia learning is drawn upon (Herrington and Oliver, 2000):

- authentic context that reflects the way the knowledge will be used in real-life
- authentic activities
- multiple roles and perspectives
- collaborative construction of knowledge
- coaching and scaffolding
- integrated authentic assessment

With these principles in mind, the efficacy of simulations in forensic science education is examined along the spectrum of mixed reality scenarios as forms of legitimate peripheral participation.

Crime Science Investigators (CSIs)

Recreations of crime scenes and real-time, real-world, 'actual' scenarios, provide perhaps the second-best standard of forensic science education, with the ultimate being one-on-one mentorship with an experienced investigator. Participation of a CSI provides an authentic context, authentic activities, collaborative investigation that is supervised and supported by the instructor and assessed according to standards in the field.

Along with the benefits to CSIs, there are considerable detractions to the format. They are extremely expensive, preparation time is prohibitive, and there is a paucity of instructors who have the level of training that is necessary to construct a legitimate, compelling and interactive scenario. Added to this is a limitation of space and a lack of appropriate facilities to accommodate the desired variations of experience that the future investigator will confront on the job.

These detractions are particularly apparent in undergraduate teaching, where large numbers of students require exercises better suited to throughput than the labour-intensive recreation of credible mock crime scenes (Figure 12.6).

Augmented Reality

The Hydra system (http://www.hydra-minerva.com/history/history.htm), while not specifically tailored for CSI scenarios, provides a tantalising preview of an augmented reality system for forensic science education. At its best, an augmented reality system would add urgency and provide detail to established scenarios, delivering a high level of authenticity through multimedia presentation.

The Hydra system adapts to situations, providing dynamism according to decisions made by students. Improvements to these systems would be in adding multiple roles available during scenarios and more variation in these roles.

The unavailability of augmented reality systems for specific forensic science education scenarios is perhaps an indicator of the downsides of the system. As with CSIs, there is a long duration required for set-up of the system and it would be prohibitively expensive to develop, maintain and deploy. There is also a heavy requirement in technical expertise, expert input from forensic specialists and appropriate pedagogical approaches; negotiating between these factors is a difficult obstacle to overcome. Still, the potential to turn classrooms into crime scenes through interactive media devices is an exciting prospect and a potential means for considerable outreach efforts.

Augmented Virtuality

There is a similar dearth in Augmented Virtuality or mixed reality systems for forensic science education, as there are no examples to draw upon. A mixed reality scenario for crime scene investigation would be highly specific, and perhaps of limited use. For instance, a mixed reality crime scene would require an actual room, much as in traditional CSI crime rooms, and a digital version of that room, constructed either through simple 3D modelling or through laser scanning. Bodies and evidence could be added to

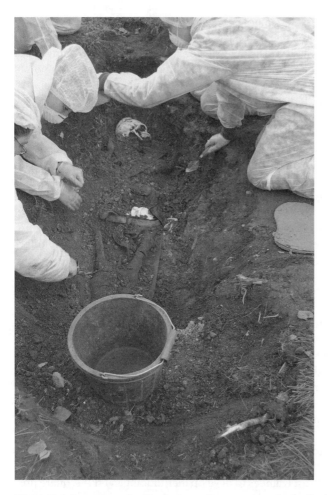

Figure 12.6   Forensic professionals excavating a mock grave; the final exercise in a four-day scenario-based Forensic Ecology training course (Courtesy of Alecto Forensics) (see colour figure in colour plate section).

the 3D model in a variety of forms, though a physical anchor would have to be provided, limiting the flexibility of the format.

Virtual Reality

While fully immersive virtual reality has been postulated since the 1980s, it has yet to come to fruition in practical terms. Mixed reality scenarios, such as those potentially provided by Google Glass (www.google.com/glass/start) (and comparable products) and smart phones have gained ascendancy. In a recent example of a video promotion created by a consortium of technology companies titled *CSI the Hague* (www.csithehague.com), an investigator would record entire crime scenes during the investigation, through a first-person perspective. Watching this record would draw students into the intimacy of the crime scene, yet would ultimately provide a passive experience, as the decisions would be made by the investigator, leaving the student uninvolved. These recordings would have to be appropriately remediated to include decision points to meet the requirements of legitimate peripheral participation.

In the examples of *CSI North Wales* and *Second Life*, virtual reality is gained through telepresence – an immersion through participation in a screen-based reality, more akin to reading a gripping novel than a full-body, goggled experience (Goldberg, 1998). While a virtual reality crime scene would not necessarily provide an authentic context, the immersive nature and the familiarity of the video game perspective and context can be incredibly evocative. *CSI North Wales* provides a large, nearly featureless field and remote sensing tools that help to disambiguate this landscape. The meticulous nature of remote detecting is evident and the scaffolding is only partially designed into the game, making outside instruction imperative for a successful result. In *Second Life* there are signs that explain different scenarios and the objects themselves are extremely interactive and can be programmed to instruct, give tours and even position and move the avatar.

Both *Second Life* and the *Unity* game engine (used to create *CSI North Wales*) are flexible enough to accommodate most of the principles of situated learning, but require forward planning and design to be fully realised within virtual worlds. To acquire a different role in *Second Life*, the avatar can simply slip into a new skin, with newly assigned roles. Students who participated in a machinima – a film made entirely within a virtual world – recreated Neolithic life by donning the 'skins' that they created, sometimes playing opposite genders and much younger or older characters (http://www.machinimaguild.com/).

By creating meaningful content in the virtual world, the students queried the nature of archaeological knowledge. The best forensic education virtual game might be the game created by the students to teach themselves. Crime scenes are dynamic complexes of activity and interactivity. Whilst they are frequently reconstructed as passive, prop-laden environments for students or trainees to develop methodological skills, or are presented in case study format by higher education lecturers with retro-fitted narratives, neither of these means of exposure does justice to the range of skills – technical, analytical and interpersonal – required of the forensic investigator at the major crime scene.

Conclusions

Establishing responsive, immersive scenarios for forensic or indeed policing students in HEIs and trainees is a long and convoluted process, which has thus far seen its greatest development emerging through senior ranks of policing and forensic professionals with decision-making exercises via the Hydra suite (Hydra Foundation, www.hydrafoundation.org). Professional CSI training in a UK context has been shown to share commonalities with these larger training suites in the importance attached to constructing and maintaining credible scenarios of crime investigation, but this same level of detailed realism appears rarely evident in similar training and teaching products currently available to undergraduate students of forensic science or forensic investigation courses.

Providers of higher education in forensic science have struggled to find robust and meaningful ways in which simulated crime scene examinations could be linked to bench-based analytical science processes, and have begun to seek ways to engage with such en vogue pedagogical concepts as immersive scenario-based learning. By contrast, the play-acting element of education, often expressed with fairly rudimentary tools, has formed an integral part of professional training for Crime Scene Investigators since it was first formalised. It is hoped that access to novel technologies will offer new opportunities for closer and more sophisticated integration of the two traditions.

References

Abt, C.C. (1970) *Serious Games*, The Viking Press, New York.

College of Policing. *CoP Training*. http://www.college.police.uk/What-we-do/Learning/Curriculum/Forensics/Crime_Scene/Pages/CSI-Stage-1.aspx (accessed 7 April 2013).

DeLucia, A., Francese, R., Passero, I. and Tortora, G. (2009) Development and evaluation of a virtual campus on Second Life: The case of SecondDMI. *Computers & Education*, **52**, 220–233.

Di Serio, Á., Blanca Ibáñez, M. and Delgado Kloos, C. (2012) Impact of an augmented reality system on students' motivation for a visual art course. *Computers & Education* **68**, 586–596.

Doak, S. and Assimakopoulos, D. (2007) How forensic scientists learn to investigate cases in practice. *R & D Management*, **37** (2), 113–122.

Forrest, A. (2004) Whither academic forensic science? *Science & Justice*, **44**, 195.

Goldberg, K. (1998) Virtual reality in the age of telepresence. *Convergence: The International Journal of Research into New Media Technologies*, **4** (33), 33–37.

Greenhalgh, P. (1989) Education, entertainment and politics: Lessons from the great international exhibitions, in *The New Museology* (ed. P. Vergo), Reaktion Books, London, pp. 74–98.

Guest, T. (2007) *Second Lives: A Journey Through Virtual Worlds*, Hutchinson, London.

Harrison, K., Martin, V. and Webster, B. (2013) Structural fires, in *Volume 9: Substantive Technologies at Çatalhöyük: Reports from the 2000–2008 Seasons* (ed. I. Hodder), Cotsen, Los Angeles.

Herrington, J. and Oliver, R. (2000) Exploring situated learning in multimedia settings. *Educational Technology Research and Development*, **48** (3), 23–48.

Huang, H.-M., Rauch, U. and Liaw, S.-S. (2010) Investigating learners' attitudes towards virtual reality learning environments: Based on a constructivist approach. *Computers & Education*, **55**, 1171–1182.

Huizinga, J. (1949) *Homo Ludens*, Routledge and Kegan Paul, London.

Hummel, H.G.K. (1993) Distance education and situated learning: Paradox or partnership. *Educational Technology*, **33** (12), 11–22.

Jones, S. (2007) Adding value to online role plays: Virtual situated learning environments. *Proceedings ascilite Singapore 2007*. Available at: http://www.ascilite.org/conferences/singapore07/procs/jones-s.pdf (accessed 26 June 2016).

Lave, J. and Wenger, E. (1991) Simulated learning in communities of practice, in *Perspectives on Socially Shared Cognition* (eds L.B. Resnick, J.M. Devine and S.D. Tesley), American Psychological Association, Washington DC, pp. 63–82.

Marsh, T. (2011) Serious games continuum: Between games for purpose and experiential environments for purpose. *Entertainment Computing*, **2** (2), 61–68.

Marsh, T., Wong, W.L., Carriazo, E., Nocera, L., Yang, K., Varma, A., Yoon, H., Huang, Y.L., Kyriakakis, C. and Shahabi, C. (2005) User experiences and lessons learned from developing and implementing an immersive game for the science classroom, in *Proceedings of HCI International 2005*.

McLellan, H. (1994) Situated learning: Continuing the conversation. *Educational Technology*, **34** (10), 7–8.

McGaghie, W.C., Issenberg, S.B., Petrusa, E.R. and Scalese, R.J. (2010) A critical review of simulation-based medical education research: 2003–2009. *Medical Education*, **44** (1), 50–63.

Michael, D. and Chen, S. (2005) *Serious Games: Games That Educate, Train, and Inform*, 1st edn, Course Technology PTR.

Milgram, P. and Kishino, F. (1994) A taxonomy of mixed reality visual displays. *IEICE Transactions on Information Systems*, **E77-D**, **12**, December 1994.

Mooney, J.S., Griffiths, L., Patera, M., Roby, J., Ogden, P. and Driscoll, P. (2012) An electronic 'eTabletop' exercise for UK Police major incident education. 12th IEEE International Conference on Advanced Learning Technologies, pp. 40–41.

Morgan, C.L. (2009) (Re)Building Çatalhöyük: Changing virtual reality in archaeology. *Archaeologies*, **5**, 468.

Ondrejka, C. (2008) Education unleashed: Participatory culture, education, and innovation in Second Life, in *The Ecology of Games: Connecting Youth, Games, and Learning* (ed. K. Salen), The MIT Press, Cambridge, MA, pp. 229–252.

Paton, G. (2009) CSI fuels forensic science degree rise. *The Telegraph* [online] 16 October 2009. Available at: http://www.telegraph.co.uk/education/6348107/CSI-fuels-forensic-science-degree-rise.html (accessed 7 April 2015).

Singhal, A., Cody, M., Rogers, E. and Sabido, M. (2003) *Entertainment-Education and Social Change: History, Research and Practice*, Routledge, London.

Swartz, R. (1974) Education as entertainment and irresponsibility in the classroom. *Science Education*, **58** (1), 119–125.

Tilley, N. and Ford, A. (1996) *Forensic Science and Crime Investigation*, Home Office Police Research Group, London.

UCLan (2011) *Crime Scene Houses*. Available at: www.uclan.ac.uk/about_us/facilities/crime_scene_houses.php (accessed 7 April 2015).

Woudhuysen, J. (2004) Education as entertainment, in *The RoutledgeFalmer Guide to Key Debates in Education* (ed. D. Hayes), Routledge, London.

13

Training Forensic Practitioners in DNA Profiling

Sue Carney

Ethos Forensics, Manchester, UK and University of Central Lancashire, UK

Introduction

DNA evidence is ubiquitous in the modern global criminal justice system. Indeed, it might be argued that DNA has become synonymous with forensic evidence. Whilst some forensic practitioners consider it the gold standard, others question its validity (Easteal and Easteal, 1990) and there is no doubt that its popularity is often at the expense of the use of more traditional forensic evidence types.

The interpretation of a DNA profile must be based on sound interpretation guidelines yet it can be subjective, especially when dealing with DNA mixtures and questions of inclusion (Budowle *et al.*, 2009). The increased sensitivity of DNA profiling techniques in recent years brings with it a selection of additional interpretational issues, as low level DNA mixtures are detected with increasing frequency and low template techniques are becoming obsolete as a result. It may not be possible to evaluate these DNA mixtures reliably, rendering interpretations even more susceptible to the risk of bias. The expression of expert opinion on DNA is sometimes contested, often controversial and, some might argue, open to debate (Balding and Donnelly, 1994). In this chapter, criteria for training and competency of forensic DNA experts will be discussed, along with an examination of how DNA evidence and its limitations fit into forensic science in the modern criminal justice system.

Prior Knowledge

Conventionally, forensic DNA reporting officers are educated to degree level as a minimum, usually in a relevant field of biology or chemistry. The benefits of a forensic science degree are debatable (see Chapters 1 and 18), some arguing that forensic science graduates have insufficient experience of fundamental scientific principles. Trainee practitioners will benefit from a thorough background knowledge of cell biology, including DNA structure and replication. An understanding of the mechanisms of mutation,

Forensic Science Education and Training: A Tool-kit for Lecturers and Practitioner Trainers, First Edition.
Edited by Anna Williams, John P. Cassella, and Peter D. Maskell.
© 2017 John Wiley & Sons Ltd. Published 2017 by John Wiley & Sons Ltd.

the diploid genome and haploid gametes is an advantage. Experience of techniques in molecular biology, including extraction processes, polymerase chain reactions (PCR) and electrophoresis, will aid in understanding the technical aspects of the DNA profiling process. A level of mathematical dexterity, especially a practical knowledge of probability theory, will assist in the principles of DNA interpretation and evidential significance. If trainees lack these basic background skills, pre-course reading or a foundation course are recommended.

Setting the Scene: Expectations

Trainee forensic practitioners fresh from their degree course might expect to routinely deal with DNA casework at an early stage. Most seasoned forensic DNA experts would disagree. Gaining an initial competency in even the most basic DNA cases should be a lengthy, structured process, including taught courses with examinations to monitor the correct application of principles learnt, followed by frequent practice casework examples, before tackling real cases under mentoring conditions. Inconsistencies in this mentoring stage are a risk since mentors, whilst typically the most experienced DNA practitioners, may not themselves be experienced at mentoring. As such, a programme for the development of mentors is recommended.

Owing to this structured approach, rates of learning might be considered slower than that expected by the trainee. Given the significant overlap in casework requirements, DNA profiling is commonly taught in parallel to body fluids, also contributing to the perceived duration of training. A fast-track course might span 18 months to sign-off, followed by a year of mentored live casework.

Most forensic practitioners would encourage exposure to casework discussions at an early stage since no expert should ever work in isolation. The endorsement of a colleague's opinion, even on an informal basis, is always welcome when dealing with a difficult interpretation. The only place where the expert witness works truly in isolation, with no back up, is in the courtroom witness box. Forensic experts from all disciplines need to be prepared for this on both a general and a case-by-case basis.

Preconceptions and Common Misconceptions

In contrast to the most commonly held misconception amongst trainee DNA practitioners, DNA evidence is rarely conclusive. The principles of DNA evidence evaluation, indeed of most forensic evidence types, might be said to call for a new way of thinking on the part of the trainee (Cook *et al.*, 1998a). A fundamental principle of DNA evidence is that its value is expressed in terms of a level of support for a particular view, usually that the matching DNA has originated from a questioned individual, as opposed to having originated from another party, unrelated to the questioned individual. As such, DNA evidence is not proof of guilt. Indeed, landmark appeal court rulings (R v Doheny, R v Adams, 1997; R v Adams, 1996), which should feature at the top of any DNA training course reading list, emphasise the DNA expert's duties in presenting DNA evidence. They also suggest that no criminal case should be decided on the basis of DNA evidence alone.

Introductory Concepts

DNA Structure and Function

The elegant relationship between the structure and function of the DNA molecule is a good starting point. Such a course should highlight those properties of DNA that are advantageous in a forensic context: that DNA is present in almost every cell of the human body, that the strands of the double helix are complementary, that DNA replicates in a semi-conservative manner, that it can be considered unique in individuals (Balding, 1999) and that it is inherited are all useful attributes.

Whilst DNA carries the genetic information, providing instructions for each individual's physical characteristics, the regions measured in forensic DNA profiling, the short tandem repeats (STRs), are non-coding regions. Recent research (The ENCODE Project Consortium, 2012) points to far more functionality across the genome – largely regulatory – than originally estimated, suggesting a new definition of the concept of the gene. Therefore, whilst it is true to state that STRs provide no information about a person's physical characteristics, practitioners should avoid stating that they are non-functional.

The Profiling Process

The DNA profiling process can be split into individual stages and a thorough 'DNA Technical' course of lectures should describe each stage in detail. This is usually a predominantly classroom-based course, but will benefit from a tour of a functioning DNA unit in which trainees are able to witness each stage of the process. With the onset of automation (Graham, 2005) of large portions of the process, there may be little to see. Too much detail of the technical specifications of the automation machinery are not relevant for the trainee reporter, but those trainees who will become analysts should be provided with more in-depth instruction on how to use the system.

Extraction

The extraction process is a chemical treatment of the forensic sample in order to break open the cells and separate the DNA. Traditional methods of manual extraction included a phenol–chloroform protocol, which has a high yield, but poses risk to the operator due to the chemicals used. Additional clean-up techniques, mostly filtering and purification steps, were often required to remove inhibitors such as excess haem from heavy blood stains and clothing dyes and, in particular, dark indigo dyes from denim. Typically, modern systems now use commercially available automated systems in which the DNA is isolated using a silica gel column or a system of magnetic beads, but the overall principle of removing the unwanted cellular components are similar. Most of the modern extraction kits are efficient at removing inhibitors or have inbuilt purification steps, meaning that re-extraction or clean-up steps are required less frequently.

There may still be some variation in the extraction protocol depending on the type of sample. A common requirement is the need for a preferential extraction in the case of a mixture of spermatozoa and vaginal cells in sexual offences cases, for example. The success of this type of extraction is dependent on a separation of the spermatozoa from the other cellular material in the sample before the DNA extraction proper. There are still inefficiencies in this separation process such that the two fractions (seminal and cellular) are rarely 100% pure, leading to the production of mixtures of DNA that may result in interpretational issues. The ratio of spermatozoa to cells has the greatest impact, especially in those samples with low numbers of spermatozoa, although recent method development has increased efficiency of spermatozoa recovery in such samples (Hulme *et al.*, 2013).

Quantification

In earlier DNA profiling systems, quantification was a separate process, usually using a hybridisation method, the results of which could be interpreted rather subjectively. Such initial quantification allowed the DNA extract to be appropriately diluted to maximise efficiency of the subsequent PCR reaction. Many modern systems use real-time PCR in which the DNA is quantified in real time during the PCR reaction. Kits such as *Quantifiler* (Green *et al.*, 2005) are able to quantify total human and total male DNA within a reaction, which is particularly advantageous in sexual offence case samples.

Amplification

In current UK DNA profiling, 16 areas of DNA (loci) plus a sex test are amplified using PCR. This replaced the formerly used Second Generation Multiplex (SGM) Plus system, which amplifies ten loci plus the sex test. Both of these profile types, and the earlier SGM system, comprise profiles held on the UK's National DNA Database (NDNAD). The US system examines 13 loci plus a sex test. This multiplex is compatible with the Combined DNA Index System (CODIS) and the National DNA Index System (NDIS).

PCR takes advantage of the properties of the DNA polymerase enzyme found in *Thermus aqauticus* (Saiki *et al.*, 1988). This microorganism is indigenous to hot springs and, crucially for the PCR reaction, its various functions can be controlled by temperature change.

Typically, 28 rounds of replication are carried out in routine profiling (Walsh *et al.*, 1992). Often 34 rounds of replication were used in specialist low template techniques, or other modifications to the profiling process were employed such as clean-up techniques or an adjustment to the voltage applied at electrophoresis, resulting in better resolution of the profile. However, current UK techniques (McLaren *et al.*, 2014) with improved chemistry, have superseded low template techniques, rendering them largely obsolete in most circumstances.

An important principal for trainees unfamiliar with DNA profiling to grasp is that each round of replication leads to a doubling of the amount of DNA, such that 28 cycles of replication will produce an exponential increase in target DNA (Figure 13.1).

Separation and Detection

The fragments of target DNA from PCR are separated using electrophoresis. This method utilises the negative charge of the DNA molecule and the speed at which fragments of different length will move through a gel matrix. Speed is inversely proportional to the length of a fragment. Shorter fragments pass more readily through the gel matrix because they are impeded to a lesser extent. Modern systems use capillary electrophoresis in which each DNA sample passes through a separate capillary containing the gel matrix, as opposed to older systems that used more problematic slab gels.

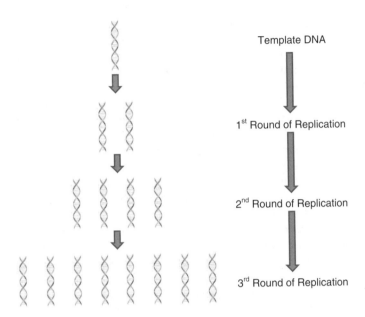

Figure 13.1 DNA replication during PCR (see colour figure in colour plate section).

Fragments are detected as they pass the end point of the gel using fluorescent markers attached to their PCR primers. Software converts these signals into an electrophoretogram (EPG) for each sample tested. Internal size standards and allelic ladders, containing all possible DNA fragments, are used to calculate the length of questioned fragments. An allele's position as a peak on the EPG indicates the length of that allele, that is, the number of repeat units in the STR (short tandem repeat).

Important learning points from this content include explanations of the features of EPGs, that peak position corresponds to length/size of a fragment and that peak height corresponds to the amount of DNA detected. Other aspects to consider are how to recognise DNA mixtures versus mutations, and recognition of stutter peaks and other artefacts resulting from the profiling process.

Mutations are infrequently seen in casework samples but can arise by a variety of mechanisms. Explanation of these, along with the expected appearance of a mutation on an EPG, if any, provides the trainee practitioner with a greater understanding of what they might expect to see in unusual circumstances.

By the end of their training, DNA practitioners will become increasingly familiar with EPGs. It may be useful during these introductory stages to supply a set number of examples of unusual outcomes so that trainees can practice their interpretations, before completing an assessed EPG interpretation. The inclusion of a *viva voce* examination with an experienced practitioner is also a useful way to consolidate this knowledge, but may be better placed towards the end of the practitioner's training.

Anti-Contamination

The explanation of anti-contamination procedures is most effectively taught immediately after the DNA technical training. By now, the trainee practitioner should be aware of the sensitivity of the profiling technique and will be able to contextualise the mechanisms of contamination. In addition to the need for protective clothing and cleaning regimes, this content should also explain the use of negative controls at extraction and PCR and the need for staff and supplier elimination databases, site visitor policies, protocols for entering DNA-clean areas and environmental monitoring processes.

Traditionally, laboratory consumables marketed as DNA-free, are batch tested to provide assurance of these claims. Data from such testing has raised concerns amongst forensic service providers since small numbers of positive findings indicate the presence of DNA on supposed DNA free items. This has resulted in a minimal number of anomalous casework results that have been successfully investigated and resolved. UK contamination incidents of a more serious nature, affecting court proceedings, have largely been due to the need for procedural improvements, and lessons have been learned from such incidents. Other countries have not been so fortunate; the infamous 'Phantom of Heilbronn' incident in Germany is a case in point. Spanning a 15-year investigation, the unidentified female 'perpetrator' of a wide variety of crimes was eventually identified as a member of staff at a swab-manufacturing company (Temco, 2008; Himmelreich, 2009).

Trainees would benefit from a comprehensive explanation of some of the contamination incidents of the past, detailing learning points and procedure improvements as a result of these incidences.

Laboratory equipment and consumables can be subject to treatment with radiation to render them DNA free and this is common practice at laboratories, particularly for non-disposable items. A new method of DNA decontamination involving the use of ethylene oxide treatment of consumables has been suggested (Archer *et al.*, 2010). This treatment does not remove contaminant DNA but breaks the nitrogen–glycosidic bond linking guanine to the sugar–phosphate backbone. This prevents polymerisation, such that any DNA present prior to treatment cannot be profiled.

Intermediate Concepts

Once trainees are familiar with the DNA profiling technical process and have gained an understanding of single source profiling results, they are ready to move on to more challenging casework examples.

Partial Profiles

Partial or degraded profiles are not uncommon when testing real forensic samples, despite the improved sensitivity of profiling techniques. Numerous exhibits have been subject to adverse conditions before arriving at the laboratory, many of which result in the degradation of DNA. It is not uncommon for degradation to occur at the higher molecular weight loci first, resulting in wedge-shaped profiles with gradually decreasing peak heights towards the higher molecular weight loci (Figure 13.2).

At this point in training, it is useful to introduce a classification system to assess the quality of profiles. A traffic light system (Buckleton, 2009) is in common use, where green profiles are well amplified and display little imbalance, amber profiles are amplified to an intermediate level with some imbalance apparent and red profiles, which can be

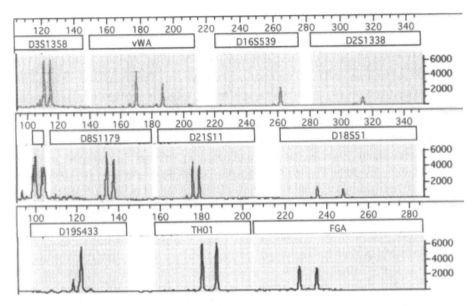

Figure 13.2 An SGM Plus profile indicating degradation at the high molecular weight loci.

considered low level, are poorly amplified and are likely to display extreme imbalance. The exact criteria for each category will vary from one forensic provider to the next, since these depend on the provider's interpretation guidelines, which in turn, are derived from the internal validation of their specific DNA profiling system. However, the principles of use of the system are similar: green profiles can be reliably interpreted with greater confidence; and amber profiles should be interpreted with less emphasis on heterozygote imbalance leading to a relaxation of the rules governing peak area difference. Caution should be exercised when interpreting red profiles, peak heights cannot be relied upon and the possibilities of drop-in and drop-out are more likely. These guidelines take on much greater significance at the later stages of practitioner development when DNA mixtures are considered.

Partial profiles, if they appear single source, may still comprise sufficient information to search an intelligence database, such as the UK National DNA Database, or the CODIS in the US, or for statistical interpretation.

Introduction to Mixtures

At this stage of training, an awareness of DNA mixtures can be introduced, rather than an in-depth knowledge of their interpretation. Trainee practitioners should be able to recognise and categorise a DNA mixture. They should learn to determine whether it can be separated into major and minor profiles, whether it can be resolved by a statistical calculation, whether it is complex, with multiple contributors, and in the case of amber and red profiles, whether caution in further interpretation is required.

These are principles that will be expanded upon during the later stages of training, but with guidance from their mentors, trainees can begin to observe the process of mixture interpretation.

Database Searches

Often, in cases where a practitioner is working in investigator mode, their purpose is to obtain a DNA profile to assist in identifying a possible offender by searching the UK National DNA Database (NDNAD) or national equivalent. There are strict criteria for profiles that are to be added to the database permanently. If they are partial profiles, they must contain greater than a specific number of alleles. Further, some of these alleles must have been detected at specific loci, termed the discriminator loci.

Profiles that do not meet these criteria can be subject to a one-off speculative search of the database instead. The fewer alleles contained in a partial profile, the more matches are expected to be generated. For this reason, partial profiles containing very few alleles must be restricted by other, non-allelic, criteria. These include specification of geographical area by police service code, or age of the individual. Race code has been removed as a non-allelic criteria for searches of the UK NDNAD because it is thought that much of the race code data held, given that it is based on offender admissions at the time of arrest, may not be accurate.

Non-allelic criteria can be useful in some cases if an offence or group of offences have taken place in a specific area or if the estimated age of the offender is known, for example, from witness descriptions. However, the possibilities remain that offenders may move around the country and witness estimations of age are inaccurate.

A reporting scientist might also choose to carry out a speculative search for ethical reasons. For example, if it is unclear whether the crime stain profile relates to the alleged incident. This might be due to case circumstance or an absence of elimination reference profiles from those who might have innocently contributed DNA to an exhibit.

Matches generated on the NDNAD to permanently loaded crime stains are communicated directly to the investigating police force by database staff. It is at a later stage that the forensic provider is contacted by the investigating officer to request the practitioner to produce a statement to report the match. Only at that stage is the name of the matching individual revealed. A learning point for trainee practitioners that should be emphasised here is that the National DNA Database, or equivalent, should not be mentioned in a forensic science evidential statement. It would be considered prejudicial to disclose to the court that the defendant had been identified via a database match since this might imply he/she holds a previous criminal record.

The results of speculative searches are treated differently to those from database loads. Depending on the search criteria (the number of alleles and any other non-allelic criteria), multiple matches are generated. The reporting scientist is sent a match list by database staff, containing all the matching profiles and their corresponding barcodes. It may be possible for the practitioner to eliminate some of the matches based on alleles in the profile that were unsuitable to search. This is particularly pertinent to profiles selected from DNA mixtures in which multiple alleles at a loci not included in the search criteria can be used to eliminate all matching profiles missing those alleles at that locus.

Speculative search results are intended as intelligence and offer little, if any, evidential significance. When reported, it should be emphasised that no evidential link to the subjects contained on the match list can be established from the search, and that it is feasible that the true offender is not included on the match list at all. Such search results are designed to provide investigating officers with further leads, and the reporting scientist has a responsibility to explain this in their report to the investigating officer.

Statistical Interpretation

The statistical interpretation (Foreman *et al.*, 1997, 1999) of a DNA match is one of the more difficult concepts that the trainee practitioner will learn. By now, the trainees should be aware that a matching DNA profile is not conclusive and they will probably have been exposed to enough casework examples to know that (in the UK) a full matching DNA profile is attributed a match probability of one in a billion.[1] Explanations of the reasoning behind this should be second nature to the DNA practitioner, but this remains a concept that many struggle with during their training.

The DNA statistics course should include a background of population genetics and probability theory (Balding *et al.*, 1986). All the factors taken into consideration during a match probability calculation need to be explained, such as allowances made for possible relatedness and a phenomenon known as the 'two trace' effect (Balding, 1995; Balding and Donnelly, 1995a, 1995b). During this course, trainees are taught how to manually calculate a match probability (Balding and Nichols, 1994).

The match probability calculation is based on the product rule (Evett *et al.*, 1996). Since alleles at each locus are inherited independently, the probability of each allele's presence in a profile is independent of any other. Therefore, the probabilities of these alleles multiplied together provides the probability of obtaining the complete profile. Allelic probabilities are obtained from allele frequency databases, comprising volunteer samples, aligned to each of the three main race codes in that country. As opposed to elsewhere in the world, UK match probabilities are capped at one in a billion, which is considered to be a fair and reasonable figure (Foreman and Evett, 2001). The convention for experts in other countries, such as the United States, is to quote the true match probability figure. The true figures, as trainees will learn from their manual calculations, are considerably rarer. In order to test the fairness of one in a billion, match probabilities were calculated for numerous example profiles, including a theoretic profile comprising the most common alleles at each locus, based on the frequency databases. In all instances, the calculated match probabilities were shown to be considerably rarer than one in a billion (Foreman and Evett, 2001; Evett *et al.*, 2000a).

A useful analogy for the practitioner to explain the product rule and match probability calculation is the 'car park' analogy. Consider the probability of observing a silver car in a large car park, such as an airport long stay car park (the UK's Heathrow airport 'parking express' has capacity for 5000 cars). Now consider the probability of observing a silver car with alloy wheels: the chances are reduced slightly. If the observed car must also have leather upholstery, this again reduces the probability and so on. Each time a new attribute is added to the description, the probability of observation is decreased. In the same way, in a DNA profile, the more alleles are added to the criteria for a match, the smaller the probability of observing a match.

The 'prosecutor's fallacy' (Balding and Donnelly, 1994) or 'transposed conditional' (Evett, 1995) is an important concept to explain here. Some practitioners seem to find this a particularly difficult concept. Practitioners must remember that their role is to address the probability of obtaining a match *if* the DNA is not from the matching

---

1 The situation in the United States is different. Experts often quote the actual match probability for the profile and, in some circumstances, may extend their interpretation to imply that, given the match probability figure, the source of the matching DNA has been conclusively identified (Budowle *et al.*, 2000).

individual but from a person other than and unrelated to them. The principles of evidential interpretation tells us that the scientist's remit to evaluate the probability of the evidence not the proposition. Conclusions must be worded carefully to avoid transposing the emphasis in this conditional probability. In other words, it's vital to place the 'if' in the right place. A useful exercise is to provide trainees with a list of variously worded DNA conclusions and ask them to state which are correct and which are transposed. The trainees should not only be able to identify correct and transposed but to explain why.

A list of commonly asked defence questions provides a useful interlude to this training course and will be useful later for witness box exercises. The practitioner should become well versed in the most commonly offered lines of defence and know how to deal with them. Examples might include:

- Comparing a match probability to the population of the United Kingdom (the defender's fallacy) to try to determine how many individuals are expected to match (Triggs *et al.*, 2004). One in a billion cannot be compared to a population. This is erroneous and a simplification.
- The brother's defence, in which it is suggested that the matching DNA is not from the defendant but from his brother (Evett, 1992).

Advanced Concepts

Practitioners reaching this stage in their development are likely to have been working on live source level DNA casework for some time, initially under mentoring conditions, then independently. There are risks to source level only reporting. Practitioners are left in a vulnerable position at court where they must be clear that they have not addressed the issues of how and when biological evidence was deposited. This is reasonable if the DNA evidence is part of a larger complex case, but in simple cases, this is dubious. Consider a case where the only evidence is a single source DNA profile from a cigarette butt for example. Is it reasonable that the source level practitioner may give their opinion on the chance of the DNA if it were from the defendant, but not on the chance of the evidence if the defendant smoked the cigarette?

Where should the line be drawn between simple and complex cases? Clearly this is one of many grey areas in forensic science. Often, simple, source level only cases can develop into complex investigations and the inexperienced practitioner must be aware of the limits of their expertise. A culture of frequent casework discussions helps here, such that practitioners are supported and rarely work in isolation, but there is another problem. Simple intelligence-type cases often contain the types of items where low level mixtures of DNA are the expected outcomes. Whilst the cases might be considered simple, the outcomes are complex. For this reason, a staged progression into activity level reporting and DNA mixture interpretation is recommended. This need not be rushed and mentors will assist in monitoring the ability and understanding of new practitioners, but the practice of leaving reporters stranded at source level is problematic and needs to be addressed by the forensic science community.

Activity Level Interpretation

Knowledge of the mechanisms of transfer and persistence coupled with casework experience are the key issues here. The practitioner will be familiar with the hierarchy of propositions (Cook *et al.*, 1998b; Evett *et al.*, 2000b) and the Case Assessment and Interpretation model of interpretation (Cook *et al.*, 1998a). Best practice suggests that practitioners address issues at activity level.

In addition to providing an opinion on a DNA match, it is of more use to the Criminal Justice System if an expert is able to provide an opinion on how and when matching DNA was deposited. Whilst addressing case issues at activity level must take into account the circumstances of the case, the DNA expert is much better placed to provide such an opinion, based on their knowledge of transfer and persistence. The alternative, in which the expert chooses only to address the source of the DNA, leaves the court to interpret how the matching DNA might have been deposited, and there is a risk that such interpretations will be based on flawed inferences.

Modes of Transfer

Expectations in relation to the quality of a DNA profile differ depend on the mode of transfer, primary or secondary, and other factors such as the abundance of DNA available for transfer. These factors can be assessed in addressing issues of contact, but it should be remembered that primary transfer does not necessarily infer contact between surfaces. Body fluids can be deposited directly onto a surface without direct contact, for example by ejaculation, spitting, blood spatter or dripping.

In general terms, during primary transfer there must be a sufficient source of DNA on the 'donor' surface and a mechanism by which transfer takes place to another surface. The particular activity being addressed within casework may indicate a suggested mechanism of transfer in the prosecution version, which must be balanced against an alternative mechanism suggested by the defence version.

Secondary transfer implies an additional interaction in the transfer process where DNA/biological material is passed from the 'donor' surface via an intermediate object or surface to the recipient surface, thus involving two mechanisms of transfer (Ladd *et al.*, 1999; Lowe *et al.*, 2002; Phipps and Petricevic 2007; Goray *et al.*, 2012; Wickenheiser, 2002). It follows that the amounts of DNA expected to be present on a surface following secondary transfer might be lower, but the question of what will be detected is heavily dependent on the abundance of DNA available to transfer in the first place (Kita *et al.*, 2008). It is also dependent upon the conditions to which the primary and intermediate surfaces/objects were subject prior to the transfer and the secondary surface/object was subject prior to sampling, since these will impact on persistence.

These issues are not straightforward because there are so many variables. A degree of casework experience helps and, again, this level of training requires mentoring and exposure to varied casework discussions. A good starting point is to assess the feasibility of the propositions. Many practitioners make the mistake of suggesting that findings are inconclusive if they describe a defence version as being possible or not excluded. But there is a difference between possible and probable. 'It is possible that I will win the National Lottery on Saturday, but it is not probable (Clayton, 2011). It is the degree of support the DNA findings provide for one version of events over the other that should be expressed. This may be quantified in a likelihood ratio or expressed in a narrative conclusion, explaining the factors considered in making the interpretation.

Sometimes findings may be too difficult to evaluate. This might be due to lack of data, lack of relevant experience (there will always be unique casework scenarios to consider) or, given the propositions being considered, the issue may be subject to too much uncertainty.

DNA Mixtures

Practitioners will by now be familiar with the 'traffic light' system of classifying profiles (Buckleton, 2009). A mixture-interpretation course should emphasise the use of this in determining which mixtures are suitable for a statistical calculation.

Mixture calculations to determine the likelihood ratio associated with a given reference profile's inclusion in a mixture are based on a probabilistic interpretation of which alleles within a mixture might be attributable to the profile of each contributor. These assessments are made based upon the relative peak heights or areas of allele pairs within a degree of tolerance dependent upon on the quality of the profile, the ratio of the quantity of DNA contributed by each putative contributor and an overview of the profile as a whole (Gill *et al.*, 1998; Clayton *et al.*, 1998). In most calculations, a number of allele combinations will be possibilities at each locus and the final likelihood ratio calculation completed by software will take account of this. The practitioner's role here is to select the allele combinations to be included in the final calculation, but the theory behind the calculation should be explained on the mixtures training course.

Many mixture calculation software packages do not take account of the probability of drop-out (R v Bates, 2006; Gill *et al.*, 2009).

Such calculations assume two contributors to a mixture. In most circumstances, any additional contributors render such calculations too difficult and much less reliable. There are a few exceptions, for example, if a third contributor is present at a considerably lower level than the two main contributors (Gill *et al.*, 2006).

Some mixture calculations allow conditioning information to be taken into account if one of the contributors is known; for example, a male–female mixture obtained from vaginal swabs where it can be assumed that the female contributor is the donor of the swabs. In such circumstances, the practitioner is faced with a simpler calculation, considering the propositions that the mixture is from the donor and suspect versus from the donor and an unknown. In an unconditioned mixture the question is different. The practitioner will likely be considering propositions that the mixture is from the suspect and an unknown verses from two unknowns.

Mixture calculations can be subjective and require a degree of judgement on behalf of the practitioner. Some practitioners will make very conservative calculations with wider acceptance criteria for the pairs of alleles they will consider as possibilities, whilst other practitioners may be quicker to rule out certain allele combinations. There is unlikely to be one correct answer in each circumstance and the value of discussion and mentored casework as follow-up to this training course cannot be emphasised enough.

In those mixtures unsuitable for calculation, it is sometimes possible to provide an opinion on the possibility of inclusion of an individual as a possible contributor, explaining that the likelihood of inclusion cannot be calculated. Again, this requires judgement on behalf of the practitioner, and care should be taken in the form of words used to describe this. Various phrases are in current use to describe these situations. Recent research (Crawford and Stangor, 2011) suggests that some forms of words are less readily understood or may be being misinterpreted by the lay reader. The issue of the probative value of matching alleles where a questioned person's reference profile is fully represented within a complex DNA mixture, in which statistical interpretation is not possible, is the subject of the Court of Appeal ruling in *Regina versus Dlugosz* (R v Dlugosz, R v Pickering and R v MDS, 2013), and makes a useful exercise for student discussion surrounding the possible approaches that may be taken in such situations. Since a likelihood ratio cannot be determined, should practitioners decide that the matching alleles are inconclusive? Alternatively, should the findings be reported as significant, with the caveat that the amount of significance (strength of evidence) cannot be determined? Other approaches include the stating of significance as being at least limited, this being the lowest and most conservative level on the verbal scale. Some practitioners advocate a subjective estimate of the level of support for inclusion, whilst others feel uncomfortable with such a qualitative evaluation of complex DNA mixtures.

To complete the practitioner's training in DNA mixture interpretation, an awareness of software packages such as *LikeLTD* (Balding, 2013) developed by Dr David Balding, which include an allowance for the frequency of drop-in and drop-out, allowing the statistical interpretation of more complex mixtures, should be included.

Specialist Techniques

A number of specialist DNA techniques are reported by experienced practitioners. Each requires additional training and competency testing.

Low Template Techniques

The increased sensitivities offered by low template techniques bring with them additional limitations. It is not possible to attribute the results of low template profiling to any specific biological material as their source. Neither is it possible to address how or when low template DNA was deposited (Hedman, 2005; Evett *et al.*, 2002).

The results of low template profiling cannot be interpreted using the guidelines applied to routine profiling results to describe peak height imbalance and artefacts. The data relating to these do not apply in low template results due to stochastic effects (sampling variation) (Buckleton, 2009; Gill *et al.*, 2009). Examples of low level profiles, run in duplicate, are a useful course material, to demonstrate the often striking differences between the two replicates due to stochastic variation (see Appendix 13.A).

A useful teaching exercise to demonstrate stochastic variation involves a large container of beads (or similar) of mainly one colour, into which small numbers of beads of differing colours in a pre-determined ratio, representing a DNA profile, have been mixed. Each trainee takes three 'samples' from the container as handfuls of beads and compares the contents of each sample. Containers of various 'dilution' can be created to represent samples with various levels of template DNA. The results of this experiment will demonstrate a greater variance in sample contents, the greater the dilution.

The phenomenon of drop-in must also be accounted for in low template profiling and samples are subject to duplicate PCRs to ensure that only repeated alleles are considered as confirmed results rather than rare drop-in events.

Given the increased sensitivity of routine DNA profiling techniques, more low level profiles are being detected than ever before. As such, some forensic providers have introduced duplicate testing into their routine profiling process, and there is an argument for treating low level profiles with the same cautious interpretation guidelines as low template results. Many samples that would have been reserved for low template techniques only a few years ago, are now yielding profiles using routine techniques, and the term 'Touch DNA' has become popular amongst police investigators and practitioners to describe the testing of these types of exhibits. This is a term that should be discouraged, since the nature of low template profiles are such that the mechanism by which the DNA was deposited cannot be determined and should not be assumed to be by touch.

Since this increased sensitivity in routine profiling is relatively new, there may be insufficient understanding amongst those practitioners who have never reported low template results. These practitioners would benefit from a low template course to explain those principles.

Relationship Testing

Another branch of forensic DNA interpretation takes advantage of the hereditary properties of DNA to address issues of relatedness. In paternity testing, the DNA profiles of a child, its mother and putative father(s) are compared. A child will inherit half its alleles from each parent and this will be manifest in its STR profile. Furthermore, if a putative father and child share less frequently encountered alleles, this gives more weight to the support for paternity. Interpretation is expressed as a percentage probability. The possibility of mutation in the father's profile is taken into account when considering exclusion. As such, fewer than a low threshold number of mismatches does not lead to exclusion, whereas, greater than the threshold number of mismatches means conclusive exclusion.

Complex relationships (sibling, half sibling, grandparent, aunt, uncle, cousin) are more difficult to establish because such individuals are not expected to share as many alleles as parent and child. Consequently, a wider selection of STRs are tested and often multiple family members' profiles are compared to address complex relationships. Results may be inconclusive and conclusive exclusion may not be possible.

Mitochondrial DNA and Y Chromosome STRs

Because of their modes of inheritance, profiling of mitochondrial DNA and the Y chromosome can assist in addressing issues of relatedness (Gill *et al.*, 2001; Jobling and King, 2003; King and Jobling, 2009).

Everyone has mitochondrial DNA, but it is inherited maternally hence only females can pass it to the next generation. This allows the tracing of the maternal branch of a family over many generations and might be applied to a complex relationship issue when testing of multiple STRs is inconclusive.

Mitochondrial DNA remains in the bones when most, if not all, sources of nuclear DNA have been lost. For this reason it is often useful in cases with unidentified remains such as mass graves or mass disaster scenarios. It may also be used in the identification of older remains.

STRs on the Y chromosome can be used to determine male line inheritance in complex relationship testing scenarios. This is also a useful test of exhibits stained with seminal fluid but where the offender is vasectomised or has a low sperm count. The technique will only provide a profile from male cells even in the presence of a higher ratio of female cells, such as might be found on a vaginal swab. As such, Y-STR analysis is increasingly considered as an option in sexual offences casework.

Familial Database Searches

The use of familial searches of intelligence databases has been pioneered in the United Kingdom, having first been used in 2002 in relation to the 1973 cold case of the murders of Pauline Floyd, Geraldine Hughes and Sandra Newton (Porter, 2011).

This technique involves the ranking of near matches to a crime stain profile, which has been searched against an intelligence database (such as the NDNAD or CODIS), not to be confused with the searching of a partial profile against a database. Near matches might indicate a biological relative of the perpetrator and ranking may be based on age and geographical location. The UK system of familial searching is based on detailed protocols and a clear approval process.

The technique is viewed as controversial in other countries, particularly the United States, where it has been legalised in a minority of states (Suter, 2010). It has, however, proved a useful tool in those states in the identification of perpetrators of high profile crimes such as the 'Grim Sleeper' serial killer case in California (Williams, 2011).

Ethnic Inferencing

Ethnic Inferencing is based on an assessment of the allele frequencies in a profile compared with those in allele databases relating to the various race codes. The feasibility of such a technique was first published as early as 1992 (Evett *et al.*, 1992). The accuracy of the technique relies on the integrity of the information contained within the racial databases used for comparison. This assumes that sample information submitted by multiple investigators is accurate in terms of the ethnicity of each sample. The technique therefore allows that this assumption cannot be reliably made and the results are probabilistic and never definitive (Lowe *et al.*, 2001).

Phenotypic Markers

Forensic DNA profiling is moving towards the analysis of genetic markers that determine physical characteristics (Kayser and Schneider, 2009). If police investigators can determine physical traits, then this has the potential to provide significant investigative information to identify an individual. These approaches are beginning to be used in criminal investigations (Soares, 2010).

In The Court of Appeal

Various questions have been asked in the UK Court of Appeal and the resultant decisions have shaped how DNA evidence is reported by practitioners in the UK Criminal Justice System. The issues range from those in the early days of DNA profiling in criminal cases, using evidence generated by techniques prior to STR profiling, when errors were made in evidential reporting, to more current issues surrounding the reporting of low level profiles and comparisons with mixtures of DNA in which no statistical interpretation is feasible. A summary of the relevant points raised in each case is presented next.

R v Deen, 1994

This rape case of R v Deen (1994) was one of the earliest challenges to DNA evidence. In the original trial, prosecuting Counsel directed the expert to commit the prosecutor's fallacy by equating the rarity of the Multilocus Probe match to the likelihood of guilt. The match was challenged – the statistical calculations being based on a false premise, leading the judge to liken the probability to a virtual certainty – as was the database upon which the calculation was based.

R v Dennis Adams, 1996 and 1997

In the original case (R v Adams, 1996), the prosecution evidence depended almost entirely on the DNA evidence. Dennis John Adams, the defendant in the case (not to be confused with Gary Adams, in R v Adams (1997), see later) was charged with rape. He had an alibi, was not picked out by the complainant in an ID parade and did not match the offender's description. The match probability of one in 200 million (in relation to a matching Single Locus Probe result) was presented as a transposed conditional. The appeal was based on the Judge's misdirection of the jury in the use of Bayes' Theorem, Adams' conviction was quashed and a retrial was ordered.

R v Doheny and R v Adams, 1997

Alan James Doheny appealed against his conviction for rape and buggery and Gary Andrew Adams appealed against his conviction for buggery (R v Doheny; R v Adams, 1997). The common grounds of appeal was the way in which the DNA evidence was presented at court. The initial DNA evidence was reported as an estimate of the relative frequency of the profile in the relevant population. This ruling coins the phrase, 'random occurrence ratio', to describe the frequency with which the matching profile is expected to be found in the general population. This was intended to refer to what is now routinely known as the match probability, which is directly derived from the Bayesian likelihood ratio, although it is occasionally referred to as the random match probability in the literature. However, the 'random occurrence ratio' is a point of contention, appearing, as it does, to encourage the practitioner to state how many people in the population would be expected to share the questioned profile. In this case, the DNA evidence was reported as an estimate of the relative frequency of the questioned profile amongst the population of sexually active males in Manchester. This commits the defender's fallacy, and such considerations risk understating the significance of the matching DNA profile.

R v Bates and Garside, 2006

In May 2005, Richard Bates and James Garside were convicted of the murder of Marilyn Garside (R v Bates, 2006). It was the prosecution's case that Garside had hired Bates to murder his estranged wife. An appeal was brought by Richard Bates on the grounds that the DNA evidence was inadmissible. The DNA evidence comprised a number of partial

DNA profiles matching Bates. At the original trial, it was explained that when calculating the significance of these partial profiles, the missing alleles had been considered to be neutral. However, the defence argued that the missing alleles should not be considered neutral, but since the frequency of drop-out of alleles could not be calculated, then neither could the match probabilities associated with the matching partial profiles. The judge rejected this argument and ruled that the DNA evidence was admissible and could be put before the jury. The Court of Appeal agreed that the approach of the judge had been correct and ruled partial profile DNA evidence admissible provided that its limitations were properly explained to the jury. It should be noted that in this case, the DNA results were low level and mixed, to the extent that the number of contributors to the mixtures could not be determined. As such, the interpretation of the matching results was agreed by the prosecution expert as being somewhat subjective. These were issues that would also be the subject of future rulings.

R v Hoey, 2007

This case concerned the low template DNA evidence in the trial of Sean Hoey, accused of the Omagh bombings (R v Hoey, 2007). When the trial collapsed due to questions about the validity of the Low Copy Number (LCN) technique, in use at the time by the former UK Forensic Science Service, the Association of Chief Police Officers announced an interim suspension of the use of LCN and the Crown Prosecution Service ordered a re-examination of pending cases containing LCN evidence. As a result, The Forensic Science Regulator instigated a review of LCN DNA, appointing Professor Brian Caddy of Strathclyde University to chair the review, supported by two DNA experts, Dr Graham Taylor of Cancer Research UK and Dr Adrian Linacre of Strathclyde University. Professor Caddy's report (Caddy, 2008) found in favour of LCN, concluding that it was a suitably robust and valid evidential technique, and the suspension of LCN DNA profiling was lifted in January 2008.

R v Reed and Reed, 2009; R v Garmson, 2010

This appeal jointly considered the reliability of LCN evidence in two cases: the murder case, R v Reed and Reed, and the rape case, R versus Garmson (R v Reed and Reed; R v Garmson, 2009). The point of contention was the stochastic threshold, that is, the amount of DNA below which stochastic effects could be expected. The Court of Appeal ruled that in cases where the quantity of DNA analysed was greater than 100–200 picograms, there should be no challenge to the methodology. In cases where DNA profiles are obtained within this range, and there is disagreement on the stochastic threshold, then expert evidence should be given as to whether a reliable interpretation can be made in the case. Low template profiles from amounts of DNA below the threshold should not be automatically considered unreliable, but it is for the defence to argue this point. It was also concluded by the Court that it was permissible for an expert to provide opinion on body fluid attribution and possible mechanisms by which the biological material might have been deposited, that is, to address activity level propositions based on low level DNA evidence, provided there was proper scientific basis for the opinion and its limitations had been made clear to the jury.

R v T, 2010

This case is not a DNA case at all, but the implications of the ruling impact on all evidence types (R v T, 2010). In the original trial, T was convicted of murder based on a matching footwear mark. The significance of the footwear mark evidence was presented in the form of a likelihood ratio (LR), providing a moderate level of scientific support for the view that the mark was made by T's shoe. T's conviction was later quashed based on the Court of Appeal's ruling on the prosecution evidence. The Court of Appeal objected to the prosecution expert using an insufficient data set, displaying a lack of transparency and using the term 'scientific support'. The prosecution expert's evidence at the original trial considered four aspects of the footwear mark: pattern, size, wear and damage. A likelihood ratio had been calculated for each aspect resulting in a combined LR of 100, equating to 'moderate support' for the view that T's shoe made the mark. The Court of Appeal considered the Forensic Science Service (FSS) database to be insufficient, that the prosecution expert had not been sufficiently transparent regarding the figures he had used and deemed that calculation of the LR had not been scientific. Despite evidence at the appeal from leading statisticians, and reports from the forensic regulator and European Network of Forensic Science Institutes (ENFSI) supporting the use of Bayes' Theorem, the Court of Appeal rejected its use in this case and ruled it unsuitable for use in further footwear mark comparison evidence. The ruling was received with dismay by the forensic science community (Redmayne *et al.*, 2011; Berger *et al.*, 2011a; Robertson, *et al.*, 2011) and a group of experts published a joint letter stating their position on the matter (Berger *et al.*, 2011b).

It was widely concluded that the court had misunderstood the Bayesian approach. They had focused on the data used to determine the LR but had criticised the LR rationale, misunderstanding that the LR reflects the fact that even for a perfect match, it does not follow that the suspect shoe made the mark, that quantification promotes transparency and that numerical quantification does not imply objectivity, rather, expert opinion requires a degree of judgement.

R v Weller, 2010

This case also challenged low level DNA evidence, but the challenge was to the mechanism of transfer of DNA rather than the profiling process, or the statistical interpretation (R v Weller, 2010). It concerned the evaluation of the activity level issue of digital penetration of the vagina rather than non-sexual contact, and the defence argued (given the previous decision in R v Reed and Reed) that in this instance there was no scientific basis for such opinion. The DNA evidence comprised a mixture of DNA from Weller's left hand fingernails, with a minor contribution of DNA matching the complainant. Various papers considering the transfer and persistence of DNA under fingernails (Cooke and Dixon, 2007; Malsom *et al.*, 2009) were cited during the trial, but the Court rejected the defence argument and concluded that it is unrealistic to provide expert testimony on an issue such as this by reference to published papers alone. Therefore, in evaluating such matters, a jury should be permitted to also take into account an expert's relevant experience. The ruling provided clarity about the information an expert can utilise, which is not limited to published work, and placed strong emphasis on the importance of practical competence, noting that the defence expert in the case was an academic rather than an expert with practical experience in this field.

R v Thomas, 2011

This is another case in which low level DNA evidence was challenged, this time involving DNA recovered from a firearm (R v Thomas, 2011). The DNA evidence comprised a DNA mixture in which the alleles in Ashley Thomas' reference profile were fully represented, but for which no statistical evaluation were possible. The point of contention between prosecution and defence was whether the evidence could be said to provide support for the view that Ashley Thomas had handled the firearm. Defence argued that the phrase 'providing support' overstated the significance of the evidence as it made the assumption that all the matching alleles had originated from one person, preferring instead, to state that Ashley Thomas could not be excluded as having contributed DNA. The prosecution expert argued that this statement, without further qualification, could be misleading and failed to provide the court with further information that could be of use to the court. An application was made to the judge to exclude the prosecution DNA evidence on the grounds that the results and opinions of the prosecution expert were unreliable. In his ruling, the judge referred to R versus Reed and Reed and allowed the prosecution expert's opinion regarding contribution to the DNA mixture. He also cited R versus Weller, in acknowledging that the prosecution expert was entitled to take into account unpublished data and expert experience.

Appeal was made on the grounds that the judge erred in refusing to exclude the DNA evidence. However, it became clear that, in the light of R versus Reed and Reed, the focus of the appeal was the use by the prosecution expert of the phrase 'provides support,' rather than the DNA evidence in its entirety. The appeal was rejected on the basis that the prosecution and defence expert's difference in opinion had been reduced to barely a distinction, the prosecution expert's concessions indicated that the evidence did not allow her to say that Thomas had handled the firearm, the judge had not erred in allowing the DNA evidence and had correctly directed the jury that it was for them to decide the weight of each expert's opinion.

R v Dlugosz, R v Pickering and R v MDS, 2013

These three cases in which each Appellant had been granted appeal based on their non-exclusion from a complex DNA mixture for which statistical evaluation was not possible, were considered together (R v Dlugosz, R v Pickering and R v MDS, 2013). The ruling did not uphold the grounds of appeal and allowed subjective evaluation of the DNA evidence in these circumstances. In an additional element to this ruling, the court decided that such subjective evaluation need not adhere to the standard verbal scale of support. The question remains as to how such subjective evaluations should be made. If experts are to use their casework experience, as previous rulings have allowed, then they should be prepared for their experience and judgement to be scrutinised.

Teaching Principles

The preparation and reporting of forensic evidence in a criminal justice system, regardless of country, is carried out within the framework of a quality management system in line with the requirements of an international quality standard, usually ISO IEC 17025:2005 (http://www.iso.org/iso/catalogue_detail?csnumber=39883). One of the requirements of the standard is that practitioners are able to demonstrate techni-cal competence within their areas of expertise. Competence is recorded and monitored in two parts. There is the gaining of initial competence and the monitoring of on-going competence. It is recommended that trainee DNA practitioners are introduced to these principles at the earliest opportunity, and understand that in training, they are working towards the gaining of initial competence. Once gained, competence is monitored at regular intervals on the basis of the ability to demonstrate the use of the skills gained at initial competence. Practitioners generally understand it is their own responsibility to monitor and maintain their competencies. The criteria for maintaining competence are based on completion of a set number of case types, as dictated by the quality manage-ment system.

Once initial competence is gained, newly qualified practitioners usually begin work on simple cases. Whilst the criteria separating simple and complex cases are not always clear, simple cases usually comprise those with small numbers of exhibits with an expec-tation of obtaining single source DNA profiles and are often reported at source level. Practitioners at this level usually go on to gain competence in mixture interpretation at a later stage. Since simple cases can readily develop into complex ones, practitioners must be aware of the limitations of their competence at each stage of their development. It is generally only those practitioners with experience of reporting complex casework who then go on to train in peer reviewing. It is also recognised by practitioners that peer reviewing, as reporting, counts towards a practitioners on-going competency.

Interpretation of casework with complex activity level propositions is time consum-ing and practitioners are encouraged to engage in regular casework discussions with colleagues. These are equally valuable for both trainee and newly competent practi-tioners to increase their exposure to the issues of complex casework at an early stage. Formalised casework reviews and workshops are also recommended for both trainees, as part of their course, and competent practitioners at all levels, in order to share good practice and discuss unusual results. These might be carried out on a regular basis within reporting teams, or as a debrief following a practitioner's recent court experi-ence, for example. Experienced practitioners should also be encouraged to take trainees to court with them, to allow trainees to observe an experienced expert deliver expert testimony.

The DNA practitioner's use of expert judgement in both investigative and evaluative case scenarios cannot be taught on a theory-based classroom course. Instead, it is learnt by experiencing a live casework environment, and for this reason, exposure to as var-ied casework as possible during both training and subsequent mentoring periods is as essential to the development of the DNA practitioner as the theoretical aspects of their course.

Appendix 13.A: Low Level Profile Examples

Example 13.A.1

A sample taken from an item handled during a robbery, profiled using ESI 17, attempting to distinguish the profile of the most recent handler, each replicate shows some variation compared with the other.

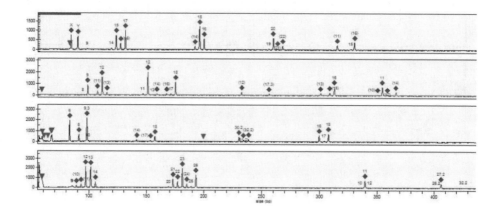

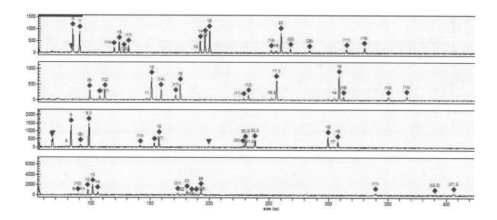

Example 13.A.2

A very low level profile at the limits of detection from a handled item. These replicates display significant drop out.

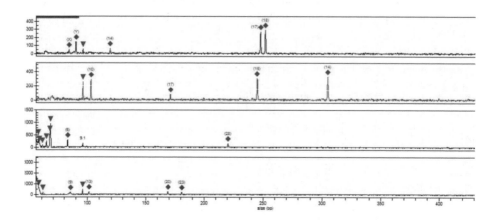

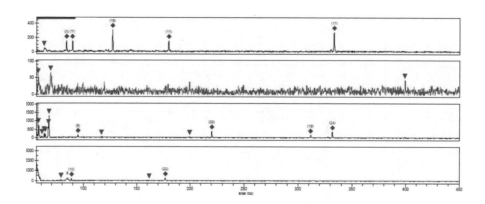

Example 13.A.3

Another set of replicates at the limits of detection, with no way to determine which, if any, of the alleles might be due to drop in events.

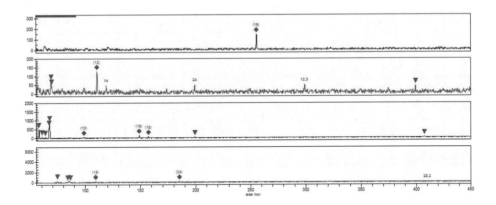

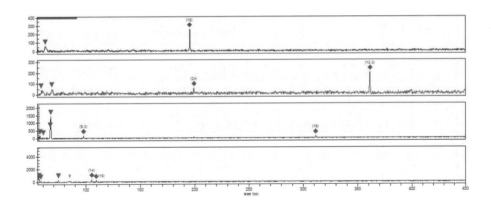

Example 13.A.4

A low level profile indicating a two person mixture.

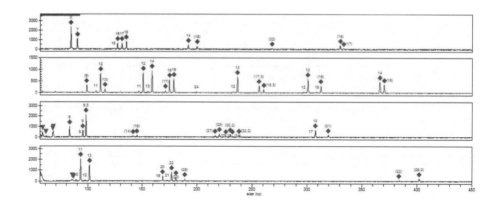

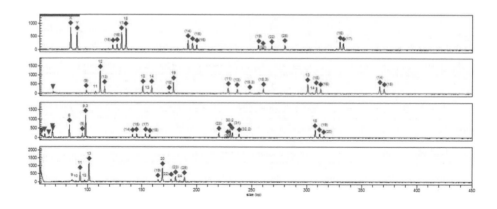

Example 13.A.5

A low level profile indicating a DNA mixture. The variation in imbalance at amelogenin between replicates means that the ratio of male to female DNA in this mixture is ambiguous.

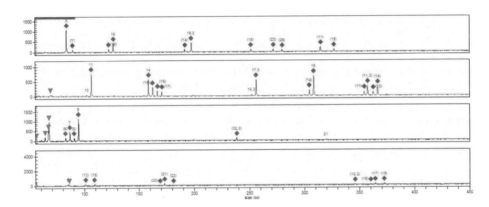

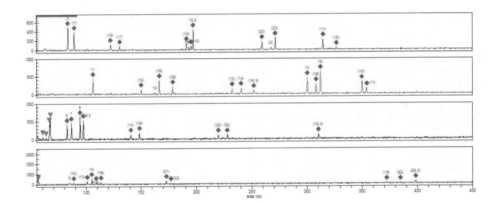

References

Archer, E., Allen, H., Hopwood, A. and Rowlands, D. (2010) Validation of a dual cycle ethylene oxide treatment technique to remove DNA from consumables used in forensic laboratories. *Forensic Science International: Genetics*, **4**, 239–243.

Balding, D.J. (1995) Estimating products in forensic identification using DNA profiles. *Journal of the American Statistical Association*, **90**, 839–844.

Balding, D.J. (1999) When can a DNA profile be regarded as unique? *Science & Justice*, **39**, 257–260.

Balding, D.J. (2013) Evaluation of mixed-source, low-template DNA profiles in forensic science, *Proceedings of the National Academy of Sciences*, **110** (30), 12241–12246.

Balding, D.J. and Donnelly, P. (1994) The prosecutor's fallacy and DNA evidence, *Criminal Law Review*, October, 711–721.

Balding, D. and Nichols, R. (1994) DNA profile match probability calculation: how to allow for population stratification, relatedness, database selection and single bands. *Forensic Science International*, **64**, 125–140.

Balding, D.J. and Donelly, P. (1995a) Inferring identity from DNA profile evidence. *Proceedings of the National Academy of Sciences USA*, **92**, 11741–11745.

Balding, D.J. and Donelly, P. (1995b) Inference in forensic identification. *Journal of The Royal Statistical Society, Series A*, **158**, 21–53.

Balding, D.J., Greenhalgh, M. and Nichols, R.A. (1986) Population genetics of STR loci in Caucasians. *International Journal of Legal Medicine*, **108**, 300–305.

Berger, C.E.H., Buckleton, J., Champod, C., Evett, I.W. and Jackson, G. (2011a) Evidence evaluation: A response to the Court of Appeal judgement in *R v T*, *Science & Justice*, **51**, 43–49.

Berger, C.E.H., Champod, J.S., Curran, C., Dawid, J. and Kloosterman, A.P (2011b) Expressing evaluative opinions: A position statement. *Science & Justice* **51**, 1–2.

Buckleton, J.S. (2009) Validation issues around DNA typing of low level DNA. *Forensic Science International: Genetics*, **3**, 25–260.

Budowle, B., Chakraborty, R., Carmody, G. and Monson, K.L. (2000) Source attribution of a forensic DNA profile. *Forensic Science Communications*, **2** (3).

Budowle, B., Onorato, A., Callaghan, T., Della Manna, A., Gross, A., Guerrieri, R., Luttman, J. and McClure, D. (2009) Mixture interpretation: defining the relevant features for guidelines for the assessment of mixed DNA profiles in forensic casework. *Journal of Forensic Science*, **54** (4), 810–821.

Caddy, B. (2008) *The Review of the Science of Low Template DNA Analysis*, UK Home Office, London.

Cook, R., Evett, I.W., Jackson, G., Jones, P.J. and Lambert, J.A. (1998a) A model for case assessment and interpretation. *Science and Justice*, **38**, 151–156.

Cook, R., Evett, I.W., Jackson, G., Jones, P.J. and Lambert, J.A. (1998b) A hierarchy of propositions: Deciding which level to address in casework. *Science & Justice*, **38** (4), 231–239.

Clayton, T. (2011) The Admissibility of Activity Level Opinions. FSSoc Body Fluids Forum, 16 September 2011.

Clayton, T.M, Whitaker, J.P., Sparkes, R. and Gill, P. (1998) Analysis and interpretation of mixed forensic stains using DNA STR profiling. *Forensic Science International*, **91**, 55–70.

Cooke, O. and Dixon, L. (2007) The prevalence of mixed DNA profiles in samples taken from individuals in the general population, *Forensic Science International: Genetics*, **1** (1), 62–68.

Crawford, C. and Stangor, C. (2011) Issues with jurors incorrectly interpreting DNA evidence. FSSoc DNA Conference, September 2011.

Easteal, P.W. and Simon Easteal, S. (1990) *The Forensic Use of DNA Profiling*, Australian Institute of Criminology, Canberra, November, ISBN 0 642 15760 X ISSN 0817-8542.

Evett, I.W. (1992) Evaluating DNA profiles in a case where the defence is 'It was my brother.' *Journal of the Forensic Science Society*, **32**, 5–14.

Evett, I.W. (1995) Avoiding the transposed conditional. *Science & Justice*, **35**, 127–131.

Evett, I.W., Pinchin, R. and Buffery, C. (1992) An investigation of the feasibility of inferring ethnic origin from DNA profiles. *Journal of the Forensic Science Society*, **32**, 301–306.

Evett, I.W., Gill, P.D., Scranage, J.K. and Weir, B.S. (1996) Establishing the robustness of STR statistics for forensic applications. *American Journal of Human Genetics*, **58**, 398–407.

Evett, I.W., Foreman, L.A., Jackson, G. and Lambert, J.A. (2000a) DNA profiling: A discussion of issues relating to the reporting of very small match probabilities. *Criminal Law Review*, May **2000**, 341–355.

Evett, I.W., Jackson, G. and Lambert, J.A. (2000b) More on the hierarchy of propositions: exploring the distinction between explanations and propositions. *Science & Justice*, **40** (1), 3–10.

Evett, I.W., Gill, P.D., Jackson, G., Whitaker, J. and Champod, C. (2002) Interpreting small quantities of DNA: the hierarchy of propositions and the use of Bayesian networks. *Journal of Forensic Science*, **47**, 520–530.

Foreman, L.A., Smith, A.F.M. and Evett, I.W. (1997) Bayesian Analysis of DNA profiling data in forensic investigation applications (with discussion). *Journal of The Royal Statistical Society, Series A*, **160**, 429–469.

Foreman, L.A., Smith, A.F.M. and Evett, I.W. (1999) Bayesian validation of a Quadruplex STR profiling system for identification purposes. *Journal of Forensic Sciences*, **44**, 478–486.

Foreman, L.A. and Evett, I.W. (2001) Statistical analysis to support forensic interpretations of a new ten-locus STR profiling system. *International Journal of Legal Medicine*, **114**, 147–155.

Gill, P., Sparkes, R., Pinchin, R., Clayton, T., Whitaker, J. and Buckleton, J. (1998) Interpreting simple STR mixtures using allele peak areas. *Forensic Science International*, **91**, 41–53.

Gill, P., Brenner, C., Brinkman, B. *et al.* (2001) DNA Commission of the International Society of Forensic Genetics: recommendations on forensic analysis using Y-chromosome STRs. *Forensic Science International*, **124**, 5–10.

Gill, P., Brenner, C.H. and Buckleton, J.S. *et al.* (2006) DNA commission of the International Society of Forensic Genetics: Recommendations on the interpretation of mixtures, *Forensic Science International* **160**, 90–101.

Gill, P., Puch-Solis, R. and Curran, J. (2009) The low template DNA (stochastic) threshold: Its determination relative to risk analysis for national DNA databases. *Forensic Science International: Genetics*, **3** (2), 104–111.

Goray, M., Mitchell, J. and Van Oorschot, R. (2012) Evaluation of multiple transfer of DNA using mock case scenarios. *Legal Medicine*, **14**, 40–46.

Graham, E.A.M. (2005) Automated DNA profile analysis. *Forensic Science, Medicine, and Pathology* **1** (4), 285–288.

Green, R.L., Roinestad, I.C., Boland, C. and Hennessy, L.K. (2005) Developmental validation of the Quantifiler™ real-time PCR kits for the quantification of human nuclear DNA samples. *Journal of Forensic Science*, **50**, 809–825.

Hedman, J. (2005) Extended Survey on LCN Analysis in DNA WG Laboratories. 22nd Meeting of the European Network of Forensic Science Institutes (ENFSI), DNA Working Group.

Himmelreich, C. (2009) Germany's phantom serial killer: A DNA blunder. *Time World*, Friday, March 27.

Hulme, P., Lewis, J. and Davidson, G. (2013) Sperm elution: An improved two phase recovery method for sexual assault samples, *Science & Justice*, **53**, (1), 28–33.

Jobling, M.A. and King, T.E. (2003) The distribution of Y-chromosomal haplotypes: forensic implications. *Progress in Forensic Genetics*, **10**, 70–72.

Kayser, M. and Schneider, P.M. (2009) DNA-based prediction of human externally visible characteristics in forensics: Motivations, scientific challenges and ethical considerations. *Forensic Science International; Genetics*, **3**, 154–161.

King, T.E. and Jobling, M.A. (2009) What's in a name? Y Chromosomes, surnames and the genetic geneology revolution. *Trends in Genetics*, **25** (8), 351–360.

Kita, T., Yamaguchi, H., Yokoyama, M., Tanaka, T. and Tanaka, N. (2008) Morphological study of fragmented DNA on touched objects. *Forensic Science International: Genetics*, **3**, 32–36.

Ladd, C., Adamowicz, M.S., Bourke, M.T., Scherczinger, C.A. and Lee, H.C. (1999) A Systematic Analysis of Secondary DNA Transfer. *Journal of Forensic Science*, **44** (6), 1270–1272.

Lowe, A.L., Urquhart, A., Foreman, L.A. and Evett, I.W. (2001) Inferring ethnic origin by means of an STR profile. *Forensic Science International*, **119**, 17–21.

Lowe, A., Murray, C., Whitaker, J., Tully, G. and Gill, P. (2002) The propensity of individuals to deposit DNA and secondary transfer of low level DNA from individuals to inert surfaces. *Forensic Science International*, **129**, 25–34.

Malsom, S., Flanagan, N., McAlister, C. and Dixon, L. (2009) The prevalence of mixed DNA profiles in fingernail samples taken from couples who co-habit using autosomal and Y-STRs, *Forensic Science International: Genetics*, **3** (2), 57–62.

McLaren, R.S., Bourdeau-Heller, J., Patel, J. *et al.* (2014) Developmental validation of the PowerPlex® ESI 16/17 Fast and PowerPlex® ESX 16/17 Fast Systems, *Forensic Science International: Genetics* **13**, 195–205.

Phipps, M. and Petricevic, S. (2007) The tendency of individuals to transfer DNA to handled items. *Forensic Science International*, **168**, 162–168.

Porter, L. (2011) *Cold Case Files*, Macmillan Publishers, 1 May 2011 pp. 41.

R v Adams [1996] 2 Cr. App. R. 467 and *R v Dennis Adams* (No 2) [1998] 1 Cr. App. R. 377.

R v Bates [2006] EWCA Crim 1395.

R v Deen, The Times, 10 January 1994.

R v Doheny; *R v Adams* [1997] 1 Cr. App. R. 369.

R v Dlugosz, R v Pickering and *R v MDS* [2013] EWCA Crim 2.

R v Hoey [2007] NICC 49, 20 December, 2007.

R v Reed and *Reed, R v Garmson* [2009] EWCA Crim 2698, [2010] 1 Cr. App. R. 23.

R v T [2010] EWCA Crim 2439.

R v Thomas [2011] EWCA Crim 1295.

R v Weller [2010] EWCA Crim 1876.

Redmayne, M., Roberts, P., Aitken, C. and Jackson, G. (2011) Forensic science evidence in question, *Criminal Law Review*, **5**, 347–356.

Robertson, B., Vigneaux, G.A. and Berger, C.E.H. (2011) Extending the confusion about Bayes, *Modern Law Review*, **74**, 430–455.

Saiki, R.K., Gelfand, D.H., Stoffel, S. *et al.* (1988) Primer-directed enzymatic amplification of DNA with a thermostable DNA polymerase. *Science*, **29**, 293(4839), 487–491.

Soares, C. (2010) Portrait in DNA: Can forensic analysis yield police-style sketches of suspects? *Scientific American*, May 2010.

Suter, S.M. (2010) All in the family: Privacy and DNA familial searching, *Harvard Journal of Law & Technology*, **23** (2), Spring.

Temco, N. (2008) Germany's hunt for the murderer known as 'the woman without a face.' *The Observer*, Sunday 9 November.

The ENCODE Project Consortium (2012) An integrated encyclopaedia of DNA elements in the human genome, *Nature*, **489**.

Triggs, C.M., Buckleton, J.S. and Walsh, S.J. (2004) *Forensic DNA Evidence Interpretation*, CRC Press, Baco Raton, p. 52.

Walsh, P.S., Erlich, H.A. and Higuchi, R. (1992) Preferential PCR amplification of alleles: Mechanisms and solutions. *PCR Methods and Applications*, **1**, 241–250.

Wickenheiser, R.A. (2002) Trace DNA: A review, discussion of theory, and application of the transfer of trace quantities of DNA through skin contact. *Journal of Forensic Science*, **47** (3), 442–450.

Williams, D.A. (2011) Recent developments in forensic DNA, *Genomics Law Report*, February 2011.

14

The Forensic Investigation of Sexual Offences: Practitioner Course Design and Delivery

Sue Carney

Ethos Forensics, Manchester, UK and University of Central Lancashire, UK

Introduction

Sexual offence cases are complex. They comprise a wide range of circumstances, exhibits and evidence types. As such, it is impossible for the forensic trainer to prepare the trainee practitioner for every scenario they will encounter. Interpretations are frequently affected by the limitations of current body fluid testing techniques, the presence of DNA mixtures and by uncertainty when crucial aspects of case conditioning information are unknown. For these reasons, the principles of forensic interpretation and exposure to a wide range of cases are crucial aspects of practitioner training in this area. Sexual offences cases are not for every practitioner. Some find the circumstances of these cases too distressing or embarrassing. The trainee practitioner must quickly become accustomed to discussing sexual acts and genital anatomy with colleagues and police officers, yet this is a hurdle that some find impossible to overcome. Some degree of sexual experience is useful in these situations. A sense of humour is essential.

Starting Points

Sexual offence casework is not for everyone. As they begin their body fluids training, some practitioners decide not to report on sex cases. This is fine. For those who do, a gentle introduction to the often disturbing and occasionally unexpected world of sexual offences casework is recommended.

Transfer is a fundamental aspect of forensic science, as Locard's Exchange Principle (Locard, 1930) that 'every contact leaves a trace,' tells us. Furthermore, in a sexual offence case, evidence is particularly time-sensitive such that issues of persistence, and the factors affecting persistence, require assessment on a case-by-case basis. Mechanisms of transfer and persistence make a good starting point for training in this area, followed by

Forensic Science Education and Training: A Tool-kit for Lecturers and Practitioner Trainers, First Edition.
Edited by Anna Williams, John P. Cassella, and Peter D. Maskell.
© 2017 John Wiley & Sons Ltd. Published 2017 by John Wiley & Sons Ltd.

detailed training in search and identification techniques for the various evidence types, and discussion of their limitations.

Evidence Types

The majority of the relevant evidence types in sexual offence cases are biological materials, commonly and sometimes erroneously referred to as body fluids. Semen is an obvious indicator of sexual activity and might be considered the evidence of choice in a rape case, but saliva is also commonly encountered when dealing with oral sex allegations or if, for example, kissing or biting is alleged. Transferred blood is a consideration if there is injury or the complainant is menstruating. There are presumptive chemical tests for all of these body fluids. Some are more sensitive than others and they are limited by common, often inconvenient, substances that also react with the test reagents.

Semen testing is generally a two-stage process. The presumptive test (Kind, 1964) indicates the presence of acid phosphatase (AP) in seminal fluid and can be used for screening clothing and bedding items. Many organisations traditionally operate a 2-minute test duration, but recent work (Redhead and Brown, 2013) suggests an extended test time may be beneficial in the screening of absorbent items.

On the identification of a stain indicating the presence of acid phosphatase, biological material is extracted from the stained fabric or swab head and viewed using high magnification microscopy, to search for spermatozoa.

Occasionally, objects on microscope slides are difficult to interpret. A microscope slide represents a three dimensional layer of material, albeit a thin layer, that is being viewed in two dimensions. If an object such as a sperm cell is rotated, for example it is perpendicular to the plane of view, then it may not display the typical characteristics of a sperm cell and may not be readily recognised when viewed.

Vaginal cells can be considered an evidence type, yet whilst they are a good source of DNA, there is no reliable chemical test in current use to identify them. This is a common limitation of sexual offence case interpretation. In terms of their appearance, vaginal epithelial cells are indistinguishable from epithelial cells from other body orifices. Therefore, in casework, the circumstances of the case play a significant role in determining the value of finding epithelial cells and how their presence can be interpreted.

Sexual assault forensic training should also consider the transfer of faeces and urine. Whilst these are less frequently encountered in practice and they contain little DNA, their chemical tests have higher specificity than those used for the commonly tested body fluids. It is a surprise to some that faeces are rarely detected on penile swabs in an anal rape allegation. Poor persistence of material transferred to the penis may be a factor.

In addition to body fluid evidence, hairs and fibres are another consideration. Traditionally, some aspects of hair identification are included in the remit of the forensic biologist, including considerations of ethnicity, type of hair and suitability for DNA profiling. Conversely, in body fluids training, fibre recovery is taught but analysis and interpretation tend to comprise a complex specialism of their own, although some forensic biologists later expand their skills to include fibre comparison.

The forensic practitioner must also have an awareness of other physical evidence types. On occasion, the presence of a footwear mark, or glass fragments for example, within a sexual assault case exhibit may call for collaboration between practitioners from multiple disciplines. As such, a detailed awareness of other evidence types should be part of the forensic biologist's training and the body fluids expert should learn when to antic-ipate these and know when consultation with a colleague is required to ensure evidence is preserved.

It is useful if these early aspects of training are conducted as a combination of lectures and laboratory practical sessions. The classroom aspects are recommended to include comprehensive knowledge of the constituents of biological materials and theory, includ-ing the limitations, of chemical testing. Many of the routine tests are presumptive rather than confirmatory. A thorough knowledge of false positives for each test should be pro-vided and details of the confirmatory tests should be learnt, despite these being rarely used.

Most UK forensic providers employ both forensic examiners and reporting officers. It is the current convention that the reporting officer is responsible for interpreting forensic findings and providing an expert opinion to the criminal justice system, whilst the examiner is a search and recovery specialist, carrying out detailed examinations of exhibits based on instructions from a reporting officer. The theory behind body fluid chemical tests, search processes and extraction techniques can be consolidated by a course of laboratory practical sessions. This is the most crucial aspect for those trainee practitioners who will become forensic examiners. However, gaining competency in these techniques is just as important for those practitioners intending to progress to reporting. An understanding of how testing is performed is critical to writing an effec-tive examination strategy. The order of examination must be carefully planned if multi-ple evidence types are expected. Many body fluid screening processes are wet tests and may impact on other evidence types. The correct order of testing avoids loss or compro-mise of other evidence. Furthermore, most reporting officers should feel uncomfortable instructing an examiner to carry out a test they do not have the ability to perform them-selves. Each process learnt in laboratory practical sessions should be subject to multiple rounds of practice before the trainee completes an assessed process that counts towards gaining competency.

The Body as a Crime Scene: Information from the Forensic Medical Examination

By now, the trainee practitioner will have a good understanding of identification pro-cesses for the major biological evidence types and an awareness of the physical evidence they must also take into account. Persistence of material on the various areas of the body and the factors affecting those persistence times is crucial in the development of a sound forensic strategy.

The Persistence Distribution

Persistence can be viewed as a distribution of frequency of evidence detection against time (Davies and Wilson, 1974). At the extremes of this distribution, there are few inci-dences of detection, the outliers. Within casework, evidence is rarely recovered at the shorter timescales, most likely due to few cases being reported that quickly, and is rarely detected as timescales begin to increase towards maximum persistence times. The spread of incidences of detection depends on the area of the body from which the evidence is recovered. For example, in the vagina, semen has been detected as long as 10 days after intercourse. However, the practitioner should remember that semen is not always expected to be found on vaginal swabs taken after 10 days. It is likely that those 10-day detection incidences are outliers, due to specific circumstances such as hospitalisation, causing decreased vaginal drainage due to the complainant lying down for a number of days, for example.

Factors accelerating drainage of semen from the vagina include washing, menstrual and traumatic bleeding, and urination. It should be remembered that semen lost from the vulva via washing and wiping may be replenished from semen that continues to drain from the internal vagina within persistence timeframes. Therefore, that washing has occurred should not be taken to mean that all the semen has been lost (Brayley-Morris *et al.*, 2015).

Details of persistence times are widely available in the literature (Davies and Wilson, 1974; Willott and Allard, 1982; Allard, 1996; Davies, 1982) and the Faculty of Forensic and Legal Medicine, in conjunction with Association of Chief Police Officers (ACPO) and the major UK forensic science providers, publish recommendations (Recommendations for the Collection of Forensic Specimens from Complaints and Suspects, 2016) for the collection of forensic specimens. These include timescales and other details pertinent to the collection of medical samples. Some of the timescales could be construed as rather optimistic, but the guidelines are formulated with the philosophy that it may be better to take a sample at the forensic medical examination just in case, rather than miss a forensic opportunity.

The FME is a Source of Information

Much of the information gained by the Forensic Medical Examiner (FME) during a complainant's forensic medical examination also conditions the interpretation of the forensic findings, so there is value in the transfer of this information from clinician to scientist. Most scientists request a copy of the FME's paperwork (usually the MEDX form) from the examination. The inclusion of the MEDX form in a sexual offence forensic submission is suggested as good practice to police forensic submissions departments.

The forensic scientist is not routinely present at the forensic medical examination, but an understanding of what takes place is vital knowledge. Input from a forensic medical examiner during practitioner training can provide useful explanations of anatomical terms commonly used by clinicians that might be unfamiliar to the forensic scientist. Use of descriptive medical terms is variable amongst FMEs. This is also a useful opportunity for the FME to learn which medical terms are commonly misunderstood, how the evidence they recover is interpreted and how effective their swabbing techniques are. Communication between the FME and the forensic practitioner may be unprecedented in the current forensic culture, but is to be encouraged to facilitate mutual understanding and sharing of best practice.

Explanation from an FME detailing exactly how and from where samples are taken will be a useful aspect of the forensic scientist's education. For example, vaginal swabs are usually taken in duplicate from three areas of the vagina: external (vulval), low and high vaginal swabs. Given that the vagina is approximately 10 cm long, the forensic scientist might mistakenly expect low vaginal swabs to be taken approximately 5 cm inside the vagina. In actual fact, most FMEs take low vaginal swabs from just inside the labia, approximately 1–2 cm internally. This detail changes most practitioners' expectations of where semen detection might be expected, particularly in a case of ejaculation outside the vagina and might affect their interpretation of the findings. That semen can transfer to the low vaginal region without ejaculation inside the vagina has implications for the evidential significance of finding semen on low vaginal swabs in the absence of semen on high vaginal swabs. These issues are best learnt through the practice of case assessment and interpretation (Cook *et al.*, 1998a) of complex sexual offence scenarios involving a number of alternative defence versions of events (refer to Appendix 14.A).

Occasionally, endocervical swabs are also taken. These are particularly useful in those cases where timeframes are at the extremes of expected persistence, perhaps due to a delay in reporting an incident. Expectations of finding semen in these cases are low.

The Speculum Issue

Other details of the medical examination can affect interpretation of forensic findings. For example, the use of a speculum during the taking of vaginal swabs can determine whether the forensic practitioner is able to interpret semen found in the high vaginal region as having been deposited there by ejaculation inside the vagina (if a speculum has been used) versus the possibility of it having been carried inside on a swab as it passes through semen-stained regions of the vulva and low vagina (if no speculum is used). The result of these variations in procedure might affect the scientist's ability to address the issue of penetration, and ultimately, in some cases might mean the difference between a charge of rape and sexual assault.

Similar considerations should be given to the use of the proctoscope for the taking of anal samples although, due to the structure of the proctoscope, it is accepted that its use may not fully prevent contamination of the rectum by semen from external regions.

Why Take Control Swabs?

In the author's opinion, control swabs are a subject of much debate amongst students and practitioners. There are two reasons for control swabs. One is to establish the DNA-free status of swabs used during forensic collections, for which a blank swab can be exhibited. The other is to establish background levels of transferred material. The selection of an appropriate control swab in these circumstances requires some thought and reference to the specifics of the case, paying particular attention to the defence version. If a defence version is not yet available, as is likely at the time of the complainant's medical examination, the medical examiner may need to anticipate the possibilities. Here is an example.

Consider a complainant alleging she was gripped on the bare arm by her attacker. Visible bruising can be seen on her arm at the site of the alleged contact. If the purpose of the forensic intervention is to identify a possible offender via recovered DNA, then the medical examiner should swab the site of the bruising to recover transferred DNA, assuming the medical examination falls within accepted time limits for persistence of transferred material on the surface of the skin – say no later than 24 hours after the alleged incident – and the complainant has not bathed/washed. However, consider the possible later, evaluative stages of this case, in which a suspect has been identified.

The value of a control swab to measure background DNA in these circumstances is dependent on the suspect's version of events. If the suspect denies any contact with the complainant, it may be that a control swab is irrelevant. However, should the suspect provide an alternative that might account for transfer of his DNA, a control swab, from a similar but unaffected area, may assist in specifically addressing this issue.

In most instances, the defence version, if any, will be unknown at the time of the medical examination. The FME is called upon to make a judgement based on what the defence version might be, in order to select the appropriate control site. It may be impractical to take a relevant control swab relative to every site of injury presented, but the FME is encouraged to discuss the options with a forensic scientist at the time. The common practice of taking a background control swab from between the shoulder blades demonstrates a lack of understanding on the part of the FME of the purpose of the control swab in the overall forensic strategy.

Setting the Strategy

For the reporting forensic practitioner, setting the forensic strategy is the most fundamental part of every case. An effective strategy can determine whether a case is worth examining and if so, the potential outcomes, and all this before any exhibits have been unpackaged.

Forensic strategy setting is much more than deciding which exhibits to examine. Yes, the forensic strategy includes an examination strategy, incorporating what has been learnt about testing and order of tests, but there are many other details to consider. The forensic strategy penetrates into the fundamental reasons for testing and dictates the purpose of the case itself.

Case Assessment and Interpretation

The case assessment and interpretation (CAI) model (Cook *et al.*, 1998a) developed by the Forensic Science Service is widely used in forensic casework. The CAI model relies on principles of transparency, robustness, balance and logic.

First and foremost, the model allows for a distinction between investigative and evaluative cases, such that practitioners can be working in one of two modes of thinking. Sexual offence cases offer a ready supply of both case types.

Investigative cases are usually those with no suspect, such as the stranger rape case. The forensic expert seeks evidence in order to postulate a suitable scenario for the incident, to explain the findings, or to identify a suspect. Evaluative cases are those with, usually, two versions of events: one describing what is alleged and the other provided by the suspect as his defence. It is worth noting here that complex cases may contain a mixture of investigative and evaluative questions. For example, those cases in which the complainant has no memory of events but there is a suspicion of sexual assault. Whilst an alternative version of events might be available from the suspect, the case can be treated as investigative if the scientist's remit is to establish what took place.

Working in evaluative mode, this Bayesian system allows forensic practitioners to use inference to determine the value of their evidence in modifying the prior probability of a scenario into a posterior probability. The weight of evidence is determined by the likelihood ratio, which can be estimated using the CAI model.

The CAI model dictates: that it is the probability of the scientific findings (the evidence) that should be considered, not the probability of a particular scenario; that the evidence must be considered in terms of two alternatives or competing propositions, and it should take into account the framework of information surrounding the case (the conditioning information).

The Hierarchy of Propositions

Selecting the most appropriate propositions can be a difficult decision. There is often more than one pair of alternatives to be considered in a case. The CAI model assists here by its description of a hierarchy of propositions (Cook *et al.*, 1998b; Evett *et al.*, 2000). Consider an alleged rape in which forensic experts have examined the complainant's vaginal swabs. The forensic practitioner, on finding semen that yields a DNA profile matching the suspect, might report these findings as support for the view that the semen on the swabs is from the suspect. Whilst this source level conclusion is a useful piece of information to the court, the forensic scientist can add another layer of interpretation by addressing activity level. At activity level, in addressing how and when evidence is deposited, the conditioning information comes into play, along with the practitioner's knowledge of transfer and persistence of evidence. In addressing whether the finding of matching semen supports the assertion that the suspect engaged in sexual intercourse with the complainant, the scientist must also consider how likely the findings are given the suspect's version of events. Moreover, the suspect's version may not always be a straightforward denial of the act and the expert must consider if there are other mechanisms by which the matching semen could have been deposited. These, if there are any, must also agree with the known conditioning information – time since intercourse, washing information, and so on, and the principles of transfer and persistence.

Frequently, the defence version is simply 'no comment.' Practitioners have previously chosen to deal with this by nominating a defence version. Caution should be exercised here. What if the chosen defence version is one that maximises the likelihood ratio? This approach would seem unfairly biased against the defendant. However, other alternatives may not be so readily apparent and it would be equally unfair to the complainant to suggest a defence version that minimises the likelihood ratio.

A different approach, and one which seems to have gained favour with practitioners in recent years, is to provide some observations in the absence of a defence alternative, making clear that the evidence has not, at this stage, been fully interpreted. The onus is then on the defence to provide an alternative to enable full evaluation of the evidence.

The highest level in the hierarchy is offence level. There are difficulties in addressing offence level in our example case. Rape is defined in The Sexual Offences Act of 2003 (UK Government Legislation, 2003), as penile penetration of the vagina, mouth or anus, where the complainant does not consent and the perpetrator does not reasonably believe the complainant consents. The scientific findings in the case do not assist in addressing consent, therefore they cannot reasonably be considered to assist in addressing offence level propositions.

Most forensic practitioners agree that activity level is the most appropriate level for expert interpretation, offence level being perceived as the sole realm of the court. The practice of reverting to source level for particularly difficult interpretations is frequently encountered. In the opinion of the author, this practice is questionable. The forensic practitioner, having a deeper understanding of the mechanisms of transfer and persistence, is much better equipped than the jury to provide a meaningful opinion on activity level questions. The alternative is to allow the court to infer activity level conclusions, but there is a risk that in such circumstances, conclusions will be reached without the proper considerations of background data or experience, and an increased risk of miscarriages of justice.

The CAI model requires careful and in-depth teaching. The CAI course is often spoken about in hushed tones by forensic practitioners. Few trainees report enjoying it and many cite it as the most difficult aspect of their training. On a more positive note, some report experiencing a 'lightbulb moment' as their understanding 'clicks.' There is criticism of the model by some practitioners and a lack of understanding amongst others, yet many practitioners are unknowingly using the principles of CAI in evaluating evidence, not realising that the formalised method provides a means of documenting their thought processes.

Why is CAI so often viewed in such a negative light? Perhaps because it relies so heavily on evaluating probabilities based on, or so it feels, little more than a whim, rather than scientific data. In actuality, these evaluations are more than whimsy. As practitioners' experience increases, so too does their ability to evaluate their expectations. Perhaps the negativity stems from what feels like documenting the obvious. In so-called 'simple cases,' practitioners often question why they need to document their expectations. However, it is these simple cases that inevitably develop into complex problems very quickly. Indeed, one of the biggest criticisms of forensic reporters is their failure to fully document and regularly revisit the case strategy.

The CAI training course (refer to Appendix 14.A) should include a thorough explanation of Bayes' Theorem, but with sufficient background explanations of probability theory. Pre-course reading with mathematics exercises is useful to ensure sufficient mathematical ability. The inclusion of break out discussion groups, each with its own tutor, is a useful way to ensure that all trainees contribute to discussion of example strategies. Course tutors are also useful in determining which trainees are struggling to grasp the concepts of CAI.

Dealing with Uncertainty

It should be accepted by the practitioner that in some sexual offence cases, there are likely to be pieces of conditioning information that are unavailable and, as such, some allowance must be made in considering expectations of the laboratory findings and evaluating the LR (likelihood ratio). Whilst such considerations in the face of uncertainty might be difficult for some students, the use of numerical probabilities should be encouraged throughout training. Practitioners who advocate the use of descriptive terms, such as low, medium and high, to document their expectations, cannot be sure of consistency, since such terms are not readily defined. One practitioner's 'medium' may not equate to another's, whereas numbers, by their very nature, readily indicate the relative magnitude of expectations.

Interpretation of Findings

Proficiency in strategy setting prepares the practitioner for making their interpretation. Indeed, a significant proportion of the hard work has already been done in estimating the LR for each potential outcome in a case. 'Simple! Plug in the relevant likelihood ratio from your strategy and there's your conclusion?' suggests the eager trainee practitioner. They are half right, but there are other factors to consider. Let us back track a little.

The Reporter–Examiner Relationship

A thorough assessment of the case has been made. The practitioner has identified whether the case is investigative or evaluative. They have identified the issue(s) to be addressed, selected the relevant exhibits and set an examination strategy. During the course of examinations there are many decisions to be made. The reporter may wish to witness some of the chemical tests, particularly AP reaction time and intensity of colour, since examination photographs are not always representative of these. The examination of some exhibits may be dependent on the condition and structure of the item. For example, identifying areas on an item of clothing alleged to have been touched by an offender, in order to sample for DNA, may take into account information provided by the complainant, usually in terms of the area of her body that was touched over clothing. Often, it is only on examination of the clothing item itself that it is feasible to try to identify those areas of the item. The type of fabric may also be a factor in consideration of which areas to sample. Cooperation and discussion between the reporter and examiner in such circumstances is valuable, remembering that all discussions should be fully documented on the case file.

Some examination strategies may be staged and conditional: if outcome A is achieved, then examine item B, and so forth. Such examinations will usually require the examiner to provide regular updates to the reporter, so that next step decisions can be made.

Stain Selection and Body Fluid Attribution

Selection of samples or identified stains for DNA testing also requires discussion. There may be a delay while the reporter and examiner assess the sperm head counts on microscope slides, for example. Factors to consider will include which samples are likely to give a good DNA result and which will be of most probative value, as dictated by the case assessment and the results of chemical testing. Anticipation of body fluid attribution is a factor here. It may be crucial to the evidential significance of a finding that the DNA detected can be attributed to a particular body fluid. This may not be possible in the event that a weak chemical reaction to a presumptive test has been obtained, when considering possible false positives coupled with the location of the stain on an exhibit. Even after these points have been considered, the results of DNA testing may also impact on the issue of body fluid attribution. Obtaining a mixture of DNA or a weak, low level DNA profile, may prevent attribution to a particular body fluid.

These issues are complex and cannot be taught. Rather, the forensic practitioner must use their knowledge of body fluid testing and CAI to determine probative value on a case-by-case, item-by-item, basis. The practitioner will learn by doing. The value of casework discussions and mentoring by senior colleagues cannot be underestimated here, and the inexperienced practitioner should be encouraged to broaden their exposure to as wide a range of sexual offence case scenarios as possible. Every case is a learning opportunity, even for the most experienced reporting scientist.

Dealing with Unexpected Results

Inevitably, there will be cases where outcomes of testing are unusual and unexpected, even when the most thorough case assessment has been carried out. Remember those outliers? It may be that an outcome at the extreme of expectations raises questions about the conditioning information, although other possible causes, such as contamination, should be ruled out first.

In some circumstances, a lack of data or casework experience may mean that expectations considered at case assessment are truly unknown. There is always the option to perform experiments on which to base expectations, if time allows. Examples might include: trying to recreate damage to clothing to address if what is observed fits with the alleged cause (in fact, this is not unusual and often forms part of a routine damage examination); and addressing issues relating to body fluid transfer and persistence, such as semen drying times on skin or assessing speed of vaginal drainage. Disclosure of such experiments in casework statements should be transparent and disclose the limitations of the study. Often, such studies are not comprehensive, focusing, as they do, on a very specific question raised by a single case. If the studies are carried out responsibly, and include suitable controls, then this should not lessen their significance to that particular case.

Negative Findings

Owing to the nature of sexual activity, an absence of evidence, as a general rule, does not translate as support for the defence proposition. Since sexual intercourse can occur without ejaculation, semen-free vaginal swabs does not infer that sex did not take place, and can be treated as a neutral outcome. However, there may be some instances when an absence of evidence is supportive of the defence hypothesis and the practitioner should evaluate each negative outcome based on their previous LR considerations. For example, in a scenario where intercourse is alleged, without the use of a condom, an absence of semen on vaginal swabs can be considered neutral, but an absence of DNA matching the complainant on the inner surface of suspect's underwear, worn immediately after the alleged incident and with no opportunity for washing, could be considered to support the defence versions, should that describe no sexual contact with the complainant.

Writing the Statement

Report and statement writing takes practice! Workshops, in which trainee practitioners have the chance to write practice statements, both individually and in groups, work well (refer to Appendix 14.B). The basics of standard statement layout are not difficult concepts to learn, but there are more subtle learning points: explaining scientific interpretation to the lay audience, writing in an unambiguous manner, the avoidance of emotive words and, perhaps the most difficult, developing a personal style of writing.

Writing for the Lay Person

Most forensic science is not hard science. The technical details of DNA profiling, body fluid testing and the principles of transfer and persistence can be explained in a technical issues section, in an appendix or via the use of footnotes. However, it's easy for the forensic practitioner to fall into the trap of using jargon. This might even include words that, to the lay person, have a slightly different meaning. Take for example the following phrase frequently used in the results section of statements to describe the process of intimate swab examination:

'The vaginal swabs were extracted and spermatozoa were found.'

To the forensic practitioner, the verb, to extract, refers to the chemical treatment of a swab or other exhibit to recover evidence, such as spermatozoa. However, to the lay person, to extract means to pull out, take out or draw out. The use of this phrase might therefore raise the question, 'What were the swabs extracted from?' Whilst this simplistic example could be described merely as a piece of pedantry, and it is unlikely in this instance that the lay reader would misunderstand the concept of swab extraction, it illustrates the point that the obvious meaning to the expert may not be so obvious to the reader. A basic principle, therefore, that must be learnt by the trainee practitioner is to say exactly what you mean. A better form of words in this example might be:

'Spermatozoa were found in material extracted from the vaginal swabs.'

Technical Explanations

The trainee practitioner should practice their lay explanations of scientific concepts. This is useful, not only for statement writing, but for presentation of evidence in court. Most practitioners build up a collection of written technical paragraphs describing mechanisms of transfer and testing processes. It's common for these to be shared amongst groups of practitioners working together, to build up a technical issues library. This can be a very useful exercise in sharing experience and good practice but there is also an inherent risk. To save time, many practitioners will search for an appropriate technical paragraph and paste it into their statement without a moment's thought. The time saving is not the issue here, but the lack of thought can have an impact. Technical paragraphs should have a specific bearing on the case. If a practitioner is writing a statement about a rape case for example, in which semen was recovered from an article of sanitary wear, the only exhibit in the case, then the semen technical paragraphs should describe recovery of semen from sanitary wear, rather than from swabs. Examination of swabs is not relevant in this case, yet the majority of 'standard' semen technical paragraphs are bound to mention swabs.

As an exercise, it's useful to ask trainee practitioners to write their technical paragraphs afresh in every case. This produces beautifully relevant technical paragraphs, and a thought out explanation of the science each time focuses the mind and can assist with interpretation. Some might argue that this would be a worthwhile exercise for experienced practitioners.

Some groups of practitioners are moving away from technical paragraphs altogether, their reasoning being that grouping a bunch of technical explanations together in a single section of a statement is tantamount to asking for them not to be read. Indeed, many barristers admit to skim reading forensic statements and jumping to the conclusions section (Ledward, 2004). Instead, practitioners have begun referencing footnotes within the body of their results and interpretation sections. It can be argued that this makes for a more readable statement, and encourages the reader to refer to the scientific principle under discussion at the most appropriate point in their reading.

The Inclusion of Conditioning Information

Transparency is a vital attribute of forensic interpretation, and in a forensic statement the scientist must outline all the information used in making the interpretation. This includes disclosure of any witness statements, interview transcripts and medical examination notes. The background information section of the statement is the obvious place for this, along with details of what is alleged and any defence version.

Many sexual offence submissions to the forensic laboratory arrive with a great deal of supplementary information, often summarised on the submission paperwork by the investigating officer. This information, coupled with that in the complainant's interview often reads like a story. Some practitioners fall into the habit of reproducing this summary, often word for word, in the information section of their statement, and worse, leaving out some vital piece of conditioning information that the officer has not included in their summary, such as timescales between alleged offence and forensic medical examination. This is extremely bad practice. This section of the forensic statement is specifically for conditioning information and should not read like a story. Furthermore, some of the extraneous detail included might be viewed as prejudicial.

A good exercise during statement writing training is to ask the trainee practitioners to review a number of forensic submissions and highlight only the conditioning information.

Choice of Words

Forensic reporting officers can spend torturous hours searching for the right form of words to describe a difficult interpretation. This is no exaggeration. Colleague discussions are helpful here and should be encouraged during mentoring of trainee reporting officers. Further, the principle of saying exactly what you mean is most relevant. As discussed, an experienced writer of forensic statements will have developed their own style and will have a variety of favoured phrases at the forefront of their mind. To the new practitioner, statement writing can be a daunting prospect, but the development of their own favourite phrases, as long as they are technically correct, should be encouraged.

An avoidance of emotive words is an important principle. Forensic science statements should be impartial. Regardless of whether written for prosecution or defence, the expert's overriding duty is to the criminal justice system (UK Government Legislation, 2015). For this reason, the use of emotive words could be viewed as prejudicial. This is particularly pertinent to sexual offence cases. The offence of rape is, in itself, a particularly emotive issue. For these reasons, practitioners should avoid the use of words such as 'rape' or 'victim'. It is much more impartial for the practitioner to discuss the fact that person A is alleged to have had sexual intercourse with person B, and to describe the victim as the complainant, or simply to use their name.

Transparency of Interpretation

In addition to the disclosure of conditioning information, stating any assumptions made during interpretation is also vital. The interpretation section of the statement should explain how conclusions have been reached and justify the strength of evidence quoted.

Subjective interpretation, based on an expert's casework experience, is not uncommon in forensic science and, on being challenged, has been allowed by The Court of Appeal (R v Reed & Reed, 2009; R v Weller, 2010).

Cognitive Bias

Issues of cognitive bias in forensic science have been in the spotlight recently. In the light of the McKie fingerprint case and subsequent public enquiry (Sir Anthony Campbell, 2011), forensic practitioners should be increasingly aware of this issue (Dror, 2014; Dror, 2015).

In sexual offence cases, practitioners are often provided with reams of information relating to both complainant and suspect. They usually need to filter through this to identify the case conditioning information, but practitioners must begin asking whether exposure to this information might cause an unconscious bias. It may be, for example, that unconscious judgements are being made, based on the appearance of the clothing worn by the parties involved, since this is often submitted to the laboratory. How can we be sure that such biases do not affect complex sexual offence case interpretations? It would be impossible to carry out a 'blind' interpretation, as some suggest, without access to the conditioning information. Awareness of the issue is a start, although conscious efforts on the part of individuals to be particularly objective have been shown only to result in greater bias (Dror and Rosenthal, 2008).

Training to Other Audiences

When practitioners are sufficiently experienced in dealing with sexual offence cases, they may wish to develop further by providing forensic awareness training to other audiences with a professional interest in sexual offence casework. Not only does this provide further opportunity to practice scientific explanations in plain English, but improves practitioners' communication skills. Different audiences require emphasis of different aspects.

Legal Professionals

Training for legal professionals may count towards their continuous professional development (CPD). Since CPD points are measured in hours, and legal types are inevitably busy people, it is likely that any forensic input will be limited to one or two hours. This provides a good exercise in prioritisation. Whilst scientific background might be interesting to legal professionals, more useful are thorough explanations of the limitations of testing and how these can impact on evidential significance in a sexual offence case. Some background on the structure of the forensic science statement can be helpful, especially to emphasise those parts of the statement, other than the conclusion, that contain valuable information. This can be linked to an explanation of how forensic interpretations are carried out. Many legal professionals are unfamiliar with Bayesian interpretation (Ledward, 2004) and are particularly interested in an explanation of the prosecutor's fallacy and how this might relate to forensic science conclusions (Balding and Donelly, 1994).

Police Officers

Forensic awareness in sexual offences for this audience should focus on the earlier stages of the case. Typically, more time can be allotted to police forensic training, providing ample opportunity to include greater detail in a half or full day course. Police are interested in choice of exhibits and their potential evidential significance, exhibit packaging best practice and anti-contamination procedure. There may be the opportunity to explain testing processes whilst providing an overview of the types of tests that are available, other than the obvious ones. It's not uncommon to find that police officers are mainly DNA-focused, so a summary of the other evidence types and their benefits is key. A useful approach is to use casework scenarios (refer to Appendix 14.A) to provoke discussion around formulating the forensic strategy. This provides an understanding of the strategy setting process, allows officers to think like scientists and prioritise exhibits according to potential evidential significance. This approach also demonstrates the vital nature of conditioning information in the case. During these discussions, the audience should be encouraged to suggest which aspects of the case information are missing and formulate questions that the scientist should ask the investigating officer. A successful outcome from this course will result in a much better quality of forensic submissions in sexual offence cases, in terms of both choice of exhibits and information provided.

Medical Professionals

The Faculty of Forensic & Legal Medicine (2016) provide guidelines on the educational requirements of forensic medical examiners. However, the mandatory requirements of UK FMEs in relation to forensic training are unclear. Some areas of the United Kingdom are fortunate to have specialist sexual assault referral centres, staffed by full-time doctors working solely in this field. Other regions use agency medical staff who, whilst being highly competent doctors, may not necessarily carry out forensic medical examinations with the same frequency. As a result, background forensic knowledge across all medical staff carrying out such examinations is inconsistent. Many FMEs are acutely aware of this, causing a small minority to have a rather defensive air. Pitching forensic awareness training as a two-way process is useful here, and there is truth in the suggestion that both forensic scientists and forensic medical practitioners can benefit from each other's knowledge.

Such a training course can provide a more technical content. As a general rule, most FMEs are interested to know the testing processes carried out on the exhibits they generate. This is a good opportunity to arrange implementation of a system of regular feedback such that FMEs are provided with details of success rates in real cases that they have worked on. The course should also focus on the details of the medical examination, highlighting commonly occurring themes such as 'the speculum issue' and the rationale behind taking relevant control swabs, as well as spreading the word about changes to best practice. Inviting comment on the practicalities of the medical examination and specific issues that arise provides a useful learning opportunity for the forensic scientist.

Conclusions

Forensic interpretation in sexual offences scenarios may be amongst the most complex facing the forensic biologist. The issues of transfer of biological evidence, its persistence on the various areas of the body, the limitations of body fluid testing and the associated interpretational issues present detailed learning for the prospective practitioner. Much of this learning is experience-based. Since each sexual offence casework scenario could be argued as being unique, each must be assessed on its individual merits, and a prolonged period of mentored work should follow formal training of the new forensic biology reporting officer. From a policing and criminal justice system perspective, success rates in sexual offence cases are low, attrition rates are high and, as a consequence, much has been written on the implementation of policy (HM Crown Prosecution Service Inspectorate/HM Inspectorate of Constabulary, 2002; HM Crown Prosecution Service Inspectorate, 2007; HM Crown Prosecution Service Inspectorate/HM Inspectorate of Constabulary, 2012; The Stern Review, 2010). Forensic evidence has a clear role to play in the successful prosecution of sexual offence cases, and as such, the place of forensic science should be presented to students in the relevant context within a functioning criminal justice system.

Appendix 14.A: Sexual Offence Case Training Scenarios

The following details a selection of sexual assault casework scenarios, based on real cases, for use in tutorials practicing case assessment and interpretation in sexual assault cases. The scenarios may also provide a useful contextual exercise for police officer training courses.

Suggested Tutorial Structure

1. Ask students to outline the conditioning information in the case scenario and to discuss which other pieces of information they would ask for.
2. When all the relevant conditioning information has been obtained, ask students to suggest the exhibits they would examine and for which evidence types, that is, to develop an examination strategy.
3. Ask students to prioritise the examinations within their strategy, justifying the priorities assigned, based on their expectations of evidential value. Even if students are not yet familiar with the Bayesian approach to CAI and the likelihood ratio, this approach introduces the concept of considering expectations in relation to alternative versions of events, using the relevant case conditioning information.
4. Discuss the limitations of each suggested forensic examination within the context of the conditioning information and the principles of transfer and persistence of biological evidence.

Scenario 1

The complainant was at a party at her friend's house. Whilst at the party she was introduced to the suspect and they were seen dancing together by witnesses at the party. At approximately 01:30 hours, the complainant went upstairs to collect her coat from the front bedroom. She alleges that the suspect followed her into the room, threatened her with a knife and forced her to lie on the bed. He then ripped off her lower clothing and forced her to have sexual intercourse. The complainant reported the incident the following evening.

Tutor Notes:

Conditioning Information, Scenario 1

- Has a suspect been identified in this case? It is vital, at the earliest stage, to determine whether the forensic scientist will be acting in an investigative or an evaluative mode.
- If a suspect has been identified, what is his version of events?
- Establish exact timescales to determine expectations of detecting the various types of evidence. No time is given for the forensic medical examination(s) (i.e. complainant and suspect) only the time of reporting. Discuss reasons for delays between reporting and medical examination.
- Discuss whether further particulars of the allegation are required. These could be obtained from the complainant's interview transcript and might include such details as whether she thought the offender wore a condom or the nature of the threat with the knife — were there any injuries that bled as a result of the knife?
- As well as timescales, discuss the information that might be gleaned from the medical examination notes: whether the complainant is sexually active; if so, whether she had any recent sexual activity prior to the alleged incident; if so, when and with whom; whether the complainant washed/bathed/showered prior to the medical examination; whether she was menstruating at the time of the alleged incident.
- If there is a suspect, has he been medically examined?
- Discuss which items have been exhibited. This leads onto discussions of an examination strategy.

Tutor Notes:

Strategy Discussions, Scenario 1

If vaginal swabs have been taken from the complainant then examination of these for semen should be the first priority in the examination strategy, provided they have been taken within a sufficient timeframe. Discussion of semen persistence times in the vagina can be entered into at this stage of the tutorial, and trainers may wish to vary their answers to the initial questions about when the complainant's medical examination took place in order to change the priorities of the case accordingly.

If penile swabs have been taken from an identified suspect, then similar discussions can be had in relation to the far shorter persistence time of cellular material on the penis. If the complainant had been menstruating, then consideration of blood testing of the penile swabs can be discussed.

In the absence of intimate swabs, discussions in relation to examination of the complainant's and suspect's underwear can be undertaken, bearing in mind that it may be unknown whether those pairs of underwear submitted are the ones worn at the time of the alleged incident. Discussion could also extend to the worth of examining the other clothing items worn by the complainant and suspect. This might include consideration of whether biological material may have been transferred to these clothing items or, dependent on the defence version of events, whether it may be worth addressing contact, in which case fibre evidence could be considered. On considering the issue of contact, prompt students to return to the case conditioning information, in which they should note that witnesses saw the complainant and suspect dancing together. Discuss how the extent of contact that might entail. Whilst dancing might result in fibre transfer to outer clothing, could it feasibly result in fibre transfer to underwear? The value of fibre evidence will also be dependent on the constituent fibres of the clothing items involved. If both parties were wearing jeans and T-shirts, for example, then transfer of such commonly encountered fibre types would likely be of little evidential significance.

Discussion amongst a tutorial group considering this scenario inevitably moves on to question examination of the bedding items. This is a good opportunity to point out the real world issue of cost in forensic examination. Bedding items are usually large and, therefore, time consuming to examine, which translates into increased cost. It is unlikely that a police force would authorise such a costly examination unless there were a reasonable chance of a useful outcome. In order to address the usefulness of this examination, students will need to return to the conditioning information and may wish to clarify further details. Whose bed is it? Who else might have slept on the bed, or had sexual activity on or in it? What was on the bed? The complainant was going there to collect her coat. Were there many coats on the bed when the alleged incident took place? If so, is it possible that there was any transfer of biological material to the bedding at all?

When all the obvious ideas from this scenario have been exhausted, students can be prompted to think about whether there are any other forensic opportunities. Has a knife been recovered? Does the suspect admit to handling it? Is it worth testing the knife for DNA that might have been deposited by whoever handled it? Was the complainant injured with the knife during the course of the incident, or did it make contact with her skin? Is it worth searching the knife for blood or swabbing the cutting edge of the blade for DNA?

As a final point, if the defence version of events contains an admission of sexual activity and it is consent that is the issue to be addressed, then given that the complainant describes the offender ripping off her lower clothing, it may be worth carrying out an examination of the complainant's lower clothing items for damage features that appear recent.

Scenario 2

The complainant was waiting for a bus following an evening at her boyfriend's. A red car stopped and the driver beckoned her over. As she approached, the driver got out and forced her into the back seat of the car. They drove around for a while, eventually stopping at a car park. The driver then got into the rear seat, pushed up the complainant's jumper and sucked her breasts. He then took a condom from his pocket and put this on before having sexual intercourse with her. The man left the complainant in the car park and drove away.

Tutor Notes:

Conditioning Information, Scenario 2
- Again, establishing whether or not a suspect has been identified is the first fact that needs to be established. This is the type of scenario that lends itself to working in investigative mode, so it may be that trainers wish to tell students that there is no suspect and their remit is to recover evidence to assist in identifying the offender.

- Establishing timescales and information from the medical examination is the next obvious enquiry. Were breast swabs taken? What happened during the alleged sexual intercourse?
- Querying which exhibits have been submitted might lead to discussion of whether a condom has been found at the location of the incident. If so, students should consider the nature of the location. Might it be the type of place that condoms from other incidences of sexual activity might be recovered? How can it be established that any condom submitted to the laboratory relates to the incident?

Strategy Discussions, Scenario 2

Given that the offender wore a condom during sexual intercourse, the most ready source of DNA from the offender in this scenario can be considered to be saliva deposited during the alleged breast sucking. The worth of examining breast swabs from the complainant will depend on the timescale between the incident and the complainant's medical examination. Should the trainer decide that this timescale is outside the window of persistence of saliva on the breasts, students should be prompted to consider screening the complainant's upper clothing for transferred saliva.

Student's expectations of saliva on the upper clothing may require some additional conditioning information. Was a bra worn under the complainant's jumper? None is mentioned in the case scenario. When was the upper clothing last washed? This will inform the students' expectations of detecting biological material from the wearer in any DNA profiling tests. If there has been transfer of the offender's saliva to clothing, a mixture of DNA matching the complainant and offender might be expected. Has the complainant engaged in any recent consensual sexual activity that might involve transfer of saliva to her upper clothing, specifically to the inner surfaces of her bra? The complainant had spent the evening with her boyfriend. If saliva from him is expected on the clothing, then an elimination DNA sample from the boyfriend should be requested.

Should no saliva be detected, discussion of other forensic opportunities can be entered into. The most appropriate strategy to determine whether a recovered condom relates to the alleged incident can be discussed. The trainer may decide that multiple condoms have been recovered and students will need to determine the most efficient system to establish which, if any, are relevant. This is also an opportunity to discuss the limitations of condom examination: that material may be transferred between the inner and outer surfaces prior to recovery; that the inner and outer surfaces may not be readily identified during the examination, since inner as recovered may not correspond to inner as worn. Further, the benefits of preferential extraction to separate seminal and cellular fractions can be explained. Time constraints versus cost is also a relevant topic here. If multiple condoms are examined and time is the most pertinent issue, it may be decided to DNA test both the cellular and seminal fractions from each surface of every condom, in the hope that the cellular profile from one of the condoms will match that of the complainant and thus, the corresponding seminal fraction might yield a DNA profile suitable to search The National DNA Database. The more condoms are examined, the higher the cost. However, if time is less of an issue, it would be cheaper to DNA profile only the cellular fractions, and if a profile matching that of the complainant is found, only then to DNA profile the corresponding seminal fraction.

Issues of contact and fibre transfer may also be discussed during the later stages of this case scenario. However, students must be reminded that fibre evidence may not provide suitable intelligence information to help identify a potential suspect during the investigative stages of the case, but might be relevant at the later, evaluative stages, should a suspect have been identified from DNA evidence, and depending on the details in his version of events, and/or should the vehicle have been identified. Since fibres are readily lost from the surface of exhibits, the value of taking contingency fibre tapings of the complainant's clothing items prior to body fluid screening tests should be emphasised.

Scenario 3

The complainant alleges that the suspect forced her into a chair, pulled down her jeans and knickers, damaging them in the process, then made her bend over a table. He penetrated her vagina with his fingers then forced her onto her back on the floor and had vaginal sexual intercourse with her. The complainant believes that he ejaculated. She was then allowed to wipe her vagina with her knickers before being allowed to leave. On being questioned, the suspect denied having sexual intercourse with the complainant but admitted digitally penetrating her vagina, stating that this was with her consent.

Tutor Notes:

Conditioning Information, Scenario 3
- Unlike scenarios 1 and 2, it is clear from the information in this case that a suspect has been identified and he has provided a defence version of events.
- Students may question whether medical samples were taken from the suspect, penile swabs being the most relevant, and if so, the timescale between the alleged incident and recovery of the samples.
- Fingernail samples may also have been taken from the suspect, but students may decide that these offer little evidential value given that the suspect admits digitally penetrating the complainant's vagina.
- Similar questions should be asked in relation to the complainant's medical samples and the associated timescale, as well as establishing the relevant details regarding her recent sexual history, washing, menstruation, and so on.

Strategy Discussions, Scenario 3
Should samples have been taken within the appropriate timescales, then penile swabs and vaginal swabs would seem to be the most relevant items to prioritise, given that the issue to be addressed is one of vaginal intercourse.

The initial laboratory findings in the case upon which this scenario is based, showed no semen on the vaginal swabs, despite them being taken within the relevant persistence time. This gives rise to an interesting discussion about the conditioning value of the information given by the complainant that the offender ejaculated during the alleged incident. It has been demonstrated in numerous cases in the author's experience, that complainants are often mistaken about whether or not ejaculation in the vagina took place. This by no means negates the view that the incident occurred, but rather illustrates the point that the details of a traumatic experience may not be entirely accurate.

The complainant described being allowed to wipe herself on her knickers after the incident. Students may wish to discuss the merits of examination of the knickers for semen, given that the offender may have ejaculated as he withdrew, depositing semen only on the external vaginal regions, which might not be expected to persist on the vulva, even in shorter timeframes.

Again, the actual findings in this case, showed low level DNA mixtures from the penile swabs, to which the complainant could have contributed, but which were unsuitable for routine statistical evaluation, such that the strength of evidence to support the view that DNA from the complainant was present, could not be calculated.

Subsequent examination of the suspect's boxer shorts yielded a major DNA profile matching the complainant, which was suitable for statistical evaluation, giving a match probability of one in a billion. Students may wish to discuss how or whether to relate this finding to an activity level interpretation, given the defence version of events and given that the DNA cannot specifically be attributed to vaginal cells, although within the framework of case circumstances, would tend to support that view. However, the suspect's admission of digital penetration gives an opportunity for secondary transfer of the complainant's cellular material from his fingers to his penis and subsequently to the inner front of his underwear. Again, students may wish to revisit the case conditioning information to determine whether there is any further detail relating to the suspect's activities between the incident and the taking of his penile swabs and underwear.

This case also provides an opportunity to discuss the process of reinterpretation, should the defence version of events change. In this case, the suspect, on being presented with the findings, gave a convoluted version of events to attempt to explain the transfer of the complainant's DNA from his fingers to his penis and underwear, which involved masturbation. However, the suspect's modified version claimed that masturbation took place several hours after the alleged incident, during which time he had carried out numerous tasks that might be expected to remove transferred cellular material from his hands before having chance to transfer it to his penis. Students should be encouraged to consider the updated defence version and to determine their expectations of sufficient cellular material remaining on the suspect's hands to allow his stated secondary transfer versus the chance of the DNA findings if penile-vaginal intercourse took place, as alleged.

Appendix 14.B: Templates for Use in Statement Writing Exercises

In using the templates included in this Appendix (Templates 14.1–14.4), students are prompted to follow the guidance included in the various sections of the statement.

The requirements of disclosure should be discussed during initial statement writing teaching and related to the Forensic Examination Record, Index of Unused Materials and Expert's Self-Certificate included in the templates. The details can be explained by referring to the relevant parts of the Criminal Procedure Rules UK Government Legislation, 2015). Parts 16 and 19 of the current rules contain guidance for the expert witness.

Disclosure Schedule Non-Sensitive Material

The list identifies material in possession of [FSP] in relation to the case referred to below, which has provisionally been deemed **Non-Sensitive**. The list is provided in accordance with the guidance given in 'Disclosure: experts' evidence and unused material'.

The purpose of this form is to inform the prosecutor of the description of all non-sensitive material relevant to the case, material that has not been examined and the location of this material. Refer to Chapter 7 of the Disclosure manual.

DESCRIPTION AND RELEVANCE (Give sufficient detail for CPS to decide if material should be disclosed or requires more detailed examination)	LOCATION State precisely where the item can be found/located	FOR CPS USE: * Enter: D = Disclose to defence I = Defence may inspect ND = Not to disclose CND = Clearly not disclosable * COMMENTS
All DNA profiles established in this case have been checked against the Staff Elimination Database. No matches have been found.	Casefile, IT	
FORMS detailing receipt and dispatch of items to the laboratory, movement of items within and between sites, submission forms detailing the nature of the offence, work required and details of victims and suspects.	Casefile	
EXAMINATION RECORDS: Details of packaging and sealing of items received at UCLAN, notes made during the examination, records of work performed, who performed the work and on what date; test results; details of quality checks.	Casefile	
Confidential commercial information, e.g. estimates, time sheets, invoices etc.	Casefile	
Notes of conversations and correspondence with Police Investigators, including minutes.	Casefile	
Records concerning other suspects.	Casefile	
Records concerning modus operandi.	Casefile, IT	
Witness statements, draft witness statements.	Casefile, IT	
Retained material from items examined has been exhibited and returned to force, with the exception of DNA extracts.	Force (details on casefile)	
Material submitted to but not examined by [FSP], details of which can be provided, has been returned to force.	Force (details on casefile)	

		SIGNATURE		CPS Reference	
CUSTOMER CASE NUMBER					
OFFICER IN CASE				Reviewing Lawer	
LGC CASE NUMBER					
LGC EXPERT WITNESS NAME	[YOUR NAME]			Date Reviewed	
DATE	[DATE]				

EXPERT WITNESS DECLARATION FORM

I am an expert in Forensic Biology and I have been requested to provide a statement. I confirm that I have read guidance contained in a booklet known as *Disclosure: Expert's evidence and unused material*, which details my role and documents my responsibilities, in relation to revelation as an expert witness. I have followed the guidance and recognise the continuing nature of my responsibilities of revelation. In accordance with my duties of revelation, as documented in the guidance booklet, I

1. (a) confirm that I have complied with my duties to record, retain and reveal material in accordance with the Criminal Procedure and Investigations Act 1996, as amended;
2. (b) have compiled an Index of all material. I will ensure that the Index is updated in the event I am provided with or generate additional material;
3. (c) that in the event my opinion changes on any material issue, I will inform the investigating officer, as soon as reasonably practicable and give reasons.

POLICE REFERENCE			
POLICE OFFICER IN CASE			
FORCE, STATION & DIVISION			
CASE TYPE			
LABORATORY REFERENCE			SIGNATURE
FORENSIC SCIENTIST	[YOUR NAME]		
DATE	[DATE]		

FORENSIC EXAMINATION RECORD

The following work was carried out by trained staff at my request using established procedures.

I reviewed the progress of the work, issued fresh instructions as appropriate and checked the findings. A case file, comprising notes made at the time of the examinations, represents a full record of the contributions of assisting members of staff.

NAME	OUTLINE OF WORK UNDERTAKEN
[names of individuals] [names of individuals]	Details of task carried out, for example: semen searching & note taking DNA Profiling
EXHIBIT NUMBER	[YOUR INITIALS/001]

POLICE REFERENCE				
POLICE OFFICER IN CASE				
FORCE, STATION & DIVISION				
CASE TYPE				
LABORATORY REFERENCE		E	SIGNATURE	
FORENSIC SCIENTIST	[YOUR NAME]			
DATE	[DATE]			

Witness Statement

(Criminal Procedure Rules 2015, r.16 & 19, Criminal Justice Act 1967 s.9, Magistrates' Courts Act 1980 s.5B)

Statement of   [First Names SURNAME]

Age of Witness   Over 18

Occupation   Forensic Scientist

Address   [Details of Forensic Service Provider]

This statement, consisting of [TOTAL NUMBER OF PAGES] pages each signed by me, is true to the best of my knowledge and belief and I make it knowing that, if it is tendered in evidence, I shall be liable to prosecution if I have wilfully stated in it anything which I know to be false or do not believe to be true.

Dated:

Signed _____

Qualifications and Experience

Paragraph to establish credentials as a credible expert witness. This could include:

– Area of expertise
– Length of experience in the field
– Details of academic/professional qualifications

Imagine that you have graduated and are employed as a forensic scientist.

Laboratory Reference:
Customer Reference:

Background Information
Set out the case conditioning information here:

Include any information upon which you have relied in making your interpretation.
Do not include extraneous details that do not affect your expectations.
Disclose any written documents relating to the case, which you have read, such as witness statements, interview transcripts, or medical examination records.

Items Received

This section is important to demonstrate chain of evidence/continuity. It may be set out as follows:

The following items were received at [details of FSP] on [date], from [police force]:

List of exhibit numbers	Description of exhibits	Who the exhibits relate to

Purpose of Examination

This section lays out the reason or purpose of the examination and should include details of the pair of propositions to be addressed.

If the case is a complex one, then it may involve more than one pair of propositions.

Use of Assistants

In undertaking the work in this case I was assisted by other members of the laboratory staff acting under my instructions. Their involvement is described in the accompanying forensic examination record, [YOUR INITIALS]/01, and I have taken their contributions into account when I prepared this statement. The involvement of other staff is recorded in case notes available for inspection at the laboratory if required.

Technical Issues

Include in here details describing all the technical procedures used in the case, for example semen screening, microscopy or DNA profiling.

Each technical note should be written for the layperson and should specifically relate to examinations carried out in this case.

If there are very length technical explanations, this section can refer to appendices containing more detailed information.

Examination and Results

Reference Samples
Detail that DNA profiles were obtained from the parties in the case for use as references.

Point out that reference profiles differ from each other.

Items From [complainant]
Detail which items were examined and what was found.

Items From [suspect]
As for items from the complainant.

Include further examination and results sections for items from any other person or location. All the items that have been examined and all the results obtained must be disclosed.

Interpretation

This is the part of the statement where an explanation of what the findings mean is provided.

Consider the strength of the evidence and which propostion(s) it supports and justify these opinions, based on the principles of transfer and persistence, and the case conditioning information.

If a number of issues are being addressed in the case, then it may be appropriate to separate the interpretation into corresponding sections.

Conclusions

The bottom line!
The writer's opinion(s) on the meaning of the evidence.
The conclusion must answer the questions (address the issues) laid out in the purpose.

References

Allard, J.E. (1996) The collection of data from findings in cases of sexual assault and the significance of spermatozoa on vaginal, anal and oral swabs, *Science & Justice*, **37**, 99–108.

Balding, D.J. and Donelly P. (1994) The prosecutor's fallacy and DNA evidence, *Criminal Law Review*, **1**, 711–721.

Brayley-Morris, H., Sorrell, A., Revoir, A.P., Meakin, G.E., Syndercombe Court, D. and Morgan, R.M. (2015) Persistence of DNA from laundered semen stains: Implications for child sex trafficking cases. *FSI Genetics*. November (**19**), 165–171.

Cook, R., Evett, I.W., Jackson, G., Jones, P.J. and Lambert, J.A. (1998a) A model for case assessment and interpretation, *Science & Justice*, **38** (3) 151–156.

Cook, R., Evett, I.W., Jackson, G., Jones, P.J. and Lambert, J.A. (1998b) A hierarchy of propositions: Deciding which level to address in casework. *Science & Justice*, **38** (4), 231–240.

Davies, A. (1982) The medical examination in cases of sexual assault. A forensic biologist's view, in *The New Police Surgeon* (ed. W.D.S. McLay), pp. 103–112.

Davies, A. and Wilson, E. (1974) The persistence of seminal constituents in the human vagina, *Forensic Science*, **3**, 45–55.

Dror, I.E. (2014) Practical solutions to cognitive and human factor challenges in forensic science, *Forensic Science Policy & Management*, **4** (3-4), 1–9.

Dror, I.E. (2015) Context management toolbox: A linear sequential unmasking (LSU) approach for minimising cognitive bias in forensic decision making, *Journal of Forensic Science*, **60** (4), 1111–1112.

Dror, I.E. and Rosenthal, R. (2008) Meta-analytically quantifying the reliability and biasability of forensic experts, *Journal of Forensic Science*, **53** (4), 900–903.

Evett, I.W., Jackson, G. and Lambert, J.A. (2000) More on the hierarchy of propositions: Exploring the distinction between explanations and propositions. *Science & Justice*, **40** (1), 3–10.

Faculty of Forensic & Legal Medicine (2016) Quality Standards in Forensic Medicine General Forensic Medicine (GFM) and Sexual Offence Medicine (SOM). Available at: http://fflm.ac.uk/quality-standards/ (accessed 11 December 2016).

HM Crown Prosecution Service Inspectorate/HM Inspectorate of Constabulary (2002) *The Report on the Joint Inspection into the Investigation and Prosecution of Cases Involving Allegations of Rape.* A HMCPSI and HMIC joint thematic inspection.

HM Crown Prosecution Service Inspectorate (2007) *Without Consent.* A report on the joint review of the investigation and prosecution of rape offences.

HM Crown Prosecution Service Inspectorate/HM Inspectorate of Constabulary (2012) *Forging the Links: Rape Investigation and Prosecution.* A joint review by HMIC and HMCPSI.

Kind, S.S. (1964) The acid phosphatase test, *Methods of Forensic Science* (ed. A.S. Curry), Interscience Publishers, New York, pp. 267–288.

Ledward, J. (2004) Understanding Forensic Evidence: Do Lawyers and the Judiciary Understand Forensic Evidence and the Bayesian Approach? QEB Hollis Whiteman. Available at: http://www.qebholliswhiteman.co.uk/articles-pdfs/understanding-forensic-evidence.pdf (accessed 11 December 2016).

Locard, E. (1930) The analysis of dust traces Part 1, *American Journal of Police Science*, 276–298.

R v Reed & Reed [2009] EWCA Crim 2698.

R v Weller [2010] EWCA Crim 1085.

Recommendations for the Collection of Forensic Specimens from Complainants and Suspects, *Faculty of Forensic & Legal Medicine* July 2016. Available at: http://www.fflm.ac.uk/publications/recommendations-for-the-collection-of-forensic-specimens-from-complainants-and-suspects-3/ (accessed 11 December 2016).

Redhead, P. and Brown, M.K. (2013) The acid phosphatase test two minute cut-off: An insufficient time to detect some semen stains, *Science & Justice*, **53** (2) 187–191.

Sir Anthony Campbell (2011) The Fingerprint Inquiry Report. Available at: http://www.webarchive.org.uk/wayback/archive/20150428160106/ http://www.thefingerprintinquiryscotland.org.uk/inquiry/files/TheFingerprintInquiry Report_High_res.pdf (accessed 9 December 2016).

The Stern Review (2010) *A Report By Baroness Vivien Stern CBE of an Independent Review into How Rape Complaints are Handled by Public Authorities in England and Wales*, Home Office, London.

UK Government Legislation, Sexual Offences Act (2003), Chapter 42. Available at: http://www.legislation.gov.uk/ukpga/2003/42/contents (accessed 9 December 2016).

UK Government Legislation, The Criminal Procedure Rules (2015) Part 19.2. Available at: http://www.legislation.gov.uk/uksi/2015/1490/article/19.2/made (accessed 9 December 2016).

Willott, G.M. and Allard, J.E. (1982) Spermatozoa—their persistence after sexual intercourse. *Forensic Science International* **19**, 135–154.

15

The Use of High-Fidelity Simulations in Emergency Management Training

Graham Braithwaite

Cranfield University, Shrivenham, Swindon, UK

The Need for High Fidelity

Forensic science and accident investigation are, by their very nature, applied and 'hands-on' subjects. Laboratory analysis is usually preceded by an intensive field phase, often without notice, and always with a range of competing priorities and pressures. These pressures come from the multitude of tasks, limited opportunity for planning and the dynamic nature of a site that often follows a traumatic event such as an accident or crime. Training for those who are to experience such a site phase needs to reflect these pressures in context whilst maximising the learning experience and minimising any risk of harm to the student.

Traditional tabletop exercises are of considerable value, but this chapter is concerned with the creation of high-fidelity simulations in which to immerse students. This does not mean a computer simulation, but rather role-play or what might be better defined as 'real-play' exercises on a mock accident site or crime scene. The examples used relate to a range of railway, marine and aircraft accident simulations that have been utilised as part of professional accident investigation training courses run at Cranfield University, UK, over a period of 35 years.

Feedback from participants and their employers consistently supports the view that the greatest training transfer has come from participation in practical, on-site training to consolidate all of the components of their new role. However, the way in which a simulation is designed and delivered has an enormous influence on the value of such training for the student. A poorly designed scenario becomes a battle of wills between students and staff as they try to outsmart each other. Worse than this, the whole endeavour can start to feel like an exercise in 'practicing bleeding' rather than the structured learning opportunity that it could be.

The need for high fidelity comes from several sources. Firstly, the participants in such training (particularly accident investigation) tend to be experienced, adult-learners who

Forensic Science Education and Training: A Tool-kit for Lecturers and Practitioner Trainers, First Edition.
Edited by Anna Williams, John P. Cassella, and Peter D. Maskell.
© 2017 John Wiley & Sons Ltd. Published 2017 by John Wiley & Sons Ltd.

are often less comfortable with a conventional classroom environment. Secondly, the role they are preparing for requires multiple tasks to be prioritised and circumstances reacted to, ranging from working with other agencies and interested parties to coping with weather conditions and interruptions. Most of the tasks are straightforward in isolation, but in practice they will rarely be experienced in isolation. Thirdly, many of the participants will move swiftly into a role where they will go to an accident site/crime scene as soon as the next working day following course completion. An example of this was an aircraft accident investigator who completed a six-week training course on the Friday and found himself recovering a wrecked Sea Harrier from the depths of the Bristol Channel by the following Monday (M. Midmore, Investigator, Royal Navy Flight Safety and Accident Investigation Centre, Yeovilton, personal communication, 2004).

Participation in a high-fidelity simulation can provide significant opportunities for reflective and peer review as well as confidence building for the participant. To what degree this is achieved is largely influenced by the design and delivery of the simulation, the willingness of the participants to engage with the simulation and the way in which the activity is debriefed.

Elements to consider in creating a teaching simulation will now be considered.

Scenario Design

The design of a scenario starts with two intended learning outcomes that would be driven by the overall learning objectives for a training programme:

1. What is it that someone should be able to do by the end?
2. How will this be assessed?

These will then need to be balanced against the limitations of budget, time and fidelity. It may well be that not everything can be covered in a single scenario, especially if it is to remain plausible to the participants.

Plausibility is an important factor to consider in designing a scenario. Real events can provide a great starting point, but caution should be exercised. Is there a danger that the participants will recognise or look-up the original scenario and therefore skip to the answer whilst missing out on the learning experience that the journey should be? Is there another danger in that an excruciating amount of effort goes into perfecting realism for limited gain?

Conversely, fictitious events can easily become contrived and open to challenge by a cynical audience, particularly when they are struggling to do their job. Whilst the use of fictitious characters, places and facts can avoid embarrassing or upsetting to real people, including victim's families, they can also make it harder for witnesses to remember detail and for the production of evidence (e.g. maps, company documentation, etc.). Bear in mind that it is hard to predict all of the evidence that a student may search out so why not use as much 'real' information as possible? Amusing place and character names can often be more a source of entertainment for the facilitators than the participants and create the impression that the topic is not being taken seriously.

Basing a scenario on a real event can provide the basic structure to build specific training experiences around. For example, perhaps the original accident featured two fatalities and no live witness? The simulation may change this to one survivor or add eyewitnesses so that the participants have a better chance of retrieving enough evidence to get to the next step. Novice investigators/scientists will inevitably make slower progress, so to keep the momentum going it may be necessary to make some evidence more readily available than it was in the real event. Scenarios can be adapted to deliver particular teaching points as well as to pace the speed of progress. For example, witnesses can be timed to arrive at certain times to drip feed information.

Another advantage of using a real scenario is the availability of photos to recreate the scene from or to prove to students that the reproduction is true to the original.

For example, in a scenario based around a mid-air collision, the wreckage trail on the ground was short. One student argued that this was unrealistic until he was shown the original photographs. In fact, the short wreckage trail was symptomatic of the very low forward speed that the aircraft had as it effectively fell from the sky following the mid-air collision. In another example, a group examining the same wreckage and observing that the aircraft was facing its own wreckage trail concluded that it had hit the ground and sprayed debris forward rather than what had actually happened, where the aircraft had tumbled along a trail before coming to rest facing the direction it had just come from. Perhaps predictably, eyewitnesses offered support for both theories!

The weather can be an aspect of realism that is close to impossible to guarantee. Such constrains can be planned for to a degree (e.g. it is unlikely to be snowing in July in England), but will need either some last minute editing of documents such as weather forecasts/aftercasts or briefing as a constraint/limitation.

Health and Safety Considerations

Introducing novices to a crime scene or accident site presents a range of hazards and the opportunity to learn how to work around them. Indeed, many of these hazards are equally applicable to experienced investigators and the 'rush to investigate' can mean that they are forgotten.

The challenge in creating a simulation is what level of realism to create and how much they manage the hazard for the participant. There is no point laying traps by way of exotic or unusual hazards for a novice, but equally there is little value in creating a benign or inert environment for those who will go out on a real investigation as their next assignment.

Hazards may fall into several different categories:

- deployment
- site hazards
- location hazards
- daily hazards
- longer-term hazards.

Deployment Hazards

These are associated with the time at which a notification is received until the point that an investigation occurs on site. Typical deployment hazards include:

- Do they know where to go?
- Will they travel individually or as a team?

- Are they fit to travel? (Tiredness, alcohol, etc.)
- How will they get there?
- How will they travel around the site?
- How will they communicate with each other and the facilitators?
- Will there be food/drink available?
- Do they need a passport, visa, currency, and so on?

Many simulations start with a 'managed arrival.' In other words, those going on site are gathered together and briefed prior to a starting point, which helps to eliminate some of these challenges. However, this is not entirely realistic and may miss aspects of planning and problem solving that are valuable intended learning outcomes.

Site Hazards

These can be categorized into five key elements, as follows.

Environmental Hazards

Accidents and crime scenes can be located just about anywhere from the depths of oceans to the peaks of mountains. Each area has its own unique set of hazards to manage.

Examples include terrain, which may be at altitude, steep, unstable, slippery or heavy underfoot (such as on sand or wet soil), leading to either a trip/fall hazard or increased fatigue on site. The benefits of simulating working at extremes such as on a cliff or a mountain must be carefully considered. Is it the sort of environment that the individual is likely to face or are the facilitators trying to hard to 'outgun' the students? What will the facilitators do if their students assess the site to be unworkable?

Similarly, certain aspects will be decided by the weather. Choice of location may help to bring a degree of certainty, but plans should cater for extremes of temperature and weather. Working in extreme temperatures, whether hot or cold, may induce stress and will necessitate increased intake of fluids/food. This will then add time to simulations as participants change in and out of personal protective equipment (PPE)/leave site, and so on. It is also worth considering that when participants come from different parts of the world, their ability to cope with extremes of temperature will vary.

Specialist clothing will help to protect the students and facilitators, although the latter may have different needs as they are often stood observing rather than exerting themselves on site (Figure 15.1).

The following may be considered:

- Base layers – to maintain warmth or wick sweat away. Generally made from man-made fibres or merino wool and not cotton, which will remain wet.
- Long work trousers with pockets for camera, gloves, and so on.
- Fleece jacket – easily washable and quick to dry.
- Bump cap – offering some head protection as well as conserving warmth.
- Breathable waterproof jacket and trousers. Consider hard-wearing fabrics such as rip-stop nylon or Gore-Tex XTR and also trousers that can be removed without having to take off footwear. High visibility markings may eliminate the need for additional tabards, and so on.

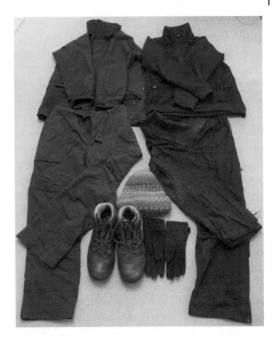

- Boots – these should be waterproof with non-slip, protected soles and toe protection. They should be easily cleaned so fabric boots may be unsuitable. Leather firemen's boots are a practical solution, but generally need wearing in.
- Socks – again man-made fibres or merino wool will help to keep feet warm and dry, avoiding blisters. A long distance hiking sock may well be the most comfortable option, perhaps with a liner sock.
- Clothes for conducting interviews – if this is a possible activity on-site and within the role, do you look professional and approachable? Could you give a news conference or speak to a relative of the deceased in what you are wearing?
- Clothes for off-site – items that can be worn in a hotel or in public where you may not want to be recognised as an accident investigator/forensic scientist, and so on. Do you have clean footwear to go into a hotel, restaurant, for example?

Local flora and fauna can present a hazard ranging from nuisance to life threatening. Stinging nettles and thorns can make life on-site unpleasant, whereas stings or animal bites can be potentially fatal. If a student has a known allergy then it is worth finding out and establishing whether they are carrying an adrenalin auto-injector (EpiPen) in case of anaphylaxis. In one example, the recipe used for fake blood on site included a large quantity of golden syrup, which in turn attracted large number of wasps to site. One student was known to have an extreme reaction to stings and therefore had to be withdrawn. Subsequent exercises needed a new fake blood recipe and a briefing about allergies.

Working in or around water needs a very clear risk management strategy.

Physical Hazards

These are usually in the form of accident wreckage, bodies, structures and vehicles. They may also be obscured, for example, by snow or fire-fighting foam or moving in the case of vehicles. Creating a realistic scene that the students can dynamically risk assess may be of considerable value, but it is also worth considering that they can quickly become immersed in the learning activity and make apparently silly mistakes. Classic traps include walking into an object that isn't normally there (e.g. an aircraft wing after the gear has collapsed), especially when wearing a peaked cap, or reversing into an object whilst trying to compose the perfect photograph.

Close supervision can help along with an agreed 'STOP' protocol or the use of a whistle. Upon hearing the command, everyone should stop what they are doing until given the all clear. In addition, students may be directed to work as a 'buddy pair' so that there is always one person looking out for the other.

Unstable structures are realistic and may need to be propped before work can continue. In designing such simulations, the trade-off is between realism and the value of any unmanaged risk.

Biological Hazards

These are a feature of all accident sites or crime scenes where injury or death has occurred. Many organisations focus their site safety training around blood-borne pathogens so the hazards are often well known. However, this may lead to a culture of avoiding working near such hazards rather than managing them to a safe level. Blood, for example, is a manageable hazard and its removal from a site may well compromise evidence collection. Appropriate PPE and hygiene can manage it and in any simulation, care should be taken to ensure that this is practiced. In particular, the removal of PPE before toilet or refreshment breaks or at the end of the site phase deserves particular scrutiny.

It is at the point that a tired person is preparing to leave site that they are most likely to exercise poor PPE hygiene and cross-contaminate. Is their PPE now contaminated? Is their footwear properly cleaned? What about writing implements, cameras, and so on?

Material Hazards

Depending on the area of concern, material hazards may include exotic metals, glass or carbon composites, wood and beyond. If a fire or severe disruption is involved then additional hazards may need to be risk assessed and managed. Without appropriate PPE there is a risk of skin irritation or damage to the respiratory system. If using 'real' wreckage, consider things like sharp metal or composites and the products of combustion (Figure 15.2). Carbon composite dust is particularly nasty so as well as using suitable respirators, it is worth wetting the site or applying a fixant/lacquer to reduce airborne particles.

The PPE needs to be used appropriately and disposed of carefully. Face masks seem to be particularly easy to either put on improperly or be tempted to be used as a chin support/hair band!

Stored energy vessels such as extinguishers, accumulators, fuel, capacitors, batteries, oxygen bottles, distress flares, oleos, ejector seats, ballistic recovery systems and tyres can remain hazardous for a long period of time so should be checked before use in a simulation. In one example, a student wanted to record that the fuel tank of an aircraft was empty and was stopped when about to take flash photographs of the contents of what was potentially a flammable vapour filled tank.

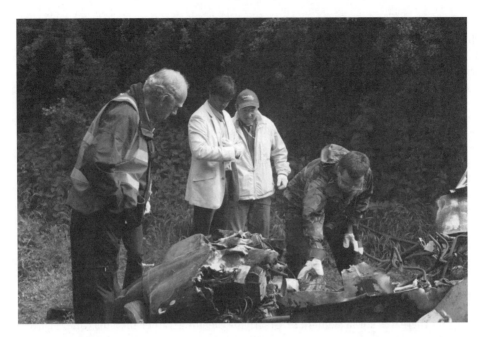

Figure 15.2 A typical light aircraft accident featuring disrupted and burnt metal and manmade material fibres (photo: author's own) (see colour figure in colour plate section).

Psychological Hazards

Even a simulated accident site or crime scene can become distressing as the fidelity increases. The use of theatrical blood can provide realism, but is enough to affect people with limited experience. In extreme cases, animal remains may be used, but this may present a real biological and psychological threat, especially as smell is such an evocative sense. This should be used with caution and the training value honestly assessed. An example was the use of a bag of old prawns on a fishing boat that had been recovered from the seabed. Keeping them in a bag meant they could be removed and disposed of safely without permanently ruining the training resource!

Where actors are used at witnesses, the psychological effect can be distinct, for example, if an actor is distressed or cries on site. Training can be stressful, especially when workload is high so suitable emotional support needs to be made available both on-site and subsequently. It may be that the student suffers a reaction based on a previous experience, which is unknown to the facilitator. In one example, a student had recently lost a family member in an accident, and in another case, a student had recently found a dead body in his garden. This made the exercise a stress point that was hard to anticipate.

Initial Response

How much the initial response is included in a simulation is likely to be governed by the training objectives. For example, an organisation may want to test its emergency response plan through a 'surprise' exercise. In other words, where staff are deployed with no pre-warning to a location that is unknown to them.

An example of this involved a Middle-East based airline where a small core team knew of, and had prepared for, an exercise that involved two investigators who were to be deployed to the United Kingdom without pre-warning. The timing of the event was such that both had worked a full day and were now at home. Traveling was realistic for them and it was predicted that they would be able to get some sleep on the flight. However, the emergency response manager had also worked a full day and ended up working through the night to prepare logistics for their arrival in the United Kingdom. In debrief, he explained that he was suffering from extreme tiredness and couldn't remember much of the exercise. There was some loss of training value and a concern about how that staff member travelled home safely.

For the two who travelled to the United Kingdom, they arrived to extreme winter weather only to discover that their own airline had lost their bags *en route*. The value of packing essential clothing in hand luggage was highlighted, but there was a further hazard that pushing on with the exercise may put them at risk of a cold-weather injury. Spare clothing supplied by the facilitation team kept the exercise on track and the luggage arrived after it had concluded.

The main beneficiaries of this exercise were the support team who were engaged with the logistics of arranging flights, transfers, accommodation, and so on. It did mean that the team arrived on site in a similar condition that they would have done in the real thing, but there was some element of 'practicing bleeding' rather than maximising their learning.

For the majority of site simulations, the starting point will be 'on-site' perhaps at the point that emergency first responders are preparing to hand over. As one experienced accident investigator described it, 'to be realistic, the investigators should arrive in the middle of the night whilst it is raining only to see a fire truck driving over the wreckage trail' (P. Claiden, Principal Inspector, Air Accidents Investigation Branch – DfT, Farnborough, personal communication, 2005). In practice, this hand over can provide an excellent opportunity to deliver key facts and safety information, although this does not remove the need for a dedicated 'exercise briefing' before starting the role-play (Figure 15.3).

Site Management

There are two elements of site management to consider:

- the management of the site by the students
- the management of the simulation by the facilitators.

The former encompasses the prioritisation of activities, liaison with other parties on site, time and workload management. Many of these activities are covered in other parts of this chapter and form an important part of the learning experience. Resources should be made available to the students subject to consideration of:

- Is this equipment that would be available to them?
- Would it be available in the timescale?
- Would they have had training to use it?
- Is it safe for them to bring these into the training environment?

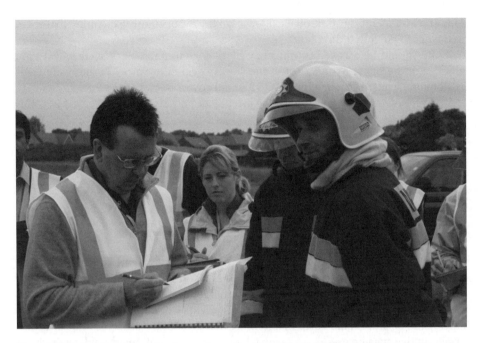

Figure 15.3 A hand over from the fire service at the start of the field phase (photo: author's own).

Examples may include vehicles, imagery tools (e.g. laser site scanner), radios, measurement tools, cones/tape for cordons, a caravan or tent to work from, portable toilets, and so on. Remember that students can be ingenious and their enthusiasm may need to be contained. In one example, a group persuaded a local helicopter company to bring an aircraft to the site for aerial photographs. However, they did not brief any of the other people on site of its arrival, which presented a physical hazard and risked blowing away evidence with its downwash.

The management of the simulation by the facilitators consists of three phases:

- planning and set-up
- delivery
- debrief and review.

The *planning phase* may take many months and should not be underestimated. Permission to use a site, for example an airport or railway, may be complex; if wreckage is to be used then its acquisition, transportation and storage needs to be arranged; if actors are to be used, their scripts needs to written, checked and learned. Whilst this may be a team activity because of the number of tasks involved, there needs to be an owner of the scenario or it will become very difficult to assemble a coherent narrative. Like the author of a novel, the owner must get to know the characters involved and how they will interact with the facts if they are able to build a believable scenario.

Equally, they must be familiar with the specifics of an accident site or crime scene and should be present throughout the delivery phase in order to deal with conflictions, errors or when students get to the edge of what has been planned for. In the last case, this may mean generating additional evidence 'on the fly' or simply explaining that there is no further to go in that direction.

Planning should also cover contingency plans for circumstances such as extreme weather. Will the scenario still work if the site is covered in snow? Is there sufficient provision for shelter? Is there appropriate first aid cover?

The *delivery phase* should start with the briefing of participants to cover:

- objectives of the simulation
- rules/limits of the simulation
- safe working rules
- roles and responsibilities
- how to ask questions of the facilitators
- timescales
- resources that are available to them
- any technical details that they must know.

This should be followed by a period of time for consolidation and group forming before going on-site. Upon arrival, the safe working rules should be reiterated, including how an exercise can be stopped, what to do in an emergency and any specific hazards that may not be part of the risk assessment that the students would do.

Supervision on site should cover maintaining the safety of the students and collecting information that may be useful in a feedback session. Interventions should generally be to keep students safe and working in roughly the right direction without turning the session into a tutorial. There needs to be enough scope to learn from mistakes without the danger of going completely off track.

The *debrief and review phase* is of enormous importance and should not be relegated to a brief chat at the end of the day. Time set aside for self- or group-reflection prior to a group debrief is a worthwhile investment. Students are likely to be exhausted at the end of a day on-site and not necessarily in the best position to benefit from a lengthy debrief. A hot debrief of instant lessons followed by a period of reflection and a longer facilitated debrief works well, although other methods such as carrying the scenario into an analysis and report writing phase can also provide good feedback to the participants (see section on Analysis and Reporting).

In addition to debriefing the students, the facilitators and actors should also be brought together to identify problems with the scenario, experiences from delivering it and suggest ways in which it could be refined. Whereas there is a danger that the next course could be made perfect for the last group of students, there is also considerable benefit to come from refining and perfecting a particular scenario. If it is to be used multiple times then it is worth asking the students not to share the scenario with others, collect in evidence such as documentation and change some key facts.

Evidence Collection

The identification, preservation and harvesting of evidence is generally the principal activity on site. In a real-play scenario, the evidence must be presented in the way it would be discovered in the real event. In other words, it may be obvious, obscured, damaged, tainted or perishable. Care should be taken to avoid over-reliance on a 'golden

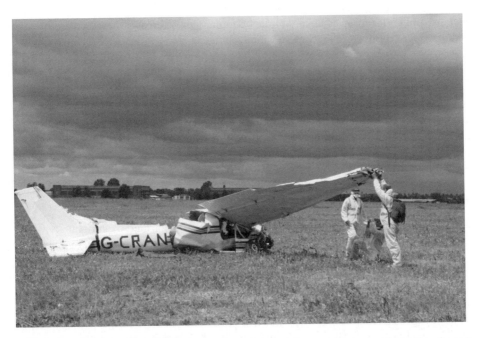

Figure 15.4 A 'real' wrecked aircraft on simulated crash site (photo: author's own) (see colour figure in colour plate section).

rivet' or single clue to solve the investigation, in case: (a) it is overlooked by the students, (b) it goes missing or is damaged, or (c) it is found in the opening stages and the rest of the allotted time is wasted.

Physical evidence such as the wreckage of a vehicle is hard to acquire and generally needs a benevolent owner or insurer (Figure 15.4). Damage to an 'un-crashed' vehicle is difficult to achieve safely for obvious reasons, but is achievable with some creativity. For example, dragging a wreck along the ground can create witness marks, but so can the use of tools, such as spades. Footprints on site created whilst laying out such witness marks may be explained as the footprints of first responders or spectators.

Marking artificialities is important to avoid confusing the student. For example, if the wreckage has been cut for moving onto the site, this may have to be marked. Participants will be aware that such artificialities are likely to exist during a simulation, but get frustrated when they pursue them as 'real' only to discover in the debrief that it was not a realistic distraction.

If multiple teams are to cycle through the accident site then ensure that evidence can be returned to its original state, especially if participants are expected to 'bag and tag' the originals. This may need multiple copies of evidence (hard with physical evidence) or an essential evidence log/photo record so that the site can be reset between groups. Resetting a site can be time consuming, but does allow smaller groups to work through the site.

The greater the realism, the easier it is for the participant to embrace the scenario. Simple touches can make a big difference: a mobile phone that rings; theatrical blood; a wallet with IDs and cash; authentic uniforms and so on. Some can be bought from specialist police/forensic science supplies companies, whereas others can be bought from eBay or scrounged from the relevant agencies.

Media Management

Crime scenes and accidents make great news and, as such, forensic scientists and investigators need a media handling strategy, even if this is within a company policy of not to speak to the media. To gain the maximum from the training experience, it is worth making their interaction as realistic as possible.

The Local Hack

Regional newspapers and radio stations will be generally manned by generalists. Their job will cover the mundane punctuated with occasional moments of excitement, the latter of which may be their opportunity to make it into 'prime time.' As a character, the local hack is likely to be keen to extract a sound bite and perhaps report in clichés. They ask leading questions and jump to conclusions – 'so would you say it was definitely murder?' Their equipment is likely to be limited to a Dictaphone and a camera.

A newspaper article put together by such a reporter is likely to be fronted by a sensationalist headline (Air crash horror, Brutal murder, etc.), include inaccuracies (e.g. name, organisation, etc.), clichés ('twenty-four hours on and investigators still don't know the cause of yesterday's accident…') and a sound bite that may well be from a witness or neighbour ('Steve Smith said he had been concerned about just such an accident' or 'Questions are now being asked about the safety of…'). An article like this can prove valuable feedback at the end of a day on site.

The Radio Interview

These can be more difficult than face-to-face interviews so should be practiced in a realistic manner. This could be as simple as sitting back to back with the interviewer or at the end of a telephone, although if a studio can be used it will only add to the realism. Live and recorded interviews have their relative merits. The former can be high pressure and capture mistakes, pauses and hesitations, whereas the latter are at the mercy of the sound editor and may have the interviewer's voice added later.

The Television Interview

A television camera can be a major inducer of stress, especially if used for a live interview. Realism can be added by briefing the camera crew that they have a deadline to meet and the only information they have is what they can gain from the scene. An edited news piece is an extremely compelling form of feedback, particularly if the editor has chosen to be mischievous. Bear in mind that the vocal track can be laid over other images to create a particular story and long-range lenses can access a site that the students thought was protected. Even a 'no comment' response can be carefully crafted into a story if the under-pressure journalist is struggling to get their story finished in time. An experienced interviewer will make the whole experience more realistic, so consider contacting a local TV station or media college.

The Press Conference

This involves a lot of resources to be realistic, but provides the opportunity to bombard the student with lots of questions. As with all of the previous scenarios, their inclusion depends on the desired learning outcomes. They add workload to a busy person on-site and help to expose them to the wider aspects of the area in which they are planning to work.

Team Management

Where several investigators/scientists are to work on-site together, the team management aspects are important and deserve attention. There is a tendency for students to want to focus on the 'fun part' of evidence collection rather than managing resources, but this is generally not the only task they are preparing for. Managing a site is not the same as leading all of the activity on the site. It may involve stepping back to retain the big picture or deal with the unexpected. The role may be assigned to a particular individual who may best benefit from the experience or be left to a team to decide, but should remain constant for the simulation to avoid confusion.

For the facilitators, this provides a clear route for information that may need to be injected into the scenario, such as information from their control centre or other agencies. It can also provide a conduit for information that the team may want to consider as part of their self-evaluation.

Multi-day scenarios may need more team management, particularly as tiredness sets in or the phase of operation moves from on-site to analysis. The people management aspects may well be as valuable as the technical aspects. Where multiple cultures are involved, for example, nationalities or disciplines, team management may need to focus on conflict resolution or extracting the best from people (Figure 15.5).

In one example, the team was being managed by a British engineer who felt that one of his Chinese colleagues had not done what was asked of him. He delivered feedback to him, but caused offence because he had done so in front of one of the Chinese delegate's colleagues, causing him to lose face. This created a level of conflict when a Libyan team member was asked to join with the two Chinese students to depose the team leader. The facilitators were aware of the situation and monitored it, but did not step in. The Libyan team member took exception to the plan and said that their role as team members was to support their team leader. The conflict was resolved internally and, upon reflection, the various team members recognised the need to manage group relations more effectively in the future.

What about interactions between experienced/less experienced students? Is that ever a source of conflict/tension? If some are condescending to others, or frustrated by others' naivety?

In a second example, the atmosphere within a group had become tense during the analysis phase due to conflicting views as to how to proceed. An experienced investigator was found outside smoking and asked how things were going by the facilitator. 'We are arguing a lot; I just needed to take a break.' When the facilitator lent a sympathetic ear, he was told 'Oh it is fine; this is the same as every investigation I have ever worked on. It is completely normal for the analysis phase.' In other words, experiencing conflict or

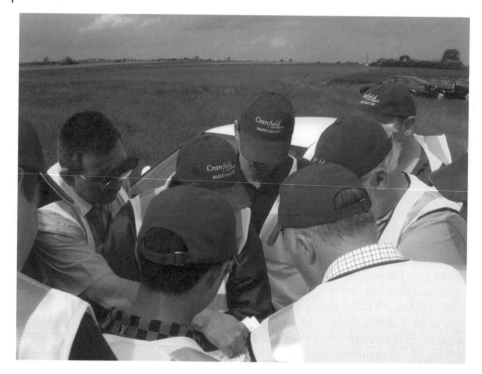

Figure 15.5 Team management across multiple cultures is a challenge (photo: author's own)!

communication difficulties is very normal and whilst it is important for a facilitator to monitor, it is not necessary to intervene to achieve the desired learning outcome. Advice may be as simple as 'why not take a break from your roles, have a coffee and come back to it in a while?'

The different experience levels of students in a team can be problematic if not properly managed. There is a risk that those with most experience will take over and the inexperienced participants will withdraw and lose out on the learning experience. Regular but informal catch-up meetings with the teams can help to capture such tendencies and encourage peer support. The focus needs to be on developing new skills rather than relying on the most experienced members of the team to deliver the 'answer' for the team.

Witnesses and Interviewing

Eyewitnesses are either a valuable source of evidence or an annoying distraction, depending on when they appear on site. Their evidence is both vulnerable and perishable, so if the student's role is to collect such evidence, time needs to be set aside to at least evaluate whether there is evidence that needs to be collected immediately. Such 'triage' activity may turn into a lengthy, unplanned interview, which may be problematic if the investigator has other tasks that they planned to achieve. Equally, a witness who is

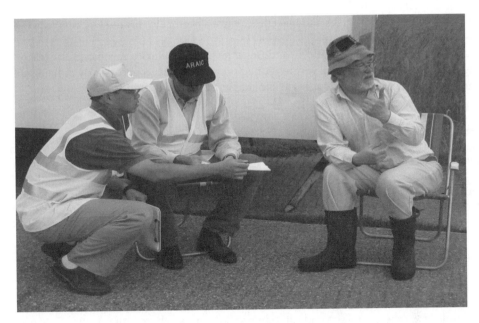

Figure 15.6 An unexpected witness interview on site (photo: author's own).

asked to come back later may well decide not to, or come back with an enhanced story based on the number of other people they have spoken to in the meantime.

To create a realistic scenario, witnesses are likely to come in all shapes and sizes. They may include: those speaking a second language; experts and enthusiastic amateurs; couples; children and so on. They may be willing and able or willing and unable. They may be in a rush or wanting their 15 minutes of fame without actually having anything useful to say. Using a variety of actors or volunteers who are not known to the students will create a high degree of realism.

To play their role requires not just the facts that they may be willing to share, but also a larger story about their character (Figure 15.6). Bear in mind that the interviewer is likely to want to build up a picture about their witness without necessarily knowing what they are looking for from them. The trade-off is between creating a complex character befitting only of a professional actor or creating enough of a character and accepting that some *ad libbing* is appropriate. For example, there is little point in asking an actor to remember a second birthday if his or hers can be written into the scenario.

Inaccuracies in a witness testimony are realistic, within reason. They should be briefed to be realistically accurate, but like all witnesses, they were not prepared for what they were about to experience so, as such, their testimony is likely to have deficiencies. They should be briefed to respond either in the way you would like them to (e.g. 'your character is angry/upset…') and/or to the way in which they are interviewed (e.g. 'if they treat you well then be more willing to give them information'). It is worth agreeing whether there is key information that the witness will give during the interview even without being directly asked – this may be important to make a particular scenario work. However, it should also be borne in mind that interviewers should only generally be rewarded for asking the right questions so the witness should not feel compelled to reel off a list of helpful facts. Irrelevancies and inaccuracies are a normal by-product of interviewing eyewitnesses.

A telephone interview can add an additional level of complexity, raising similar teaching points to the radio interviews mentioned previously. This is particularly difficult for those using their second language, so should be used with caution.

Coaching Techniques

Simulations can vary from the simple 'site tutorial' where students are walked through the activities that they might do on-site, to a real-time simulation where they effectively run the site phase shadowed by facilitators (Figure 15.7). In the case of the latter, the facilitators provide supervision, advice when requested (e.g. through a 'time-out' system) and manage the available time.

A site tutorial may be based on either a specific scenario or a showground of evidence types to work through. The student must be clear which it is, as the temptation will be to try and solve what is in front of him/her. The latter is a good way of covering lots of things in a short amount of time without the need for a complex or contrived scenario, whereas the former has a higher degree of realism. The showground technique allows for multiple groups to be on-site and rotating between tasks, whereas the specific scenario requires consecutive scheduling.

An example of the showground technique allowed four facilitators to cover risk assessment, evidence identification, photography and sampling in one site by rotating the groups, whereas the specific scenario technique required an ordered walk-through with a larger group.

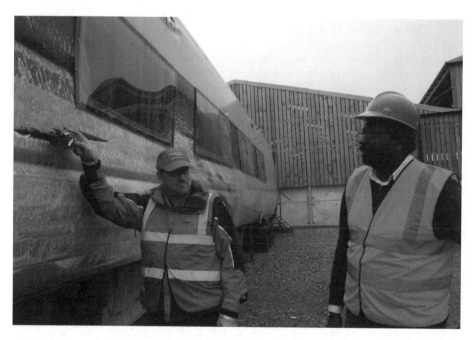

Figure 15.7 A tutorial on-site led by an experienced facilitator (photo: author's own).

The real-time simulations are harder to organise, but can deliver a richer learning environment, especially if used as a next step following a site tutorial. Participants are introduced to a scenario at a particular point in time and then asked to work in real-time from that point on.

Analysis and Reporting

Whilst for many, the use of simulation will focus entirely on practical activities, it is worth considering extending the scenario into the analysis and reporting phases. Many analysis techniques are taught in class using theory or case studies, but few start with the students actually collecting and reviewing their own evidence.

Completing an investigation – whether a crime or an accident – depends upon collecting enough evidence to withstand rigorous analysis. Experienced scientists and investigators would realise that this involves reviewing evidence for its quality and reliability. Evidence may be misleading or ambiguous; witnesses may be vague or contradictory and so analysis must withstand these limitations. In many cases where the end of the field phase may bring apparent certainty about what has occurred, the analysis phase generally starts with the realisation that there are multiple interpretations amongst the team. Indeed, for many, the analysis phase starts with a diminishing level of confidence until key facts can be bottomed out (Figure 15.8).

Approaches to analysis are varied both in terms of formal tools and more fundamentally, personal preference. Some will like to broaden their thinking through mind mapping or brainstorm, whereas others will prefer a more procedural approach such

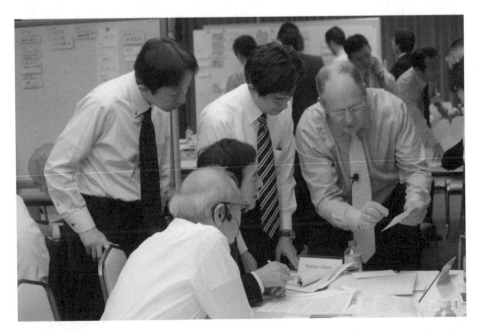

Figure 15.8 The analysis phase is an intensive learning phase (photo: author's own) (see colour figure in colour plate section).

as working with logic trees or timelines. It is a process that needs close management to avoid the discussion becoming personality-driven or feeling too personal. This role generally falls to the team leader, but the facilitator can play a vital role in keeping people on track.

Analysis generally needs space and access to resources. This may be as straightforward as access to a room with plenty of table space, blank walls or whiteboards, stationery and refreshments. Some have found that access to a computer and projector allows the analysis and report to be authored by a larger group more easily.

Feeding back the results of the analysis through a presentation provides a useful opportunity for peer review. However, as many roles would ultimately require a written report, there may be considerable educational benefit in taking the simulation through to the completion of a final report. This takes time and may extend any conflicts experienced during the analysis phase, but is able to demonstrate some of the practical problems that come with multi-author reports, especially when preparing for a deadline.

To make the experience as close to real life as possible, the feedback is then provided on the basis of the written report alone. This could be from peers, a facilitator, industry expert or perhaps legal counsel. A mixture of more than one type of feedback may highlight the different audiences that many reports are attempting to communicate with.

Summary

The simulation of accident sites or crime scenes creates a fantastic learning opportunity for students planning to work in such environments. It is an approach that according to Woodcock *et al.* (2005) is '…well accepted by participants and shows flexibility for a range of uses.'

There are many aspects to consider in setting up such training experiences, but with good planning and facilitation, the educational value is unparalleled.

Reference

Woodcock, K., Drury, C. G., Smiley, A. and Ma, J. (2005) Using simulated investigations for accident investigation studies. *Applied Ergonomics*, **36**, 1–12.

16

Police Training in the Twenty-first Century

Mark Roycroft

University of East London, University Way, London, UK

Introduction

The changing face of policing provides an opportunity for police training and education to be totally professionalised within a Higher Education backdrop. This could instil an element of mentoring and evaluation of policing services for all police and staff from the time of joining through the spectrum of a lifetime career. The wider context of how to police a particular community and the unique challenges that provides can be incorporated into the wider training and education of officers and staff. This will then become an integral part of the police culture and training, providing additional transparency and accountability. The police can thus be seen as a 'true' profession, on a par with established professions such as law and medicine without losing the Peelian concept of policing, where the police are an integral part of the community. The UK Police are facing the 'perfect storm' of crime investigation and policing issues. There is increased scrutiny of investigations along with changes in law enforcement organisations, which contribute to a metaphorsis in the policing milieu.

The Police Service and forensic staff will have to adapt to the new politics while retaining a quality service for the public. Using the concept of 'new institutionalism' (Scott, 2004), the emergency services will have to analyse the new rules and procedures and provide an 'interaction between organisational context and action' (Greenwood and Hinings, 1996). This chapter hopes to address how the impact of community policing can be effectively monitored and how any improvements can be quickly introduced into the organisation. In Australia, the police have reformed substantially over the last decade and this was done eventually on an incremental basis, rather than a constant 'big bang' (Marks and Sklanksy, 2011).

Learning styles are changing – particularly in policing. The Winsor (2011) and Neyroud (2011) Home Office Reports into Police entry requirements and promotion have highlighted the need for a more professional approach to internal promotion and initial training. They also discuss the direct entry at different ranks within the police service. This, along with the creation of the upcoming Police Professional Body, has caused

Forensic Science Education and Training: A Tool-kit for Lecturers and Practitioner Trainers, First Edition.
Edited by Anna Williams, John P. Cassella, and Peter D. Maskell.
© 2017 John Wiley & Sons Ltd. Published 2017 by John Wiley & Sons Ltd.

a sea change in police education and training, which places the emphasis on the individual officers. Higher Education will play a vital part in this environment.

Neyroud (2011) talks of a police service that should move from a 'service that acts professionally' to a 'professional force'. The idea of police professionalism and policing as a bona fide profession are discussed in this chapter. Sklansky (2012) sets out four meanings of police professionalism, one of which is the idea of 'self regulation' in the manner of the legal profession. The other three concepts are 'high expectations,' internalised norms and professional policing. He states that this should be 'reflective and knowledge based, a matter of expertise rather than common sense, intuition or innate talent.' This could be enabled by the work of academics while not neglecting the 'street skills' that are required for all emergency services.

Academia and policing skills are not mutually exclusive; research can in fact enhance the decision making of the practitioner. The author's PhD research (Roycroft, 2009) looked at this aspect of policing providing in depth analysis of Senior Investigating Officers (SIO) in 166 cases in the Metropolitan Police. This emphasised the benefit of experience mixed with 'naturalistic' decision-making that enabled the SIO to identify the type of murder quickly and therefore select solving factors for that particular case. One of the principal solving factors identified by quantitative research was the management of witnesses and the early selection of particular lines of enquiry. Forensic strategy emerged as the leading solving factor. The forensic strategy meetings with the SIO and forensic experts remain one of the most important aspects of SIO strategy. The research was intended to add academic rigour to the experience and ability of the 34 SIOs interviewed to provide a reflection on what works and what does not.

Tilley and Laycock (2014) describe the police as professional problem solvers. All emergency services deal with a vast array of troublesome situations, they argue that it is time to refocus on what the police should do and understand the core business. This affects all aspects of policing and introduces the need for collaboration and interoperability between forensic staff and police investigation teams.

In addition, Tilley and Laycock (2014) add that 'a professional organisation is also concerned with continuous improvement and continuing professional development of its members,' and the maintenance of high standards and non-discrimination along with valuing research, and separate different 'professions.' The creation of the new Policing College is one step towards that professional development. Practitioners can draw on a body of established research, which has academic rigour and a high status of ethics. The maintenance of a code of ethics allows members to take a break for personal development or domestic reasons but maintain their professional status. It states that it will work with universities to share and develop the underlying evidence base for policing practice. It will work with the private sector to access training from outside the police service and work closely with international partners.

The Policing Higher Education forum is a good example of a body that can assist in moving this debate forward. The universities involved in policing-type degrees have formed a body that wishes to benchmark and provide quality assurance in the courses provided by their institutions, it is hoped that they will become an integral part of the new Policing College. The issue of quality assurance in policing degrees and courses is paramount to ensure a uniform standard of education and training for potential and current police officers and staff.

The current economic climate could act as a driver for closer operation in police terms and is leading to greater collaboration and shared services with Forces. It could also lead to improved joint working as different organisations will need to consider sharing services, responding to critical incidents and being first at the scene of emergencies, highlighting similar issues for all services. Training should include not only technical skills but 'soft skills', such as group work and communication skills, to equip the practitioner with the requisite skills to integrate with the community. This correlates with the demands of general employers from all walks of life who are asking universities to equip their students with 'life skills'. Employers value interpersonal skills, integrity and communications skills (Santella and Emery, 2007). Yorke and Knight (2006) developed their USEM model of employability, where USEM is an acronym for four inter-related components of employability:

- Understanding of the subject
- Skills
- Efficacy skills
- Meta recognition strategic thinking and self awareness.

The traditional training school, with didactic rote type learning, is being replaced by a more Open University type of teaching process. This could encompass the best of the old traditions allowing the individual to develop their skills in a reflective manner. The new style of training would enable the individual to work towards a recognised qualification that would have currency outside the organisation and would allow the individual to pursue specialisms and share best practice. Specialist degrees should prepare the practitioner for a career in Policing and Forensic Science, while allowing the student to pursue specialist interests in an environment with academic rigour and mentoring. The mentoring could be provided by ex-practitioners with an academic background and could concentrate on the principles of dealing with critical incidents and explaining the context of how the individuals should respond. The emphasis on inter-operability and multi-agency working informs the student that they do not operate in a vacuum, but are part of a wider organisational network safeguarding and working for members of society.

Training of Future Police Detectives

The Winsor report (2011) lays out different pre-join and entry pathways for future police officers and detectives. Future Detective Inspectors and Chief Inspectors could in theory be in place after three years' service. While this may lead to a cross-fertilisation of certain skills that would be advantageous to the police and investigations, it may also reduce the experiential base of senior detectives. It might enhance high-tech crime investigations and certain specialised crime types, but will it make the investigation of Category A crimes (major crimes with implications about society) more efficient? Future police training under the new Professional Policing Body (PPB) could see providers outside the police running training courses, such as detective courses. While recognising the need for change and transference of necessary skills, the detective career path, as shown by Roycroft (2009), must be maintained and developed to ensure that these investigations are managed correctly. The traditional career path may be outdated but the essential skills required to lead major investigations must be developed and enhanced.

Detective training could be further professionalised and as Blair Gibbs (Research Director for Crime & Justice) stated in 2012 (personal communication) there is a 'dearth of detectives at Chief Constable level.' Officers' crime fighting abilities and, more crucially, investigation management skills should be acknowledged and given credence over other 'softer' competencies needed for promotion. This professionalisation could take the form of a Masters' degree, acknowledged within British Universities as a gold standard for the world. Its completion should be upheld as the benchmark.

Cassella and McCartney (2011) state that 'there needs to a broadening of forensic science education to incorporate those who have to understand forensic evidence including lawyers… and more importantly the Police.' The Neyroud Home Office report (2011) on Police Training called for a central governing body along the lines of a Royal College of Policing in the United Kingdom, which is now in place. This raises the issue of how detectives and senior detectives will be selected and trained. A new qualification will support and recognise developing expertise amongst neighbourhood officers, response officers, investigators and specialists. Cassella and McCartney feel that plans to incorporate police officer training within this 'flawed model' may not professionalise, but could build upon the problems inherent in legal and forensic training. They state that such developments will work against the aim of preventing miscarriages of justice and enhancing investigative capacities, and believe that the risks associated with the current deficit in trans-disciplinary learning and teaching, such as an increase in miscarriages of justice and failed investigations, will then be broadened and deepened. With no embedded policing discipline within universities it may prove difficult to find the right educational mix. It is important that the training and education of all ranks is implemented thoroughly and correctly from the start.

This provides an opportunity to open police courses to the best outside influences. The training and education of police officers of all ranks could be broadened and expanded to improve critical thinking and decision making skills. A review of 40 years of inquires into high profile police investigations (Roycroft, 2009) revealed seven distinct themes that affected the police:

- clarity and leadership among senior officers
- skills of SIOs
- systematic failures
- phasing of enquires
- the role of the major investigation room
- information management
- individual investigative strategy failures that prevailed in each investigation.

The challenge for the police is to 'train' these deficiencies out of police practice if possible. This requires a national 'library' of police responses to investigation and analysis of the solving factors on a continual basis.

The twenty-first century investigator will have to be much more aware of global issues. Advances in information technology have meant that criminals can operate from anywhere and the police have to react accordingly. Geographical jurisdictions are now global and present particular problems for the police.

Despite criticisms, the British Police are still seen as the 'gold standard' for serious crime investigations. The constitutional position of the UK police allows a high profile within law enforcement and peace keeping within the United Kingdom. Unlike their European neighbours, the British Police Service holds a prominent position within the Criminal Justice System. This has been diluted in part by the Crown Prosecution Service (CPS) and could be further watered down by elected Crime Commissioners. To maintain this prominent position, the police need to build on a largely respected standing, by ensuring the quality and perceived quality of all levels of investigation. The integrity of those in charge of investigations needs to be maintained and will be subject to increased scrutiny. The police ought to enhance the review process of enquiries both internally and if requested make them a matter of public record (excluding sensitive material).

Evaluation of Police Performance

Thirdly, this chapter looks at the means to measure and evaluate police performance and how best to measure and evaluate the impact of training on improving community safety. There are many different types of evaluation tools and they can be used in a variety of ways. Although these tools are related, the different terminologies employed by evaluation practitioners can lead to confusion. The tools all address performance measurement, ongoing monitoring and performance indicators, along with project and programme evaluation. All of these measures are there to elicit responses from the community to assist the police in their deployment of resources.

Some of the methods of evaluation are as follows:

- polls of police performance carried out by an independent company
- victim satisfaction surveys
- crime rates
- accident and emergency admissions
- false arson/fire calls
- less property damaged
- community meetings
- websites
- social networking
- forensic results
- impact of forensic examinations on clear up rate.

Avoiding Miscarriages of Justice

The maintenance of investigative quality will assist the police to maintain public confidence and funding. Cassella and McCartney (2011) state that miscarriages of justice result not from a single error but a compounding of issues associated with police investigations, forensic evidence reporting and the subsequent legal use of these materials. The police have paid compensation to victims' families in poorly managed cases; this may prove the next testing ground for investigations as victims' families challenge poor investigations. In recent years, the rights of victims within the justice systems of the

United Kingdom have been considerably extended, with the creation of new organisations and procedures and the provision of greater funds (Lewis and Ellis, 2006).

Convictions and police enquiries are subject to scrutiny from various bodies, such as the Independent Police Complaints Commission (IPCC) and the Criminal Cases Review Commission (CCRC). Between 1997 and 2005 the CCRC had received over 8500 referrals of cases of suspected miscarriages of justice: 318 of these had been referred to the Court of Appeal, of which 266 had been fully considered. In 187 cases the original conviction was quashed and of the remaining 79, the conviction was upheld. Past inquires can help inform present or future investigative strategies by providing best practice and highlighting potential pitfalls. There is a need to catalogue and find a suitable repository for how cases are solved. This should be held centrally (by the Association of Chief Police Officers (ACPO) or the Home Office) and be made available to all investigating and senior investigating officers (SIOs). This would be of particular benefit to multi-victim murders and those low incidence murder types such as contract killings. This database could help avoid miscarriages of justice or failed investigations by highlighting the pitfalls of certain types of investigation. The police need to develop a repository for the skills and solving factors used in these enquiries to inform a new generation of senior detectives. This library of cases, which could then be indexed, and the creation of this 'super' database would enable SIOs to have access to a diagnostic tool that could influence their decision making. Jones *et al.* (2008) discuss this in terms of 'capturing the learning.' Software packages could be written to assist in the diagnostic decision making of investigating officers and senior investigating officers. The police still lack a national 'library' of case solving and the material on the Home Office Large Major Enquiry System (HOLMES) is not routinely analysed and stored after analysis. If HOLMES was developed to automatically download the requisite solving factors, the resultant material could be analysed by experts in the Force along with academics to improve the quality of investigations. This would also afford SIOs a diagnostic reference tool to augment their decision making during investigations. Police services would also be assisted in public inquiries or reviews, and it would illustrate the depth and breadth of decision making. The United Kingdom lacks a facility to formally debrief all cases of murder and thus opportunities are being missed to collate this information nationwide. There is a need to debrief all aspects of murder investigation nationwide and code the responses.

Maintaining and Developing the Role of the Senior Investigating Officer (SIO)

Looking across the historical pattern of enquiries (see Table 16.1), it appears that at particular historical moments certain high profile major crime investigations come to be seen as problematic in some way or another. At such times, the conduct of the investigation itself is reviewed, either through a public enquiry, some other framework, or internally, with the result that some reform in policing practices is recommended. The introduction of significant reform is not a continuous progression and development; rather, it tends to occur in 'fits and starts.' The plethora of changes provide a 'once in a lifetime' opportunity to look at not only how crimes are investigated, but how investigators are selected and trained. The National Police Improvement Agency (NPIA) are now proposing training SIOs towards a Professionalising Investigation Programme (PIP)

Table 16.1 Skills of the Senior Investigating Officer.

Skills of Senior Investigating Officer	Relevant Inquiry
1 Effective decision-making. The SIO should 'exercise critical faculties'	Macpherson Report (1999)
2 Planning the phasing of inquiries	Climbie Inquiry (2003); Taylor Review (2002); Byford Report (2006)
3 Scene management/understanding 'critical incident' management including forensic strategy	HMIC Soham Report (2002)
4 Witness management	Macpherson Report (1999)/ HMIC Soham (2002)
5 Strategic investigative awareness/ability to manage investigations	Macpherson Report (1999)/HMIC Soham Report (2002)
6 Experience of major investigations	Shipman Inquiry (2003)/ Taylor Review (2002)
7 Management of the Major Investigation Room (MIR)	Macpherson Report (1999)
8 Leadership	Byford Report (2006)/ Macpherson Report (1999)

level 4, with the intention of making senior officers aware of the strategic issues involved in investigations. This will engender an understanding of the implications for officers and Forces involved in major enquiries.

Greater Manchester Police (GMP) have appointed their first SIO to deal with domestic murders, and the Winsor Report (2011) advocates direct entry to inspector and superintendent level, meaning that future SIOs could be officers who have little experience of running investigations. This lack of experience may cause difficulties, and while direct entrants may bring other valuable skills to the Service, they will lack the depth of experience required to manage major enquires. The police need to maintain and develop the skillbase developed over a long period of time. The Lawrence case and the Leveson Inquiry (2012) illustrate the damage done to victims' families and the reputation of the Force when incorrect decisions are made throughout investigations.

The ACPO (2005) Core Investigative Doctrine states that flawed decision-making has been responsible for failed investigations. The doctrine further mentions 'verification bias' where the detective allows their early assumptions in a case to determine their investigative strategy. Jones *et al.* (2008) describe this as being where the investigator adopts a hypothesis as to what has happened and then finds the evidence to support his/her hypothesis and excludes contradictory evidence. This was very evident in the persistence of the Yorkshire Ripper investigators to build their enquiry around the tape of 'Wearside Jack,' which later was established to be a hoax (Byford Report, 2006). Stelfox (2009) defines the qualities required of an investigator as follows: 'knowledge of the law, information profiles, human behaviour, investigative techniques and investigative strategies.' and Flanagan (2000) also described five stages in investigative techniques:

- initial crime scene assessment.
- assessing incoming information
- selecting appropriate lines of enquiry
- case development
- post charge management.

These key skills should be augmented and developed within the proposed new training regime with universities. SIO training should be a prerequisite for promotion to the highest ranks to emphasise the key skills of prioritisation, phasing of enquires and correct decision making. The proposed PIP level 4 training should give ACPO officers an awareness of how investigations of this type should be run and therefore highlight the resources needed over the lifetime of such an enquiry. An awareness of how to manage the 'phasing' of an enquiry over the long periods that Category A (the most difficult high profile case) and Category B (not necessarily high profile but difficult case) cases last for is essential to ensure that the correct number of resources are deployed at the right time.

Expert Witnesses

Expert witnesses have become a fixture in global criminal justice systems. As trials become increasingly more scientifically complex, Casella and McCartney (2011) state that it becomes difficult to challenge their expertise and opinions, that checks and balances are required and there is a danger of creating a 'battle of the experts'. The management of expert witnesses will become a growing issue for senior investigators. Shanteau (1992) states that 'Experts are operationally defined as those who have been recognised within their profession as having the necessary skills and abilities to perform at the highest levels'. The use of expert witnesses has been an issue in child protection cases and with other forensic experts.

The Compartmentalisation of Investigative Skills

The compartmentalisation of investigative skills is a major concern. Canter (2012) stated that 'now that every aspect of policing has become a sophisticated speciality', that the day of the generalist police officer is over. The specialism of many investigations, with the larger Forces having separate murder, rape and fraud teams, means that career detectives may not get the 'rounded experience' that they require. Can any senior investigator be expected to be a master of all these different 'trades'? The cross-tabulation of skills may stretch the reserves of investigators and in turn the responsible Force to the limit. The Police Service has to ensure that the individual specialisms are maintained and developed along with the quality of more mundane investigations. Succession planning is a key issue. The Home Office A19 regulations (officers have to retire on 30 years' service) have seen some Forces denuded of swathes of experienced officers. It is therefore more important than ever that the UK Police Force Library records the experiences of past investigations and develops a HOLMES database for the twenty-first century, which acts not only as a storage and retrieval system but as a 'neural network' type package. This database could inform investigators about gaps in their investigations. Similarly, police intelligence systems must routinely be developed to cope with organised crime and changes in crime types.

The use of police analysts and analysis must be developed to become an integral part of police investigations and the SIO training of the future would benefit from taught modules in this area. Crime scene examiners with a deep skill base should be in place to advise SIOs and senior officers. It is perhaps time to look again at the role of the traditional 'Lab Sergeant' role in the Metropolitan Police, which acted as a nexus between the investigation team and forensic providers. The 'Lab Sergeant' was an advisor to the SIO and provided a valuable understanding of police procedure and forensic strategy.

Forensic Provision

An HM Inspectorate of Constabulary (HMIC) report (2012) discussed 'serious' failings in police (rape) investigations. The HMIC report stated that cases were not being linked, DNA samples were being used incorrectly and correct checks were not being carried out. Streamlined forensic reporting (SFR) has been introduced and involves better assessment of the evidential value of forensic evidence at court, which saves resources and delays at Court. Although there is concern that SFR may lead to more miscarriages of justice (Zenith Crime Blog, 2015). The challenge for the police is linking similar cases and ensuring that both detectives and forensic scientists have consistent forensic strategies. The Lawrence trial of 2012 illustrated the following points:

1. The need for a thorough preliminary examination in any given set of circumstances.
2. The importance of accurate and full notes.
3. The need for case material to be properly preserved and kept.
4. The need for a careful examination of all items including packaging.
5. The importance of contamination avoidance procedures
6. The dangers of making assumptions and cutting corners.

There have been calls for a public enquiry to discover if private providers were fit for purpose following the unexplained death of the MI5 employee Gareth Williams. During the Coroner's inquest (The Independent, 2012), disquiet was expressed about the contamination of forensic material.

Silverman Report on the Closure of the Forensic Science Service

In January 2011, Professor Bernard Silverman, Home Office Chief Scientific Adviser, was commissioned by Home Office ministers to conduct a review of research and development relevant to forensic science (Silverman, 2011). This review demonstrates the very wide range of research and development relevant to forensic science, carried out by forensic science providers, universities and laboratories associated with Government. It was informed by widespread consultation, with over 80 respondents, including over 40 universities identifying research relevant to forensic science. The review makes recommendations to policy makers and others in the forensic science community. It particularly underlined the crucial role that representative organisations, learned and professional societies have in providing a forum for the communication, development and validation of ideas, to act as advocates and representatives of the field, and to be a focus for the relevant research and development communities.

The consequent likelihood of fragmentation of analysis between the police and forensic service providers (FSPs) risks a decline in:

- Effective use of forensic science in the courts, through loss of context in the development of forensic strategy, analysis and interpretation of results in complex cases.
- Quality of the forensic science delivered to the Criminal Justice System (CPS).
- Public confidence in impartiality.

Ethical Issues

There are privacy issues raised by the retention of DNA samples and profiles by the police, and not with the conditions under which they were taken. This is an important distinction since it precludes any interrogation of the legitimacy of the legislation which allows the police to breach bodily integrity to obtain non-consensual samples without consent. Cassella and McCartney (2011) state that it seems generally accepted in UK jurisprudence that police should have the right to obtain DNA samples for comparison on the National DNA database (NDNAD), at the point of charging an individual whether or not DNA evidence relevant to the investigation of the offence for which the individual is being charged exists. Article 8(2) of the European Human Rights Act (ECHR) states that any breach of the right to respect for private and family life must be 'in accordance with the law.' A central feature of these considerations, about whom should be sampled and profiled, what type of information samples and profiles currently and potentially provide and how such information should be used to support criminal investigations, is that they circulate continuously between two different, but social and organisational 'sites.' These are: sites of operation (e.g. criminal investigation departments, police forensic science units, etc.) and sites of deliberation (e.g. government departments, judicial committees, government advisory commissions, independent social and human rights groups). In each jurisdiction that possesses a national DNA database, it is possible to discern various key organisations and agencies within each of these kinds of sites that contribute to the co-production and co-development of the large number of material and discursive practices that together make up the appropriate and legitimate uses of these technological resources. Therefore, the existence and continued operation of any national DNA database relies upon a series of continuous considerations and negotiated agreements amongst a range of actors seeking to satisfy different aims, expectations, ambitions and relevant expert and lay constituencies.

High Volume Crime

As discussed earlier, compartmentalisation affects the rounded experience of detectives in major forces and ensures that different levels of resources are deployed to different crimes. The high volume crimes, such as burglary, robbery and assault, form the basis of performance figures for any operational command unit commander. The investigation of these offences along with autocrime, domestic disputes and minor frauds, form the backbone of any CID 'office' in a Police Borough. These offences face scrutiny from senior managers in the Force and the HMIC, along with the demands of victims. The HMIC Report (2014) into reporting crimes looked at all 43 forces and found that most forces should work towards 'improved compliance,' improved call handling systems and maintain regular contact with the victims. In one major force, the IT system was described as 'outdated with limited capability.' Tighter result codes were called for and systems should be in place to monitor repeat victims and vulnerable victims. This is particularly pertinent after the Pilkington family tragedy in Leicestershire after the suicide of Fiona Pilkington, 38, and 18 year old Francesca in October 2007. The home of single mother Ms Pilkington was repeatedly targeted by groups of up to 16 youngsters, with stones, eggs and flour thrown at the house. Police were contacted 33 times in ten years but the family only received eight visits from officers. The inquest jury returned verdicts of suicide and unlawful killing, and said the response of the police and two local councils had contributed to the deaths.

Many critical incidents and high profile cases begin their investigative life on a police local 'Borough' and then, as their importance becomes more apparent, they are transferred to a specialist team. The need to maintain this 'golden hour' (Winsor Report, College of Policing, 2015) principle of investigative ability is important for the reputation of forces. The golden hour is the term used for the period immediately after an offence has been committed, when material is readily available in high volumes to the police. Positive action in the period immediately after the report of a crime minimises the amount of material that could be lost to the investigation, and maximises the chance of securing the material that will be admissible in court. The need for urgent and effective forensic analysis of such incidents is critical. There are many crimes that slip between the criteria of specialist teams and these 'mini major' investigations swamp borough resources and experience while remaining critical enquires. The balance in the future will be between maintaining the gold standard on major police investigations and ensuring the quality of high volume crime investigation.

New Investigative Challenges

The British Police will have to contend with new challenges that in some cases will physically stretch them across international boundaries and internally will change the culture and manner of operation.

Eco-terrorism

The Federal Bureau of Investigation (FBI) defines eco-terrorism as 'the use or threatened use' of violence of a criminal nature against innocent victims or property by an environmentally orientated sub-national group for environmental political reasons, or aimed at an audience beyond the target, often of a symbolic nature. Groups such as the Animal Liberation Front or Earth Liberation Front present a challenge to law enforcement in the United Kingdom and United States. In the United Kingdom, groups have targeted the Huntington Life Sciences, car dealerships, forestry companies, corporate and university-based medical research laboratories, restaurants, medical-supply firms, fur farms and other industries. These political groups, which draw in members of the public, will pose a challenge for investigators in the future. Once again these organisation and movements are driven by social networking.

In London, on 1 April 2009, the Metropolitan Police faced a demonstration of anti G20 protestors. The 'Camp in the City' aimed to draw attention to carbon trading, claiming that it was far from being a way of reducing release of climate change gasses in the atmosphere. The camp took place outside the European Climate Exchange in Bishopsgate. In the resulting demonstration a member of the public, Ian Tomlinson, died and the police faced severe criticism over its tactics of 'kettling' and the way they dealt with Ian Tomlinson (IPCC Report into Death of Ian Tomlinson, 2010). The Metropolitan Police Authority Civil Liberties Panel was set up as a result of this death and exemplifies the scrutiny that investigations of this type will face.

Cybercrime

These are crimes that primarily target computer networks or devices and include computer viruses, cyberstalking, and fraud and identity theft. Other criminal offences include Phishing scams and information warfare along with online fraud. The next big challenge for investigators is forensic cloud investigation, which will involve multiple jurisdictions. There are high volume cyber crimes such as child pornography, which know no international boundaries and involve multiple jurisdictions. Osterburg and Ward (2010) state that investigators face 'the increasing problem of not being able to present a case that can be understood by the jury.' The Royal United Services Institute (Quintana, 2012) speak of cyber situational awareness where intelligence officers will use all 'source intelligence' including open source material. They quote the example of the NATOs Operation Unified Protector, where Jordanian officers were monitoring social network sites on behalf of NATO and British intelligence officers were contacting Libyans to direct trusted sources inside the country. Such information was fused with information from other sources to gain a richer picture of what was happening within the country. This example shows one way in which intelligence can be augmented by open source material and then used in a pro-active manner. A multi-disciplinary methodology will be needed to exploit the layered approach to building intelligence. The need for specialist investigators and digital forensic provision is of the utmost importance. This topic is discussed in more detail in Chapter 6.

Domestic Terrorism

Beeson and Bisley (2010) state that there will continue to be a 'trade off between civil liberties and national security.' This will mean that the police are restricted in how they investigate and collect intelligence on terrorists. Awareness training is needed for police officers to gain the trust of all communities and spot the early signs of radicalisation. There is a need for outreach programmes to be extended while maintaining a robust investigative response to prevent terrorist attacks. Police tactics will have to adapt to the new threats. They will have to disrupt potential attacks, arrest suspects and gather intelligence simultaneously. Forensic analysis of terrorist cases, especially bomb scene management, will remain a critical skill. As groups like Al Queda become a global franchise then international co-operation between law enforcement agencies will be critical.

Passive Data and Social Networking

The two elements of 'passive data' and social networking have led to changing patterns in crime generation and in the investigative strategies used. The evidence gathering involved in trawling databases, close circuit television (CCTV) cameras and bank accounts has 'grown' investigations enormously. They generate a huge number of 'actions' for the police to deal with. Furthermore, juries now expect, as do the Courts, to see a physical manifestation of evidence and this puts extra pressure on the police to produce evidence in a physical form. The use of social networks during the summer riots of 2011 has been described as the infrastructure for the spread of the riots. Following major incidents, the UK Police need to ensure that they have an adequate route for the public to forward video and photographic images, from a range of personal electronic devices, in incidences where these images may help in a large-scale investigation, such as in the Boston marathon bombings. The police will also have to ensure that there is digital provision for local authority CCTV to be downloaded in real time.

Recommendations

In light of these challenges faced by twenty-first century investigative teams, it is suggested that a suite of changes be implemented in modern policing strategy.

1. The police should create a library of murder cases that could be accessed via a software package to assist SIOs in solving hard to solve cases. There is a need to debrief all aspects of murder investigation nationwide and code the responses.
2. Thorough investigative training and mentoring for SIOs and ACPO officers to ensure a consistent standard of investigation across the United Kingdom.
3. The broadening of forensic science training to ensure an overlap between police, forensic and legal training.
4. Devising a structure to enable scrutiny of social networking sites during critical incidents.
5. Creating new databases and neural networks to analyse all information on current investigative databases such as HOLMES, to enable the police to understand all the facts in a case and linked cases.
6. Adapting investigative databases such as HOLMES for the twenty-first century.
7. The management of witnesses to be maintained and developed during the lifetime of an investigation, taking cognisance of different populations.
8. Developing the Family Liaison Role in a changing population and managing the expectations.
9. Developing international cooperation in transnational enquires and a multi-agency approach to global enquires such as child abuse and fraud enquires.
10. Developing the management of expert witnesses and the regulation of experts to support investigations and court cases.
11. Developing skills to fight the threat of Organised Crime Networks (OCNs) at all levels of policing.
12. Creating the right structure and response to deal with rapidly changing disorder.
13. Ensure the quality and timeliness of community impact assessments in the light of the Duggan Inquest (2011).
14. Overcoming the compartmentalisation of skills in investigations to maintain consistent quality in high and low volume crime investigations.
15. Creating a new national intelligence model for the twenty-first century will mean less bureaucracy and an ability to respond to rapidly changing circumstances.
16. Ensuring adequate measures in place to ensure the linking of cases forensically.
17. Managing cybercrime.
18. Combating eco-terrorism.
19. Combating the threat of home-grown terrorism.
20. Understanding the significance of passive data and developing methods for the collection of passive data during investigations.
21. Developing the investigative review (of individual cases) process to ensure consistency and independence.

22. Maintain and develop manuals within the new Police Professional Body. There is a need to maintain guidance and mentoring for all detectives, especially SIOs. A more interactive mentoring system should be developed to ensure a consistent standard.

Conclusions

The perfect storm that the UK police face has stirred debate on the principles and aims of policing and investigation. This has been a perennial debate, but these seismic changes forced by cultural and economic circumstances may lead to developments in the recruitment, training and organisation of British detectives. The range of threats that they face has been discussed and the police's response to these challenges against a gloomy economic backdrop will test the Home Office and Chief Constables. The detectives of the future will need to be better equipped to deal with the range of challenges and maintain their respected standing.

Glossary

ACSO Assistant Commissioner Specialist Crime Directorate
ACPO Association of Chief Police Officers
CPIA Criminal Procedure and Investigations Act 1996
HOLMES Home Office Large Major Enquiry System
HMIC Her Majestys Inspectorate of Constabulary
DC Detective Constable
DS Detective Sergeant
DI Detective Inspector
DCI Detective Chief Inspector
DCS Detective Chief Superintendent
FLO Family Liaison Officer
IO Investigating Officer (deputy SIO usually a DI)
MIT Major Investigation Team
MIR Major Investigation Room
Murder Manual ACPO Police Murder Manual
MIMI Murder Information Murder Index
MIRSAP Major Incident Room Standard Operating Procedure
NDNAD National DNA Database
NPIA National Police Improvement Agency
PITO Police Information Technology Organisation now NPIA
PACE Police and Criminal Evidence Act 1984
SIO Senior Investigating Officer

References

Association of Chief Police Officers (ACPO) (2005) *Core Investigative Doctrine* 2005:72. http://library.college.police.uk/docs/acpo/Core-Investigative-Doctrine.pdf (accessed 11 January 2017).
Beeson, M. and Bisley N. (2010) *Issues in 21ˢᵗ Century Politics*, Palgrave Macmillan, 2010.

Byford Report (2006) Sir Lawrence Byford report into the police handling of the Yorkshire Ripper case. Home Office. Available at: https://www.gov.uk/government/publications/sir-lawrence-byford-report-into-the-police-handling-of-the-yorkshire-ripper-case (accessed 26 June 2015).

Canter, D. (2012) Policing is no longer a general-purpose job. *The Times* 6 March 2012. Available at: http://www.thetimes.co.uk/tto/opinion/columnists/article3341200.ece (accessed 10 January 2017).

Cassella, J.P. and McCartney, C. (2011) Lowering the drawbridges: Legal and forensic education issues in the 21st century. *Forensic Science Policy & Management: An International Journal*, **2** (2), 81–93.

Climbie Inquiry (2003) THE Victoria Climbie Inquiry. Available at: https://www.gov.uk/government/uploads/system/uploads/attachment_data/file/273183/5730.pdf (accessed 10 January 2017).

Duggan Inquest (2011) The Mark Duggan Inquest. Available at: http://webarchive.nationalarchives.gov.uk/20151002140003/http://dugganinquest.independent.gov.uk/ (accessed 10 January 2017).

Greenwood, R. and Hinings, C.R. (1996) Understanding radical organizational change: Bringing together the old and the new institutionalism. *Academy of Management Review*, **21** (4), 1022–1054.

HMIC Report (2012) Forging the links: Rape investigation and prosecution. Available at: https://www.justiceinspectorates.gov.uk/hmic/media/forging-the-links-rape-investigation-and-prosecution-20120228.pdf (accessed 10 January 2017).

HMRC Report (2014) Crime-recording: making the victim count. Available at: https://www.justiceinspectorates.gov.uk/hmic/wp-content/uploads/crime-recording-making-the-victim-count.pdf (accessed 10 January 2017).

IPCC (2010) Investigation into the Death of Ian Tomlinson. Available at: https://www.ipcc.gov.uk/sites/default/files/Documents/investigation_commissioner_reports/inv_rep_independent_investigation_into_the_death_of_ian_tomlinson_1.pdf (accessed 26 June 2015).

Jones, D., Grieve, J. and Milne, B. (2008) The case to review murder investigations. *Policing*, **294**, 470–480.

Leveson Inquiry (2012) Report into the Culture, Practice and Ethics of the Press. Available at: http://webarchive.nationalarchives.gov.uk/20140122145147/http://www.levesoninquiry.org.uk/rulings/ (accessed 10 January 2017).

Lewis, C. and Ellis, T. (2007) *Criminal Victim Support Study*, (ed. Z. Wei), People's Court, China.

MacPherson Report (1999) MacPherson Report on the death of Stephen Lawrence. Available at: https://www.gov.uk/government/uploads/system/uploads/attachment_data/file/277111/4262.pdf (accessed 10 January 2017).

Marks, M. and Sklansky, D. (eds) (2011) *Police Reform from the Bottom Up: Officers and their Unions as Agents of Change (Police Practice and Research)*, Routledge, London.

Neyroud Report (2011) Home Office, on Police Training. Available at: https://www.gov.uk/government/publications/review-of-police-leadership-and-training (accessed 10 January 2017).

Quintana, E. (2012) Securing the Fifth Environment: The RAF and the Importance of Cyber. Available at: https://rusi.org/publication/rusi-defence-systems/securing-fifth-environment-raf-and-importance-cyber (accessed 10 January 2017).

Santella, A.P. and Emery, C. (2007) *Turbocharge Your Undergraduate Business Curriculum Using Enterprise Systems and Action/Problem Based Learning.* Allied Academies, Tallahassee, FL.

Scott, W.R. (2004) Institutional theory: Contributing to a theoretical research program, in *Great Minds in Management: The Process of Theory Development*, (eds K.G. Smith and M.A. Hitt), Oxford University Press, Oxford.

Shanteau, J. (1992) Competence in experts: The role of task characteristics. *Organizational Behavior and Human Decision Processes*, **53** (2), 252–266.

Silverman, S. (2011) Research and Development in Forensic Science: A Review. Available at: https://www.gov.uk/government/uploads/system/uploads/attachment_data/file/118916/forensic-science-review-report.pdf (accessed 10 January 2017).

Sklansky, D. (2012) The Persistent Pull of Police Professionalism. National Institute of Justice. Available at: https://www.ncjrs.gov/pdffiles1/nij/232676.pdf (accessed 10 January 2017).

Smith, N. and Flanagan, C. (2000) The Effective Detective: Identifying the skills of an effective SIO. Police Research Series, Paper 122. Available at: http://library.college.police.uk/docs/hopolicers/fprs122.pdf (accessed 10 January 2017).

Soham Report (2002) A report on the Investigation by Cambridgeshire Constabulary into the murders of Jessica Chapman and Holly Wells at Soham 4th August 2002, Sir Ronnie Flanagan, HMIC. Available at: https://www.justiceinspectorates.gov.uk/hmic/media/investigation-by-cambridgeshire-constabulary-20040530.pdf (accessed 10 January 2017).

Stelfox, P. (2009) *Criminal Investigation*, Willan, Milton.

Taylor Review (2002) The Damilola Taylor Murder Investigation Review. The Report of the Oversight Panel. Available at: http://library.college.police.uk/docs/met-police/Damilola-Taylor-Murder-Investigation-Review-2002.pdf (accessed 26 June 2015).

Tilley, N.J. and Laycock, G. (2014) The police as professional problem-solvers, in *The Future of Policing*, (ed. J. Brown), Routledge, London, pp. 369–382.

Osterburg, J.W. and Ward, R.H. (2010) *Criminal Investigation*, Library of Congress Publishing.

Roycroft, M. (2009) PhD thesis, Surrey University.

The Independent (2012) Calls for inquiry into 'astonishing' DNA error. Independent 31st March 2012. Available at: http://www.independent.co.uk/news/uk/crime/calls-for-inquiry-into-astonishing-dna-error-7604130.html (accessed 26 June 2015).

The Shipman Inquiry (2003) 2nd Report The Police Investigation of 1998. Chairman Dame Janet Smith OBE HMSO. Available at: https://www.gov.uk/government/uploads/system/uploads/attachment_data/file/273226/5853.pdf (accessed 11 January 2017).

Winsor Report (2011) Independent Review of Police Officers and Staff Pay. Part 2. Available at: College of Policing 'Golden Hour' https://www.app.college.police.uk/app-content/investigations/investigation-process/#golden-hour (accessed 10 January 2017).

Yorke, M. and Knight, P.T. (2006) Embedding employability into the curriculum. Learning and Employability. Series 1 No. 3. Higher Education Academy. Available at: http://www.employability.ed.ac.uk/documents/Staff/HEABriefings/ESECT-3-Embedding-employability_into_curriculum.pdf (accessed 10 January 2017).

Zenith Crime Blog (2015) Wither now for forensic science? Available at: https://zenithcrime.wordpress.com/2015/10/06/wither-now-for-forensic-science/ (accessed 10 January 2017).

17

The Design and Implementation of Multiple Choice Questions (MCQs) in Forensic Science Assessment

Claire Gwinnett

Staffordshire University, Department of Forensic Science and Crime Science, Faculty of Computing, Engineering and Science, Science Centre, Stoke on Trent, UK

Introduction to Multiple Choice Questions (MCQs)

Multiple Choice Questions (MCQs) are a type of objective test question that involve an answer to be chosen from a list of possible responses (McKenna and Bull, 1999). Multiple choice questions can be very varied and may include multiple answer questions, true and false questions, matching words and phrases and inserting answers into sentences. This list is not exhaustive and is really only limited by the creativity of the designer. MCQs are commonly used within education for both summative and formative assessments, as they are a practical and efficient means of assessing large groups of students (De Milia, 2007). Much research has been completed upon MCQ use, design, management and implementation and due to this there are an abundant number of resources that can be used by academics if they wish to use this type of assessment within their own teaching.

Before introducing some of the literature surrounding MCQs and their design and implementation, certain key terms must be understood and defined. These definitions can be found in Box 17.1.

Box 17.1   Key terms

Item – the overall individual MCQ
Stem – the text of the question
Lead-In Information – background information required to answer question(s); may include photos, case study information, graphs, crime scene sketches and so on
Options – the choices of answer provided
The Key – the correct answer in a list of options
Distractors – the incorrect answers in the list of options

Forensic Science Education and Training: A Tool-kit for Lecturers and Practitioner Trainers, First Edition.
Edited by Anna Williams, John P. Cassella, and Peter D. Maskell.
© 2017 John Wiley & Sons Ltd. Published 2017 by John Wiley & Sons Ltd.

There is a large body of research into MCQ use, for example, studies completed by Carneson *et al.* (2003), Schultheis (1998), Fellenz (2004) and McCoubrie (2004). MCQs are a universally used assessment technique, and literature surrounds the use of MCQs in many disciplines, including veterinary studies and medicine (Head and Ogden, 2006). Within this literature there have been attempts to produce guidelines for academics in the production of MCQs, including McKenna and Bull (1999), Atkinson (2002) and Higgins and Tatham (2003). The fundamental theories behind such guidelines will be discussed further here. Studies by Collins (2001) and Lorusso (2004) discuss the importance of constructing questions that reflect the material being taught, using consistent writing styles and the correct construction of the stem and the options. In addition to the construction of the MCQ test, the important issue of marking schemes is also well documented in the literature; examples of these will be provided in the section on Marking Methods for MCQ Assessments.

In addition to publications, there are readily accessible databanks of MCQs for other subject areas, such as the OCTAVE database (for veterinary science education) (Head and Ogden, 2006), but unfortunately there is no national database of forensic science related MCQs available for academics to use currently. MCQ examples for forensic science education remain primarily within private collections in forensic science departments and published examples by forensic science organisations, such as the Chartered Society of Forensic Sciences (CSFS) (CSFS, 2015).

The Benefits and Limitations of MCQ Use in Forensic Science Assessment

In 2009, Hannis and Welsh conducted research into the provision of forensic science education across UK Higher Education Institutions (HEIs) for the Skills for Justice Forensic Science Occupational Committee. In this report they highlighted particular skills that forensic science employers required from graduates, these included problem solving, application of forensic principles and understanding of forensic techniques, evidence interpretation, laboratory skills and communication skills. For HEI forensic science course providers to engage with this report and address the needs of potential future employers of their students, learning, teaching and assessment material must reflect these highlighted key skills. Varied assessment schemes are generally seen in forensic science degrees due to the diverse and practical nature of the subject, however academics face the on-going challenge of creating course assessments that assess important skills whilst engaging the student body, but at the same time balancing available resources and teaching loads. This challenge has been amplified as courses with forensic science in the title have increased in student numbers (Higher Education Statistics Agency, 2015; Mennell, 2006). A rise in student numbers is obviously not a negative for a university but the marking time for essay style questions, portfolios and other open-ended assessments is considerably increased and reduces the time available for other important academic activities. An increase in marking time also impacts upon the time interval in feedback provision. These problems can be overcome by using close-ended assessment types such as MCQ tests. The increase in productivity and efficiency in marking and feedback provision has been widely acknowledged as the main strength of MCQ tests (Bleske-Rechek *et al.*, 2007; Nicol, 2007; Williams and Clark, 2004) but other strengths have also been identified. Nicol (2007) describes the advantage of MCQs when using computer networks for computer assisted assessment (CAA), which allows flexibility in delivery times and addresses modern student learning needs. This is particularly true when describing distance-learning courses that are being undertaken by overseas forensic science students. As stated by Collins in 2006, MCQ tests can be shown to have a high degree of validity if the questions are 'drawn from a representative sample of content areas that constitute predetermined learning outcomes' (Collins, 2006). In addition, the marking of such an assessment will not fall prey to the subjectivity of the marker due to the predetermined marking system, unlike that of essay style assessments in which subjectivity can sometimes inadvertently occur.

When discussing MQC use, there are many arguments against their use. A key debate within MCQ use is the reliability of this assessment method, with critics claiming that they are 'too easy', they allow participants to pass through guesswork and do not test higher order cognitive skills that other assessments such as essays and laboratory write-ups are able to (Fellenz, 2004; Welsh, 1978). Although these comments are relevant, there are published ideas and methods that address these issues. Bloom, in 1959, published a taxonomy of hierarchical cognitive learning that is regularly used by MCQ designers to test knowledge, comprehension, application, analysis, synthesis and evaluation. Bloom's approach will be discussed further in the section on The Development of More Sophisticated MCQs. With this in mind, MCQs can now be designed to assess a range of different module objectives beyond just the recollection of facts.

A summary of the arguments that are raised in the literature about MCQ assessments can be seen in Table 17.1.

Forensic Science Students Perceptions of MCQs

Interestingly, forensic science students also agree with many of the comments in Table 17.1. Eighty-six second year students studying for a forensic science, forensic investigation or policing and criminal investigation degree at Staffordshire University were asked to complete a questionnaire about their perceptions of using MCQs as summative and formative assessments and their preferences in terms of implementation of MCQ tests within their course. The results from this questionnaire will be discussed throughout the chapter. Of these students, 100% had heard of MCQ tests before and only 4.65% had not participated in an MCQ test before university. Many student perceptions of assessment types can be formed early in their academic careers (Dorman and Knightley, 2006) and it is useful to identify students' perceptions of MCQs in HE when they have already experienced this assessment type prior to university. The students were asked for their thoughts on the use of MCQs for summative assessments using a five-point Likert scale, where 1 = strongly disagree, 2 = disagree, 3 = neither agree nor disagree, 4 = agree or 5 = strongly agree. They were asked to comment about the following statements:

A. MCQs are more enjoyable than essay style questions in exams
B. MCQs require more revision than other exam types
C. MCQs can test knowledge only and do not test other skills important to forensic science and policing, such as problem solving
D. MCQs can be used to test evidence analysis skills
E. MCQs can be used to test ability to interpret criminal cases

Table 17.1 A summary of the criticisms and defences of MCQ tests.

Criticisms of MCQs	Defences of MCQs
Encourage only factual recall and do not test higher cognitive skills, such as critical analysis skills (Paxton, 2000; Scouller, 1998)	Allow higher cognitive skills such as comprehension, application, analysis, synthesis and evaluation to be tested if correctly constructed (Bloom, 1959; Cox, 1976)
Feedback is limited and is not personalised as it is predetermined during test development (Nicol, 2007)	Provide instant feedback to the participant if computerised
Do not allow the participant to take a more active role in assessment by clarifying own goals and self-regulating their own performance, as described by Boud (2000)	Can be easily automated and delivered online (Bull and McKenna, 2004)
More sophisticated MCQs can be time consuming to produce (Miller *et al.*, 1998)	Marking is quick and easy and removes subjectivity
Encourages a surface approach to learning rather than a deeper approach (Entwistle and Entwistle, 1991)	Can test a broad coverage of concepts consistently and quickly (Collins, 2006)
Allows guessing of answers (Biggs, 1999)	Robust marking systems can be utilised to prevent/reduce guessing and are also not subjective unlike some other forms of assessment
Participants do not prepare for MCQ tests as effectively as other forms of assessment (Scouller, 1998)	Confidence based marking schemes allow insight into the thought processes of the participant and can provide information about their perceptions of their competency (Bush, 1999)
	Allow more questions to be asked in a test on a greater number of topics than standard tests

The mean scores for each of these statements can be seen in Figure 17.1. Table 17.2 shows the responses to individual statements pertaining to MCQ assessments.

It was interesting to see that the students generally agreed with Scouller 's (1998) views that MCQs do not test higher cognitive skills, such as problem solving, with lower mean scores for statements D and E compared with C. The lower mean scores for D and E showed that the majority of students either disagreed or were noncommittal about whether MCQs were able to help test forensic science and policing skills such as case interpretation or evidence analysis skills. This is a common misconception and it is easy to think that the complex nature of criminal cases and results from evidence analysis can only be assessed using more open ended assessment types such as essays or reports. Although MCQs should not entirely replace these assessment types, they can be used in conjunction with the more traditional assignments. It is clearer to see that students find MCQ tests more enjoyable than essay style questions with a mean score of 4.11. One student who supplied a score of 4 to statement A also stated 'MCQs are good starter questions to an exam. They get you in the exam mood and calm nerves.' This 'less stress' style of exam question may be the reason why the forensic science, investigation and policing students sampled prefer these to essay style exams, but it was also clear that

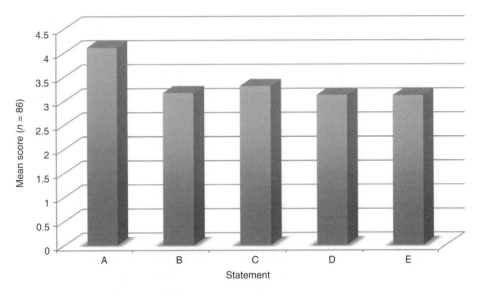

Figure 17.1 Mean scores for second year students' perceptions of MCQs ($n = 86$).

some students also feel that essay questions require more skill and demonstrate knowledge better, with a student who stated that they strongly disagreed with statement A noted that 'Essays are more difficult but you get to put across the knowledge you have learnt in the module more effectively. MCQ feels like "guess the answer" and therefore no skill is required.' The idea that MCQs encourage guessing and do not reflect

Table 17.2 Responses to individual statements in questionnaire ($n = 86$).

Statement	Strongly disagree 1	2	Neither agree nor disagree 3	4	Strongly agree 5	Mean	SD
MCQs are more enjoyable than essay style questions in exams	1	6	14	26	38	4.11	1.00
MCQs require more revision than other exam types	4	17	33	23	8	3.16	1.01
MCQs can test knowledge only and do not test other skills important to forensic science and policing, such as problem solving	5	13	28	29	10	3.31	1.06
MCQs can be used to test evidence analysis skills	7	15	31	25	7	3.11	1.06
MCQs can be used to test ability to interpret criminal cases	6	17	32	22	8	3.11	1.06

a student's true knowledge has been explored by Bleske-Rechek *et al.* (2007) and Cox (1976), and more sophisticated marking schemes that discourage guessing have been developed and reviewed; these will be discussed in the section on Marking Methods for MCQ Assessments. The effect of chance and answer guessing in MCQ tests and test reliability has been explored by Burton (2001). Burton shows methods for quantifying the effects of chance so that appropriate test length and number of answer options can be more reliably designed, this will be discussed further in the section on Designing MCQs for Forensic Science. Overall, it is important that participants in MCQ tests understand the validity of such tests so that they engage appropriately with them and recognise their value.

MCQ Testing in Forensic Practitioner Competency Testing

Skills that are being assessed in undergraduate and postgraduate students also require assessment in practicing forensic scientists. This requirement stems from the need for validation in court and to demonstrate an appropriate level of competency. It is widely known that the quality of forensic and expert evidence must be assessed in an unbiased fashion and prove to be of a suitable standard. This standard setting can be seen with the UK Forensic Regulator requiring forensic science providers to be accredited to the international standard ISO 17025 (Science and Technology Committee, 2011). 'Competency' is a key performance criterion within the forensic investigative process for all forensic practitioners and proving competency in a UK Court is an important aspect of the legal system. Many professionals within the forensic arena have a variety of qualifications, but they all need to demonstrate 'continuing professional development' and continuous professional competency. Since the Council for the Registration of Forensic Practitioners (CRFP) ceased operating in March 2009, there has been an imperative to provide a quality control system, which will help maintain public confidence in forensic practice in the United Kingdom and to provide assurance to the UK Criminal Justice System. This is especially important for forensic practitioners who are from smaller laboratories that do not have ISO standard accreditation or those who are infrequently required to act as a forensic expert due to the very specialist nature of their expertise.

Where the CRFP essentially based their accreditation of forensic experts on peer review (CRFP, 2008), a new method for assessing competency in forensic experts has been developed by the Royal Chartered Society of Forensic Science (CSFS) (CSFS, 2015), which includes a pre-assessment evaluation of the practitioner, a practical based proficiency test and an MCQ test. MCQs are used for the testing in professional competency outside the United Kingdom, with the American Board of Forensic Toxicologists using MCQs to assess competency (http://www.abft.org/). As the outcomes of such assessments allow a practitioner to describe themselves as competent, the MCQ tests are designed to be a robust assessment strategy that allow the level of knowledge and understanding across a broad range of forensic science topics to be identified and quantified and allow the use of learning outcomes and assessment criteria to provide quality assurance and academic rigour. This successful testing scheme, organised by the CSFS, highlights the versatility of integrating MCQ assessments within important competency testing schemes and should be seen as an example of best practice in MCQ design for forensic science.

Designing MCQs for Forensic Science

When designing a set of MCQs to be used to assess competency in forensic science, it is important to firstly outline what you want from your MCQs. To aid this decision, you may want to consider the following:

1. Do you want to use your MCQs as a formative or summative assessment?
2. Do you want participants to answer the MCQs in examination conditions or use them to gain feedback in taught sessions or guide group work?
3. What level of expertise, experience or skill is expected of your participants?
4. Do you want to test purely knowledge and recollection skills or more sophisticated skills such as problem solving?
5. How much time has been allocated to test your participants?

Once you have addressed these questions you will have an outline of the depth and breadth of the MCQ test that you want to produce. This may just be a basic, knowledge based test that is seen as more of a quiz type of test at HE level but is useful for revision sessions, in-lecture feedback and end of module reflection, or a higher level test for end of year summative assessments. Regardless of the type of MCQ or the level, there are some basic principles that must be adhered to when constructing MCQs to avoid misinterpretation and therefore negatively affecting pass rates. Much of the disapproval surrounding MCQs is not actually attributed to the weakness of the assessment type but in the construction flaws of the test questions (Collins, 2006). Bearing this in mind there are a number of basic design features that must be abided by; these will be discussed further in the following sections on Basic MCQ Design Principles and The Development of More Sophisticated MCQs.

With all types of MCQ, whether basic or more sophisticated, the first stage of writing a good MCQ is the construction of learning objectives and defining the levels of learning (Collins, 2006). As stated by Collins (2006) there should be a direct relationship between the instructional objectives and the test items. To achieve this, focus should be upon the most important skills and knowledge that are expected from your participants, whether this is lower level knowledge about forensic science principles or a particular skill such as the comparison of footwear impressions. When deciding on the topics of the MCQs it is important to avoid controversial topics that may have many answers and that can't clearly be articulated in an MCQ. Some topics within forensic science are constantly changing due to technological advances, casework or government stipulations. MCQs can address new technology, new interpretation methods and new government protocols but should avoid controversial issues where knowledge is currently incomplete or being debated. Whereas essay style assignments can lend themselves nicely to the discussion of controversial new protocols or rulings within forensic science, this does not apply to MCQs. The nature of MCQ options can allow participants to assess a series of facts and judge levels of correctness by using terms such a 'most' and 'best' in the stem, but these should still be facts that can be written as declarative sentences and should be unbiased and not be based on the views of a subset of the forensic population. To encapsulate such topics, a hybrid approach to assessment is advised; for example, the mixed use of MCQs and assignments that allow some flexibility in the answers, such as live debate and essay style assignments.

Basic MCQ Design Principles

There are many types of MCQ that can be used such as true/false, multiple correct answers (keys), matching questions and MCQs that require the options to be placed in order. McKenna and Bull (1999) provide a list of different types of objective question that can be used for assessment, particularly in computer assisted assessment (CAA). This chapter will focus upon MCQs that require one or more options to be selected by the participant. The design features for this type of MCQ can be applied to other forms but it must be noted that there will be some differences when evaluating the results and robustness of these types of test item. MCQs that require only either true or false to be selected have issues with robustness due to the reduced number of options (two) and therefore the greater effect of chance and guessing upon the results. For summative assessments it is the opinion of the author that these types of test item are not used. For MCQs that require ordering of answers then these require slight variations on the different marking schemes available, and are discussed in the section on Marking Methods for MCQ Assessments, to allow credit to be given for partial correct orders.

It is important for the creator of any MCQs to fully understand the foundations of MCQ design and to avoid the common item-writing flaws, described under Designing the Stem and Designing the Options. Interestingly, reviews conducted by Tarrant *et al.* (2006) of MCQ collections used for undergraduate nursing assessments showed that high proportions of MCQs (49.4% of 2770 MCQs observed) contained design flaws, indicating the need for further training for assessors in MCQ design.

Designing the Stem

It is maybe easier for the academic new to MCQ design to identify flaws within an MCQ than to create a flawless MCQ the first time. Example 1 demonstrates an MCQ that contains many of the faults that can be accidently incorporated into the stem of a question.

Example 1 How NOT to construct an MCQ stem

Fibres examination is an important part of CRIME SCENE ANALYSIS. Which of the following analysis methods is seldom used in fibres analysis?

(a) **Microscopy**
(b) **Melting point**
(c) **FTIR**
(d) **Microspectrophotometery**
(e) **Crime scene reconstruction**
(f) **Fingerprint dusting**
(g) **None of the above**

Focusing on the stem of Example 1 only, it is important to note that the stem should be clear, grammatically correct and complete (McKenna and Bull, 1999). The stem should contain all relevant information but should not contain unnecessary material that is not directly linked to the question, for example, in Example 1, the first sentence is not necessary and is not required for the actual question. As stated by Collins (2006), the stem should not be an opportunity to teach or create red herrings; the participants should be tested upon their knowledge and skills, not on their ability to understand a riddle.

Capitalisation of letters within the stem should be used only to emphasise an important point, not randomly as seen in Example 1. This includes highlighting the number of options that should be selected or key words such as 'most' or 'best'. For example, an appropriate use of capitalisation in a stem may be:

'Which ONE of the following techniques is used for the analysis of paint samples?'

It should be noted that Example 1 does not stipulate the number of options that should be chosen. If an MCQ test has been designed so that all of the questions require only one answer then instructions stating this can be given at the beginning of the test, but if MCQs requiring more than one answer are also included, each question should instruct the participant on how many answers should be selected.

In Example 1, the term 'seldom' is used. Vague terms such as 'rarely', 'frequently' should be avoided where possible unless clearly defined. Using vague terms can lead to participants who think deeply about each question to become stressed and choose the incorrect option even though they know the correct answer. Equally, terms such as 'always', 'never', 'all' or 'none' should be used with care with some academics stating that they should not be used in any form (Collins, 2006), as very few situations are universally true or absolute. In some situations of forensic science, the use of these absolute terms can be robustly used, for example, in situations where incorrect/correct procedures are standardised or where law or accreditation stipulates a certain procedure without variation. For example, the following question during the time of this book being published can be used in the United Kingdom for forensic science teaching:

Which ONE of the following documentation methods is ALWAYS carried out at a major crime scene in the UK?

(a) **Topographical surveys**
(b) **Photographs**
(c) **3D scanning**
(d) **Aerial imaging**

Answer = (b)

This last question is correct for all police forces in the United Kingdom as of 2015 for major crime scenes, but if protocols differed across police forces this MCQ would disadvantage participants from certain geographical areas. In questions where you use absolutes, care must be taken as to make sure the MCQs are kept up-to-date with any changes in law or protocols and that the MCQ clearly states any exceptions or particular specifications, for example, if the question only refers to a particular country (or police force), this should be included in the stem.

Negatively phrased questions should be avoided, but if they must be used, capitalise, underscore or use an appropriate method to highlight the negative phrase (McKenna and Bull, 1999).

Designing the Options

Using Example 1 as seen in the previous section, but now focusing upon the options for this MCQ, it is clear to see that some of these options are poorly designed.

Example 1 How NOT to construct options

Fibres examination is an important part of CRIME SCENE ANALYSIS. Which of the following analysis methods is seldom used in fibres analysis?

(a) **Microscopy**
(b) **Melting point**
(c) **FTIR**
(d) **Microspectrophotometry**
(e) **Crime scene reconstruction**
(f) **Fingerprint dusting**
(g) **All of the above**

It has been stated that the best number of options is three to five (Collins, 2006), with three options proving to be as effective as four when tested by McKeachie in 1986. Collins states that producing more than five options is sometimes difficult as the nature of many topics do not have more than four plausible distractors, and by creating more, these options are flawed and obviously incorrect. Burton, in 2001, quantified the reliability of multiple choice tests and concluded that four options are too unreliable for tests that use several grade bands rather than a simple pass/fail result. Burton states that reliability can be increased by increasing the number of options but in ≥60 question tests, the reliability is very similar to using four option questions. Burton recommends that to improve the reliability of tests then guessing needs to be discouraged, which can be achieved by using appropriate marking schemes, such as negative marking; this is discussed further in the section on Marking Methods for MCQ Assessments. If a more sophisticated marking scheme is utilised, this removes the need to create a long list of options, as seen in Example 1. As stated previously, all of the options should be plausible and each of the distractors should be accurate but do not fully meet the requirements asked of the question (McKenna and Bull, 1999). Creating distractors that have a certain level of correctness can be arduous but the designer should still avoid using obviously wrong answers such as options (e) and (f) in Example 1. 'All of the above' should not be used as a way to increase the number of options or to make constructing the stem easier. When using 'all of the above' as the key, the participant needs only to identify that two or more of the options are correct and will then be able to choose the correct answer even though they may not fully understand all options. Alternatively, when using 'all of the above' as a distractor, the participant needs only to note that more than one option could potentially be correct, which then leads to a dilemma for the participant who has to second guess the MCQ designer to whether one answer is more correct than the others or all of the options are of equal correctness and then 'all of the above' should be selected.

When creating distractors the designer should consider the following questions:

1. What do participants normally get incorrect when asked this question?
2. What are the common misconceptions in this topic area?
3. What options are incorrect but would seem correct to the participant?

The correct answer should not be highlighted in the list due to grammatical errors and all of the options should be in the same tense as the stem. The designer should not try to 'conceal' the correct answer by using abbreviations or acronyms (seen in option (c) in

Example 1) as the options should be clear as to exactly what they mean. Clarity in the options is especially important if there could be more than one meaning, for example, in option (a) in Example 1, 'microscopy' does not provide the participant with enough information as this could mean stereomicroscopy, polarized light microscopy, comparison microscopy or scanning electron microscopy, and without this extra information, the participant has to make a guess as to the meaning.

Options should be listed in a logical order where possible, this does not necessarily mean in alphabetical order but if numbers are used these should be in either descending or ascending order and if dates are used, these should be in chronological order.

Ultimately, it is not possible for a participant to correctly answer weakly designed MCQs without guessing. This is seen in Example 1, participants with no forensic fibres knowledge would be able to eliminate options (e), (f) and (g) and the more competent participants would also be able to eliminate option (a) as in its simplest form, microscopy would not be 'seldom' used. This would then leave the participant to subjectively decide what 'seldom' means and relate it to the use of the techniques stated in (b), (c) and (d). As any fibres analyst knows, the use of these techniques depends upon the individual laboratory, fibre type, whether the fibre is dyed, the controls available and the information required in the case. Without this information being provided to the participant, it is not possible for the correct answer to be accurately identified. An improved version of Example 1 would be:

Which ONE of the following analysis methods is the BEST for providing information about the dyes present in synthetic fibres?

(a) Stereomicroscopy
(b) Melting point
(c) Fourier Transform Infrared Spectroscopy (FTIR)
(d) Microspectrophotometry (MSP)

Answer = (d)

As part of any MCQ design, the creator will quickly review the MCQ for any obvious errors or problems. A checklist is a useful tool to compare the MCQ with and to allow no obvious errors to slip through. Box 17.2 shows a quick guide/checklist that can be used when constructing MCQS.

Box 17.2   A Quick Guide to Creating MCQs

When putting together Multiple Choice Questions (MCQs) for testing, the following should be considered:

Guidance on the Production of a Stem (the Question)
1. Stems should be clear and concise.
2. Try not to use imprecise terms such as 'seldom used,' 'rarely seen' …
3. If more than one option has an element of truth ask participant to select 'the best.'
4. If the correct option is not the only possible response (there are others but they are not listed in the options), include, the phrase 'of the following' …..

5. Start the question with, for example: Which of the following is **not** required to...? Which of the following **best** describes... ? Which **one** of the following is the most important reason why... ? Which **one** of the following reasons is the most important? Which **one** of the following is the **most** important reason? Which **two** of the following statements are true? Which **one** of the following sequences is correct?

6. Try to include some questions which involve the participant to analyse a scenario, some case information or a principle before answering the question, for example, provide some details of a piece of evidence and then ask them questions based on them having to interpret the results. In these questions make sure that the stem contains enough information for the participant to actually answer the question, that is, try not to miss out some crucial fact.

Guidance on the Production of the Options

1. Distractors should be designed by asking:
   I. What do people normally confuse this answer/statement with?
   II. What is a common error in the interpretation of this finding?
   III. What are the common misconceptions in this area?
2. DO try to make all options linked in some way to make them more plausible.
3. Normally each question should have a choice of four options.
4. DO try and make all of the distractors reasonably plausible.
5. DO try to keep all options approximately the same length.
6. DO alter position of correct answer.
7. DO keep the options in the same tense as the stem.
8. DON'T make the correct answer so obvious with three really silly answers!
9. DON'T use 'All of the Above' as an option.
10. When providing feedback for your MCQs, do make clear which is/are the correct answer(s), for example, the correct answers can be in red font.

The Development of More Sophisticated MCQs

Unless basic forensic knowledge recall is all that is required to be tested, an assessor will want to also test for a range of skills that are pertinent to being a forensic scientist. These skills, which may include critical thinking, problem solving and interpretation skills, are regularly and simultaneously tested in laboratory write-ups and essay style questions, but may also be tested via MCQs. This idea may sit uncomfortably with assessors that have traditionally used other forms of assessment but with careful planning and design, MCQs can be highly successful and drastically reduce marking time. For MCQ competency testing schemes for forensic practitioners, it is essential that these high-level MCQs be included so as to test the specific skills expected in a forensic expert who presents evidence in court.

The creation of such MCQs still uses the underlying principles previously discussed but have different aims in regards to their learning outcomes and levels of understanding being demonstrated by the participant. The learning outcomes for such MCQs can be categorised nicely utilising Bloom's Taxonomy (1959). Bloom's Taxonomy originated from Bloom's classification of the goals of the education process in which the Cognitive Domain was identified as a category of educational activity along with two

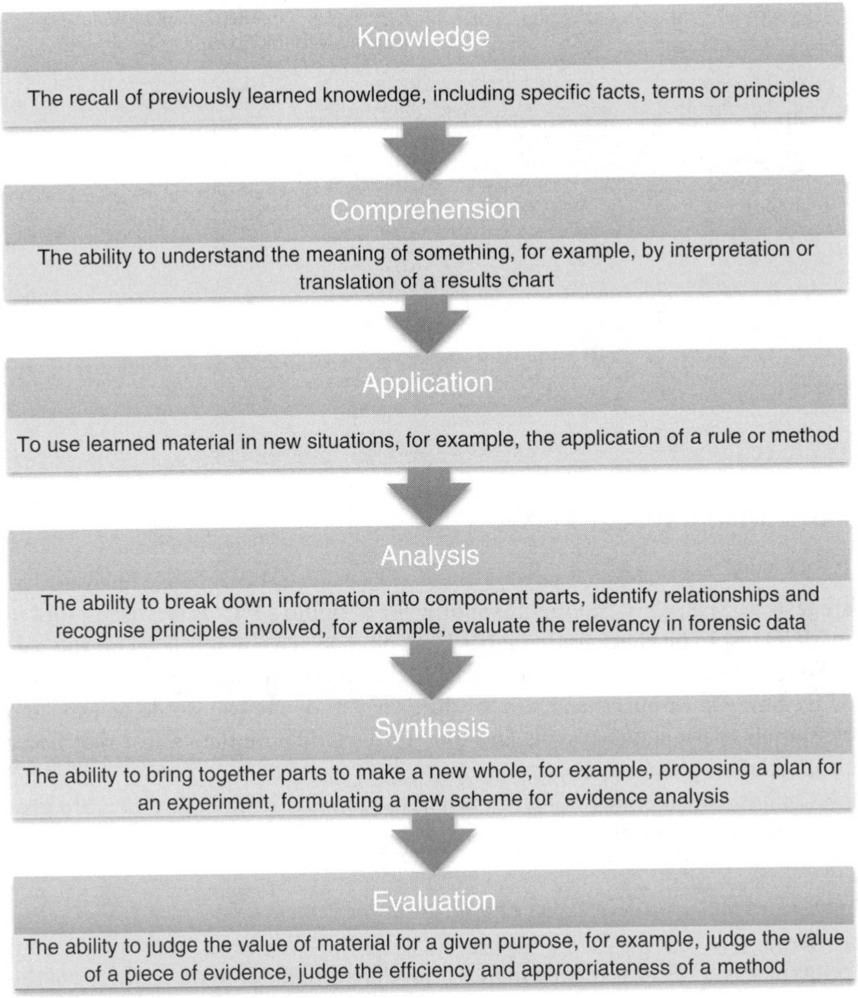

Knowledge

The recall of previously learned knowledge, including specific facts, terms or principles

Comprehension

The ability to understand the meaning of something, for example, by interpretation or translation of a results chart

Application

To use learned material in new situations, for example, the application of a rule or method

Analysis

The ability to break down information into component parts, identify relationships and recognise principles involved, for example, evaluate the relevancy in forensic data

Synthesis

The ability to bring together parts to make a new whole, for example, proposing a plan for an experiment, formulating a new scheme for evidence analysis

Evaluation

The ability to judge the value of material for a given purpose, for example, judge the value of a piece of evidence, judge the efficiency and appropriateness of a method

Figure 17.2 Bloom's hierarchy of educational objectives (Bloom, 1959).

others: the Psychomotor Domain and the Affective Domain. Investigation into cognitive skills within this Cognitive Domain led to a six level hierarchy of educational objectives, also known as Bloom's Taxonomy. The six hierarchical levels described by Bloom can be seen in Figure 17.2 with brief descriptions of each level.

Bloom's Taxonomy is arranged so that it starts at the most simplest level (Knowledge) and proceeds through skills that become more sophisticated and challenging. In terms of MCQ development, many academics have simplified the hierarchy seen in Figure 17.2 (Collins, 2006), as it can sometimes be difficult to design an MCQ that fits only one of Bloom's educational objectives. This simplified version, as seen in Figure 17.3, combines comprehension and application and also combines analysis, synthesis and evaluation to create 'problem solving.' This more streamlined version enables MCQ developers to more easily categorise their questions for testing and understand to what level their

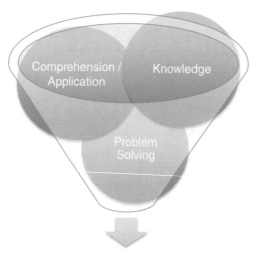

Figure 17.3 Simplified version of Bloom's taxonomy for MCQ use.

Bloom's Taxonomy for MCQs

MCQs are testing. The use of Bloom's taxonomy for designing MCQs is a useful tool to enable an MCQ test to be checked that it has been pitched at a suitable level for the participants. For example, a first year undergraduate test may contain a greater proportion of knowledge based questions than a test for third year students who would be expected to demonstrate higher cognitive skills and therefore would complete a test that had a greater proportion of problem solving MCQs.

Examples of how to generate MCQs at each of the levels seen in Figure 17.3 are provided in the following sections.

Design Features of MCQs Testing Higher Cognitive Skills

The basic design features for MCQs still hold true when creating more sophisticated MCQs, but typically questions testing higher level skills will differ in one or more of the following ways.

1. Stems will utilise phrasing that elicits the participant to make judgments based upon experience and application of existing knowledge. This may be seen by MCQs asking for the 'BEST', 'MOST COMMON' or 'PREFERRED' methods or ideas.
2. Stems may include additional information for the participant to scrutinise and interpret. This may range from a simple photograph to a full text, series of papers or actual evidence exhibits.
3. Have a series of linking questions surrounding a particular scenario, topic or item of material. This allows depth to be generated in the questioning of the participant's understanding of the additional information.
4. May change the delivery of such a test. For example, an MCQ test that requires background reading of additional information may need participants to receive the additional information in advance, have access to particular software or equipment for analysis and/or require the participant to create a report, product or artefact prior to the MCQ test in order to correctly prepare.

Owing to these potential differences, MCQs that test higher cognitive skills may have longer stems and subsequently take much longer to complete. The provision of background information allows huge breadth in the types of MCQ that can be subsequently asked and this information may only be limited by the creator's imagination. The designer should avoid using red herrings within this background information and extraneous material (Collins, 2006) unless the learning outcome is asking for participants to demonstrate their ability to identify the key information in a given case scenario. If this is required, the information should be tightly controlled by the designer. Further discussion of using background information is described in the section on Problem Solving Based MCQs.

How to Convert Knowledge Based MCQs to Test Higher Level Skills

A simple method to start creating MCQs that test higher cognitive skills is to take an existing knowledge based MCQ and convert it into a more sophisticated MCQ. Example 2 shows a typical format of a knowledge based MCQ that can be used in forensic science assessment.

Example 2 Typical format of a knowledge based MCQ

What is the common term used to describe marks that are invisible until chemically or physically developed?

(a) **Latent**
(b) **Patent**
(c) **Obscure**
(d) **Concealed**

Answer = (a)

This MCQ is purely asking the participant to remember the meaning of the word 'latent' in terms of marks found at a crime scene, this is obviously important but does not reflect all of the skills needed of someone involved with mark development or interpretation. If the examiner required MCQs that asked for deeper thinking on this topic, the question could be changed to include a description of a scenario in which a fingermark is present on a particular object and then ask 'what is the best method for enhancing a mark on this surface?' This would then require the participant to have knowledge of latent marks, the development techniques available and their relative effectiveness and to then apply this knowledge for this particular scenario. Although care must be made in the construction of this type of MCQ, for example, to make sure that the stem is clear and contains all the relevant information needed to correctly answer the question and the distractors are all plausible and accurate but do not fully meet the criteria for the correct answer, the production of these are not too onerous (Collins, 2001). Problematically, the nature of forensic science is that many crime scenarios involve complex relationships between evidence, require research to answer particular questions and interpretation is generally not straightforward. A set of MCQs testing multiples skills is therefore required. Examples of comprehension and comprehension/application MCQs are discussed next with design features noted where appropriate.

Comprehension Based MCQs

Comprehension based MCQs are relatively easy to create as they are the natural next step from a knowledge based question. An example of such a question can be seen in Example 3.

Example 3 Typical format of a comprehension based MCQ – courtesy of Professor Wesley Vernon OBE

Which ONE of the following would potentially represent the MOST stable feature in the identification process for a forensic podiatrist?

(a) **A single heloma durum**
(b) **A Beaus line**
(c) **Halluxrigidus**
(d) **Plantar callus**

Answer = (c)

Example 3 requires the participant to firstly have knowledge of each of the features that are listed in the options but then they must identify which is 'MOST stable'. All of the options are plausible but the participant must show comprehension of what is meant by 'stable' in the context of identification and then choose the answer that is the greatest in terms of stability. Example 4 provides a further MCQ that would be classed as a comprehension based question.

Example 4 Typical format of a comprehension based MCQ

Which ONE of the following is the MOST appropriate order of analysis for a glass shard found on a suspect when trying to identify the source of the glass?

(a) **Hot-stage microscopy, stereomicroscopy, density determination, trace elemental composition analysis**
(b) **Stereomicroscopy, hot-stage microscopy, density determination, trace elemental composition analysis**
(c) **Stereomicroscopy, trace elemental composition analysis, hot-stage microscopy, density determination**
(d) **Density determination, stereomicroscopy, hot-stage microscopy, trace elemental composition analysis**

Answer = (b)

Example 4 may initially look like it could be a knowledge based MCQ but, in fact, a participant must understand the relative merits and limitations of each of the techniques in order to identify the 'most appropriate' sequence of methods.

Combined Comprehension and Application Based MCQs

MCQs that ask for application skills as well as comprehension require the participant to use existing knowledge in a new way, for example, the application of an idea, rule or method to a new but concrete situation. Example 5 shows an application based MCQ in the area of forensic fibres examination.

Example 5 A combined comprehension and application based MCQ

If a fibre found at a crime scene has an Optical Path Difference of 250 nm, a thickness of 63 μm and a negative sign of elongation, what is the MOST likely fibre type? Please choose ONE option.

(a) **Modacrylic**
(b) **Acrylic**
(c) **Triacetate**
(d) **Diacetate**

Answer = (b)

Example 5 is one type of an application based MCQ where a participant is required to calculate the birefringence of a fibre and then based upon these results interpret that data into fibre type, which would involve the ability of being able to apply extant knowledge of fibre properties and apply it to this piece of evidence. As many birefringence values overlap between different fibre types, participants would be expected to take these data, along with other known information about fibres, and determine the 'most likely' fibre type. Other examples of application-based questions may be a description of a particular crime scene and then a question asking about what procedure would be best to retrieve certain evidence types. These types of questions expect a breadth of knowledge and understanding about existing forensic science protocols and procedures and the ability to implement these in new crime based scenarios.

Problem Solving Based MCQs

The simplified version of Bloom's (1959) hierarchy of cognitive learning combines analysis, synthesis and evaluation to form problem solving. It is sometimes easy for the designer to believe they have created a true problem solving MCQ (where all three cognitive levels have been combined), when in fact it only tests one of these (usually analysis). This of course is not a problem if you want to create an MCQ that only tests one of these levels but it is important for the designer to know what they are creating. Medical teaching has perfected the design of problem solving MCQs and the forensic science assessor can learn from this. Collins (2006) clearly stated the difference between MCQs testing lower level cognitive skills and problem solving MCQs within medical teaching. For example, an MCQ that asks a student to identify a particular characteristic on a medical scan is not a true problem solving MCQ. However, an MCQ that provides specific patient information and imaging data and asks the student to choose the most appropriate course of action does test problem solving skills. With that in mind, single MCQs, or a series of MCQs, can be designed for the investigation of a particular evidence type or criminal case. In order to identify the difference between just analysis MCQs and problem solving MCQs, examples have been provided as follows.

Example 6 An analysis based MCQ

What animal has the hair in photo 1 originated from?

(a) Cat
(b) Deer
(c) Horse
(d) Mouse
(e) Dog
(f) Rabbit

Answer = (e)

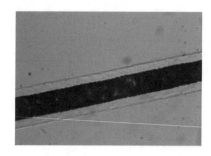

This type of MCQ requires the participant to carry out measurements and make judgments based upon the results in order to identify the species of animal that this hair has originated from. The analysis type has not been stated, therefore participants would need to know that medulla distribution type and medulla index (or medulla ratio) are the two best characteristics that can be observed on this particular photo for species identification. The participant may use other visible characteristics such as cuticle scale profile and scale margin to help identification. Participants would have to measure the medulla index taking into account the size of the photo and then apply this knowledge to animal hair characteristics in order to identify the species. For these types of question the participants should be informed as to what equipment to bring, that is, a calculator, ruler or information charts such as a medulla ratio graph for cat and dog hair could be provided by the assessor in the test. Other examples of analysis based MCQs could include the comparison of a footwear mark/fingermark from a crime scene to a control sample and then questions being asked surrounding the participant's conclusions.

Evaluation MCQs are easier to differentiate from analysis based MCQs as they are particularly asking for the participant to pass a judgment upon a conclusion, idea, experimental opinion or interpretation of data. Evaluation based questions in forensic science assessment may include the participant passing judgment upon the accuracy of an expert witness statement or quality of a fingermark.

Example 7 Example of Background Information Provided for a Problem Solving MCQ

A single suspect hair was found at the scene of a crime (BGD/01). Three suspects were taken into custody and control hairs were taken from each suspect's head and were analysed (HGS/02), (HGS/03) and (HGS/04), respectively. Ten width measurements were taken from each hair.

Evidence List
BGD/01 = hair retrieved from the crime scene
HGS/02 = hair retrieved from suspect 1
HGS/03 = hair retrieved from suspect 2
HGS/04 = hair retrieved from suspect 3

Width measurements of hair samples (μm)			
BGD/01	HGS/02	HGS/03	HGS/04
54.2	63.2	55.3	67.5
54.8	64.2	55.9	68.1
55.3	64.3	54.2	67.3
55.2	63.8	54.1	66.9
54.1	63.7	56.3	66.2
54.7	63.1	56.2	69.6
53.6	65.7	54.3	68.5
53.2	57.3	54.2	68.1
54.6	63.4	54.9	66.8
54.7	64.2	53.3	67.4

Investigate the data provided in the scenario using an appropriate statistical software package and answer the questions provided to you in the exam based upon your investigation.

It is common to see background information provided in problem solving MCQs in medical education being based around details of a medical scenario, including patient details, symptoms and medical records. This type of background information can easily be utilised in forensic science questions. However, details may include suspect information, case history, details of the crime scene or data from the analysis of evidence.

Example 7 is an example of background information that is based upon the data from samples analysed from a case. Example 7 only includes one set of quantitative data for each sample, that is, width measurements. Despite this, it could be extended to multiple datasets for further characteristics, include further control samples or added evidence. The scenario details in Example 7 are basic but could be extended by providing additional information about the suspects, where the crime scene hair (BGD/01) was found, and population information regarding the characteristics prevalence in the general population.

The background information seen in Example 7 allows the participant to demonstrate their ability to identify what would now be the best procedure to handle these data in order to gain information about the case. No instructions on how to handle the data have been provided, leaving it to the participant to decide the next sequence of steps. These may include gaining descriptive statistics from each of the datasets, error analysis, significance testing or application of the Bayesian Approach if population statistics have been provided. In order to allow the participant to fully investigate the data, this background information might be provided to the participant in advance of the MCQ test (therefore be designed as partially seen exams) or additional time and resources provided within the test to allow the participants to carry out their analysis. It is very important to increase test timing if the latter approach is used, as the participant may have a large amount of material to read (and *re-read*) before making a response.

One advantage of providing the question before the test and allowing the participant to bring along their notes and results to the test (checking notes prior to examination is advised), is that the participant is not prompted by the questions in what to potentially do with the background information, for example, what tests to carry out. The MCQs surrounding the background information may question any aspect of the data or the scenario, including the processes that should be employed to investigate the case. It is very common to have a series of questions that in their entirety test the range of skills which constitute problem solving rather than just one question. Example 8 demonstrates one of the MCQs that may be asked regarding the data in the scenario.

Example 8 Possible MCQ for a Series of Problem-Solving Questions

Which ONE of the following statements regarding the width measurements of the hair evidence (BGD/01, HGS/02, HGS/03 and HGS/04) are TRUE?

(a) BGD/01 and HGS/02 are normally distributed datasets.
(b) HGS/03 only is a normally distributed dataset.
(c) BGD/01, HGS/02, HGS/03 and HGS/04 are all normally distributed datasets.
(d) BGD/01, HGS/03 and HGS/04 are normally distributed datasets.

For the participant to answer this question, they may have chosen to utilise a Kolmogorov–Smirnov test to indicate the distribution of the data, the use of histograms and skewness or a combination of multiple approaches to answer the MCQ in Example 8. This problem solving to decide the most appropriate approach tests participants beyond just their ability to analyse the data.

Tests that have questions which feed from one or more particular crime scenario and combine evidence, procedures and ideas that require the student to have completed research prior to their answer are recognised to be time consuming to produce (Miller *et al.*, 1998) but are interesting for students to complete and test higher cognitive skills effectively. Research conducted by Williams and Clark (2004) observed that students rated the effort they exert before an MCQ test higher than their actual ability or teacher input. This study showed that students perceive their input towards the preparation of an MCQ test, such as note-taking, reading and so on, as being very important leading to deeper learning prior to the tests. By providing case scenarios and information about forensic evidence before MCQ tests, this will encourage the desired deeper learning as an outcome. This type of MCQ test could be expanded further, instead of only providing a case summary or a description of the evidence, video recordings, for example, simulated CCTV scenarios or actual evidence (for practical assessments), could be used as a lead-in to the questions. Collins (2006) stated that if background information in stems of problem solving questions is in a less interpreted form, this creates a more difficult question.

The potential difficulty when designing MCQs that provide a lot of prior information as part of a crime scene scenario and are lead-ins for more than one question, is to avoid producing questions that cue a response to subsequent questions relating to that scenario (Gwinnett *et al.*, 2011). Careful writing of the stems and ensuring that each question is as independent as possible reduces the risk of giving the participants 'clues' to the subsequent questions. The effect of cueing has also been discussed in MCQ use for clinical nursing practice, which also attempts to provide 'real-life' scenarios to test participants' higher learning skills (Brady, 2005).

Creating Whole Tests of MCQs

When designing summative assessments, the overall assignment should be viewed with question level and question type in mind. How MCQs are integrated into exams should reflect participant preferences on question type, level of exam, length of exam and academics' preference on marking scheme and marking time. When designing MCQ tests, it can become apparent that a designer should not become bogged-down with attempting to make every question test higher cognitive levels. There is a tendency, once fully aware of the potential to test skills such as problem solving, to design all of the questions in an assessment to meet this level. In reality, the level must take into account the subject matter as well as the level of understanding that is required from participants. For example, in an assessment covering general forensic science principles, questions can legitimately be centred mainly on factual issues such as expert witness duties, continuity of evidence and court conduct. In order to make sure that the balance of different MCQ levels is appropriate for a test, assessors should categorise each question into the appropriate Bloom Taxonomy education objectives and calculate the proportions of each. This categorisation can be very useful when generating a pool of MCQs in which to choose questions for future tests and also aids any justifications for test design to external examiners or validators.

Integrating MCQs into Forensic Science Education and Assessment

Designing a collection of questions for MCQ formative and summative assessments is only the first step towards implementation. The next stage is to identify where, when and how you are to use them. The forensic science academic has many opportunities to integrate MCQs into their teaching and assessment but where and how much they are utilised should be the choice of the academic and the students and should be fit-for-purpose for a particular subject area or HE institution. When identifying the best manner to integrate MCQs into a curriculum, the following questions must be considered:

1. Should assessments be 100% MCQs or should they be blended with other forms of question?
2. Do you want to use MCQs for purely summative assessments or as an aid in other learning and teaching activities?
3. When do you want to implement the MCQ tests, for example, beginning, middle or end of a module?
4. What method do you want to use to implement the MCQS, for example, online, paper based or other commercially available method?
5. How do you want to manage and organise your MCQs?

Each of these points will now be addressed in the following sections.

MCQ Test Formats – The Blended Approach

The nature of forensic science means that the vast breadth of subjects, skills and ideas may not all be fully suited to the MCQ format. In addition to this, the potential for students to adopt a surface learning approach in MCQs, if not designed to be more sophisticated as described by Scouller (1998), could mean that the assessor may have more confidence if a blended approach is utilised. Traub and MacRury (1990) have indicated that if participants expect a test that has open-ended questions rather than MCQs, students will prepare more effectively and perform better in both types of question, which may make a blended test more attractive to the assessor. The blended approach may utilise a mix of MCQs, short answer questions and essay style questions within a single exam. A common approach is ask a participant an MCQ regarding a particular topic and then follow that with a question asking for a justification of the participants choice of answer. This approach allows the participant to demonstrate further knowledge about the topic and provide a deeper answer. It also provides the assessor with an insight into the confidence of the participant in their answer, although it must be noted that certain MCQ marking schemes can also provide this information. A blended approach may also be employed to allow the participant to choose a topic to further demonstrate their skills. For example, in a test with two sections, the first section may include MCQs on all aspects of a topic, scenario or item of evidence, and then a second section may provide the participant with a choice of essay style questions that focus on a particular area of the topic being assessed. This combined approach, provides some reduction in marking time when assessing the topic as a whole but still incorporates an essay style question for the academic that is reluctant to test with MCQs alone. The blended approach is a useful step towards using full MCQ tests and is particularly useful for assessors inexperienced in MCQ design, as any small errors in the stem or options may be offset by the opportunity for the participant to explain their answer.

Different Uses for MCQs

As every HE academic knows, assessments are not just for summative analysis of a student's ability but can be used creatively to provide feedback, engage students with their own progress and to create interesting learning environments. MCQs are well suited for all of these approaches and there has been much development in methods for delivering MCQs in different situations (please see the later section on Methods of Implementation for a further discussion of these). The MCQ questionnaire delivered to 86 forensic science, investigation and policing students at Staffordshire University investigated students' preferences for MCQ use. Students were asked that if they were to have MCQs integrated into their curriculum, which methods of MCQ test use did they perceive to be valuable to their learning? Figure 17.4 shows the range in responses from these students.

It is interesting to identify that students value the use of MCQs as a revision aid as well as a formative test. The use of MCQs in lectures as a method for self-reflection and knowledge evaluation is a relatively easy and fun method to implement. 'Quizzes', quick fire questions and voting systems are interactive methods that can be utilised in lectures, either at the beginning of a session as a recap on the previous week's work, at the end of the session as a reflective method for students to identify the effectiveness of their learning, the teaching and the topic covered, or dotted throughout the session. The last is a useful way to keep students engaged and increase the student activity within the lecture. MCQs, like any other question activity being introduced into a lecture, should not just be there arbitrarily. The academic should decide what the planned outcomes of the lecture should be and relate the use of MCQs to these. For example, if an outcome of the lecture is for students to be able to identify different fingerprint patterns and ridge characteristics, then MCQs could be based around a practical activity where students

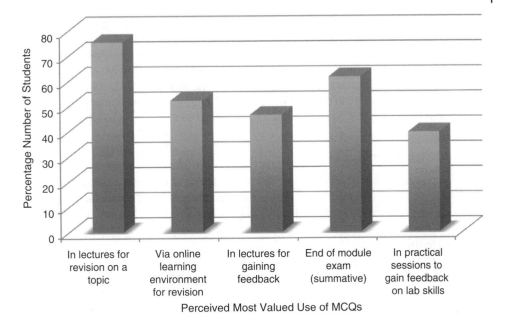

Figure 17.4 Students' most valued uses of MCQ test ($n = 86$).

observe a fingermark and control prints and answer MCQs regarding pattern type, number of particular ridge characteristics and the students' conclusions about which suspect the fingermark can be attributed to. These MCQs will quickly identify the students' skill in fingermark analysis and comparison within a lecture environment. If MCQs are to be used in lectures, the academic must plan in advance the method of delivery and feedback dissemination. There are many methods to suit all levels of technology competence; some of these will be discussed in the section on Methods of Implementation. As seen in Figure 17.4, the use of 'self-tests in practical sessions' was also seen as valuable to 39.5% of the students questioned, which highlights the need for forensic science academics to think about how feedback can be given in different ways in laboratory sessions as well as lectures or tutorials. It is common practice for short answer questions to be included into laboratory schedules for the students to answer based upon their results generated in the laboratory, but also utilising MCQs could be a quicker and more effective way of quickly providing feedback within the session so that lessons can be learnt before the next session.

Positioning MCQ Tests Within a Teaching Programme

Depending upon the intended use of the MCQs, the assessor may wish to generate a schedule of MCQ implementation. Not only is it necessary to identify where the MCQs are placed within a session, it is important to identify where in the teaching programme MCQ tests can be most effectively implemented. At the beginning of a course or module of study, MCQs can provide the teaching team with an indication of the students' existing knowledge and skills and therefore enable the course content and delivery to be made fit-for-purpose for each cohort. Formative and summative MCQ tests delivered mid-way within the teaching of a course can provide participants with feedback on their progress and highlight areas needed for improvement. Mid-way positioned MCQ tests also help encourage students to engage with revision strategies in a timely manner, reducing last minute cramming for final assessments. MCQ tests used at the end of a module are commonly used as the final summative assessment, although a series of MCQ tests in the final quarter of the course can help escalate revision before the final assessment (even if that final assessment is not MCQ based).

Methods of Implementation

There are a variety of methods that can be used to deliver MCQ tests to students, which each have positive attributes. Many of these are technology based implementation systems that are either freely or commercially available to assessors. It is beyond the scope of this chapter to discuss each of these methods but an overview of selected methods is provided in this section.

Traditionally, MCQ tests were implemented in a paper-based manner, where participants would select their answers upon a hard copy of the test sheet. As technology in education has advanced, there are now more efficient and sophisticated methods for delivering MCQ tests. However, paper-based tests still have their advantages for locations that do not have access to the Internet or adequate computers. Issues with 'timing-out' of sessions and poor Internet reception do not affect paper-based tests and therefore information about the assessment location is required prior to planning the test.

The marking of paper based methods has become more advanced over the years, with electronic automated scoring systems being put in place that use imaging technology to allow quick scanning and marking of answers on specific forms, for example, Scantron's Remark Classic OMR (Scantron, 2015). These systems have the advantage of taking paper-based answer sheets and generating results akin to computer-based testing systems, albeit much less sophisticated. DiBattista *et al.*, in 2004, investigated the use of the Immediate Feedback Assessment Technique (IF-AT), which is an inexpensive waxy-coated form in which participants scratch off the coating and reveal whether they have chosen the correct answer. This type of form allows the participant to continue answering the question until the correct answer is achieved, earning partial credit depending on the number of attempts used (Epstein Educational Enterprises, 2015). Dibattista *et al.* (2004) found that this system was accepted positively by undergraduate students and had some advantages over other forms, such as its ability to provide immediate corrective feedback, shown to enhance learning in multiple ways. The IF-AT system has also been shown to enhance learning in a laboratory setting, a place where computer devices for the completion of MCQs may not be accessible in some institutions delivering forensic science (Epstein *et al.*, 2002).

Technology enhanced testing systems range from very popular, commercially available and robustly tested systems that are either stand alone or are embedded within a virtual learning environment, such as Blackboard, to smaller, bespoke made systems designed for particular testing schemes. Testing systems such as these have the advantages of being able to provide instant feedback to students, and allow assessors to interrogate the results quickly and effectively. Many systems allow the generation of question banks, collaborative authoring of questions, a range of delivery methods on different devices and provide a series of reporting options. For example, QuestionMark®

Perception (QuestionMark®, 2015) allows full management of the entire assessment process and allows assessors to create detailed reports, such as assessment performance over time, frequencies of option choice, comparisons of different test centres and question type and status of the MCQs in the question banks. ClassMarker (ClassMarker, 2015) is also an online test implementation system that enables the creation of custom tests but also the integration of test results back to assessors' systems.

A popular method of implementing MCQ tests is utilising institutionally purchased virtual learning environments, for example, Blackboard, and there inbuilt test and survey features. These virtual learning environments have a range of template MCQ structures such as 'fill in blanks' and ordering questions ready for the assessor to populate (Jennings, 2012). These systems allow the upload of documents and background information but maybe lack some of the tailored features that systems purely dedicated to testing have.

The OCTAVE database of MCQs for veterinary schools is an example of a bespoke system that has readily searchable questions, which have been meta-tagged by subject area so that students can search for questions that are most applicable to their studies (Head and Ogden, 2006). Students can select either to complete the MCQ testing in either an assessment, assessment/revision or revision/instant feedback mode that determines how the answers and feedback are presented. Feedback for both correct and incorrect answers provides a reference for further study, which encourages deeper learning and stimulates student reflection.

Management and Organisation of MCQs

Part of the work of integrating MCQs into a curriculum involves the management of the questions and development of robust quality control procedures. This is especially important if designing MCQs for the assessment of forensic practitioners that must potentially stand-up to scrutiny in a UK Court. If a collection of MCQs is being developed over many years, will be re-used in different tests and are being created by a group of designers, then a continuity trail is desirable. This continuity trail allows information such as when, where and how MCQS have been previously used. This is particularly useful when teaching a large number of students that may also be from a range of different courses, schools and faculties, as quality control procedures will avoid accidentally using questions already seen by a particular cohort. This trail can most easily be provided by utilising a database that states the name of the MCQ designer, any changes made by external examiners and when and how the questions have been used. In HE, an MCQ database containing forensic questions would benefit from the ability to be updated by multiple designers and to audit the evolution of questions over time. This feature is useful when showcasing a course's assessment methods to University External Examiners. The use of educational technologies, such as Blackboard (Jennings, 2012) and ClassMarker, are very useful tools for storing and implementing MCQ tests, but it may be beneficial to develop your own software program that combines both a testing facility and also a management system. This would allow the user to not only store and search for MCQs based on topic, type and level of cognitive thinking being tested, which is similar in style to other extant databases of MCQs, but would also allow the evolution and quality control procedures to be viewed for each individual question. A bespoke MCQ testing software system for more sophisticated, large-scale schemes could allow multiple users to view developing MCQs and provide revisions and comments regarding design and validity, all of which is logged providing a trail of continuity. This means that the test creator is not limited to the structure of a pre-made online learning environment software and can make bespoke tests for different purposes without the need for copying and pasting MCQs from other areas. For example, the OCTAVE MCQ database allows easy scrutiny of the answers given in an MCQ test, such as generating frequencies of response to different options and the effectiveness of each question (Head and Ogden, 2006). This may be particularly useful for HE institutions who deliver bespoke courses to external companies.

Marking Methods for MCQ Assessments

Whilst standard (traditional) marking schemes (where a correct answer is awarded equal marks and these are totalled for the final score with no partial credit given) are still very popular, alternative scoring processes, such as negative marking, confidence based marking, the 'hedging' format and 'value exam' format are available to reduce guessing and encourage participants to identify their level of confidence in their answers, which promotes deep thinking (Walker and Thompson, 2001; Burton, 2004). Alternative marking schemes also provide benefits to the assessor in being able to gather feedback from students in terms of their choices, confidence in their understanding and knowledge and insights into their attitudes to risk. In order to help assessors choose which marking method is most appropriate for them, Table 17.3 outlines the most common methods and their relative advantages and limitations.

Before choosing a marking method, it may be useful for the assessor to consider the following questions:

1. **Am I going to use an online computer based implementation system?**
   If no, many of the alternative marking schemes are time consuming to calculate by paper-based methods, therefore standard marking or negative marking may be preferable.
2. **Do I want to investigate the risk preferences of the participants?**
   If yes, consider using the 'hedging' or 'liberal test' method. Risk preferences of participants in MCQ tests have been investigated by Walker and Thompson (2001).
3. **Do I want to get a clear idea of the confidence that participants have in their answers?**
   If yes, consider using the 'value choice' method.
4. **Do I want to gain an insight into the participants thinking when responding to the question or in the effectiveness of the distractors?**
   If yes, consider using the 'order-of-preference' method.
5. **Do I want to penalize incorrect answers in some manner?**
   If yes, consider how severe the penalty should be and consider choosing negative marking or other form of correction. Any form of correction due to incorrect answers should be carefully considered, as it has been indicated in a study conducted by Betts *et al.* (2009) that participants have shown to score higher and leave fewer questions unanswered when there is no correction due to incorrect answers compared with those that had.

Table 17.3 Examples of MCQ marking schemes.

Marking method	Overview	How it works	Is this method for me?	Limitations
Negative marking	A simple method that reduces guessing by fixing a small penalty to incorrect answers.	For each correct answer, 1 point is awarded, for each incorrect answer −1 point is awarded.	An easy method to employ that is easily understood by participants.	Participants may end up with overall negative scores (Bush, 1999).
Order of preference	Allows participants to assign an order of preference to their answers and gain partial credit for a second choice or third choice evidence.	Participants rank their answers in terms of preference and 4 points are awarded if the correct answer is their first choice, 2 for their second and 1 for their third.	Provides insight into the thought processes of the participant when considering the different options.	Allows participants to gain partial marks for 'almost' getting the correct answer – this only works if the options have been correctly designed and all have different 'levels' of correctness.
'Hedging'	Each question is asked twice and participants have the option to try for partial marks by choosing two different answers if uncertain of the answer.	If the participant is confident, they will choose the same option twice and receive full marks. If they are not confident they will choose two different options and receive only half marks if one answer is correct. Participants may also opt to take a standard test by only selecting one option once (Walker and Thompson, 2001).	Provides some knowledge about the participants' confidence in their answers but also helps identify the participants' risk preference without requiring extra work for the assessor in setting this system up.	This method depends upon a participant's preference for risk and therefore a knowledgeable but unconfident participant may end up with no higher than 50%.
Liberal tests (Bush, 1999)	This method is the same as the 'hedging' method but allows participants to choose up to three answers to spread the risk. Scoring is based upon the probabilities of the answers chosen being correct.	If the participant chooses only one answer and it is correct, they receive 100% of the marks for that question. If two answers are chosen, one of which is correct, 67% of the marks are awarded and if three options are chosen, one of which is correct, they are awarded 33%.	Very attractive to participants as they have the opportunity to express partial knowledge and may attain some marks for each question, even if unsure of the answer.	More lenient than the 'hedging' method, which may come under scrutiny.

Table 17.3 *(Continued)*

Marking method	Overview	How it works	Is this method for me?	Limitations
Value choice (Walker and Thompson, 2001)	Participants have the option to place a weighting upon their answer; 1–3 points, which are awarded if correct.	The participant's score is a percentage of correct points (number of correct points divided by total number of points attempted) (Walker and Thompson, 2001). Participants who are confident will give greater points value to their answer but can also express uncertainty by choosing 1 point. If no weighting is chosen, the points for that question default to 2.	A clearer method for obtaining knowledge about the participants' confidence in their knowledge of the material being tested. Participants have a sense of control as they are helping to determine their own grade.	This method is more time consuming to mark if paper based but can be overcome with a computer based implementation system that allows this form of marking. Does not provide any information about a participant's attitude to risk although this is to the benefit of obtaining information about confidence levels.
Confidence assessment (Bush 1999)	This method is the same as 'value choice' but also incorporates different severities of penalty if the incorrect answer is chosen based upon the original confidence of the answer.	Same as 'value choice' but when 1, 2 or 3 points are given to an incorrect answer, the resulting marks awarded are 0, −2, −6, respectively.	This method is particularly useful for MCQs that are highly important and require a penalty if incorrect.	May lead to very low or even negative overall scores.

6. **Do you want to assess the tests reliability in some way?**
   If yes, consider using a model based measure, as investigated by Burton (2004), that takes into account test length, number of options per question and marking scheme (negative marking in the case of Burton's 2004 work).

Whichever marking scheme is chosen, instructions must be clearly described and this is especially true when the students must actively participate in the scheme. Walker and Thompson (2001) indicated that there can be some negative feelings from students when they do not understand the instructions as they feel like they were at a disadvantage.

Conclusions

Multiple Choice Questions are a popular and efficient method for educational assessments but have been criticised by academics in the past. The knowledge of how to create more sophisticated MCQs along with robust implementation schemes and suitable marking methods now mean that MCQ tests can be usefully employed to test higher cognitive skills, gain student feedback and improve the learning experience. The variety of uses and design features that are offered by MCQ assessments means that they are very useful in forensic science education and can be robustly utilised to assess the skills desired from an individual required to work in the criminal justice system.

References

Atkinson. M. (2002) Writing effective multiple choice exams, *The Successful Professor*, **1** (6), 2–4.

Betts, L.R., Elder, T.J., Hartley, J. and Trueman, M. (2009) Does correction for guessing reduce students' performance on multiple-choice examinations? Yes? No? Sometimes? *Assessment & Evaluation in Higher Education*, **34** (1), 1–15.

Biggs. J (1999) *Teaching for Quality Learning at University*, Society for Research into Higher Education and Open University Press, Buckingham.

Bleske-Rechek, A., Zueg, N. and Webb, R.M (2007) Discrepant performance on multiple-choice and short answer assessments and the relation of performance to general scholastic aptitude. *Assessment and Evaluation in Higher Education*, **32** (2), 89–105.

Bloom, B.S. (1959) *Taxonomy of Educational Objectives. Vol I: Cognitive Domain*, McKay, New York.

Boud, D. (2000) Sustainable assessment: rethinking assessment for the learning society, *Studies in Continuing Education*, **22** (2), 151–167.

Brady, A.-M. (2005) Assessment of learning with multiple choice questions. *Nurse Education in Practice*, **5**, 238–242.

Bull, J. and McKenna, C. (2004) *Blueprint for Computer-Assisted Assessment*, Routledge Falmer, London.

Burton, R.F. (2001) Quantifying the effects of chance in multiple choice and true/false tests: Question selection and guessing of answers, *Assessment and Evaluation in Higher Education*, **26** (1), 41–50.

Burton, R.F. (2004) Multiple choice and true/false tests: reliability measures and some implications of negative marking, *Assessment and Evaluation in Higher Education*, **29** (5), 585–595.

Bush, M. (1999) Alternative Marking Schemes for On-Line Multiple-Choice Tests. 7th Annual Conference on the Teaching of Computing, Belfast. Availbale at: http://www.caacentre.ac.uk/dldocs/BUSHMARK.PDF (accessed 12 December 2016).

Carneson, J., Delpierre, G. and Masters, K. (2003) *Designing and Managing Multiple Choice Questions*, Southrock Corporation Ltd, Australia.

ClassMarker (2015) Quiz API and Integration Options. Available at: http://www.classmarker.com/online-testing/integrate/ (accessed 10 December 2016).

Collins, J. (2001) Writing Multiple Choice Questions for Continuing Medical Education Activities and Self-Assessment Modules. Available at: http://www.arrs.org/uploadedfiles/arrs/publications /writingmultiplechoicehandout.pdf (accessed 12 December 2016).

Collins, J. (2006) Writing Multiple-Choice Questions for Continuing Medical Education Activities and Self-Assessment Modules. *RSNA Radiographics*, **26** (2). DOI: http://dx.doi.org/10.1148/rg.262055145.

Cox, K.R. (1976) How did you guess? Or what do multiple choice questions measure? *Medical Journal of Australia*, **1**, 884–886.

CRFP (2009) CRFP's Submission to the Forensic Science Regulator's Review of the Optimal National Approach to the Registration of Forensic Practitioners. Available at: https://www.gov.uk/government/publications/forensic-practitioner-standards-review-appendix-ii-crfp-submission (accessed 10 December 2016).

CSFS, The Royal Chartered Society of Forensic Sciences (2015) Certificate of Professional Competence – Components. Available at: http://www.csofs.org/Certificate-of-Professional-Competence-CPC (accessed 12 December 2016).

De Milia, L. (2007) Benefiting from multiple-choice exams: The positive impact of answer switching, *Education Psychology*, **27** (5), 607–615.

DiBattista, D., Mitterer, J.O. and Gosse, L. (2004) Acceptance by undergraduates of the immediate feedback assessment technique for multiple choice testing. *Teaching in Higher Education*, **9** (1), 17–28.

Dorman, J.P. and Knightley, M. (2006) Development and validation of an instrument to assess secondary school students' perceptions of assessment tasks. *Educational Studies*, **32** (1), 47–58.

Entwistle. N.J. and Entwistle, A. (1991) Contrasting forms of understanding for degree examinations: The student experience and its implications, *Higher Education*, **22**, 205–227.

Epstein Educational Enterprises (2015) What is the IF-AT? Available at: http://www.epsteineducation.com/home/about/ (accessed 10 December 2016).

Epstein, M.L., Lazarus, A.D. and Calvano, T.B. (2002) Immediate feedback assessment technique promotes learning and corrects inaccurate first responses, *The Psychological Record*, **52**, 187–201.

Fellenz, M.R. (2004) Using assessment to support higher level learning: the multiple choice item development assignment, *Assessment and Evaluation in Higher Education*, **29** (6), 703–719.

Gwinnett, C., Cassella, J. and Allen, M. (2011) The trials and tribulations of designing and utilising MCQs in HE and for assessing forensic practitioner competency, *New Directions*, The Higher Education Academy, 7, 72–78.

Hannis, M., Welsh, C. (2009) Fit for purpose? Research into the provision of forensic science degree programmes in UK HE, a report for the Skills for Justice Forensic Science Occupational Committee.

Head, S. and Ogden, C. (2006) Development of a Searchable Database of Veterinary MCQs with Educational Feedback for Independent Learning, in *10th CAA International Computer Assisted Assessment Conference Proceedings* (ed. M. Danson), Loughborough University, Loughborough, July 2006, pp. 213–224.

Higher Education Statistics Agency (HESA) (2015) Statistical Release 210, Available at: https://www.hesa.ac.uk/free-statistics (accessed 10 December 2016).

Higgins, E. and Tatham, L. (2003) Exploring the potential of multiple-choice questions in assessment. *Learning and Teaching in Action*, **2** (1), 1–12.

Jennings, D. (2012) The Design of Multiple Choice Questions for Assessment, *UCD Teaching and Learning Resources*. Available at: http://www.ucd.ie/t4cms/UCDTLA0042.pdf (accessed 10 December 2016).

QuestionMark® (2015) QuestionMark® Perception. Available at: https://www.questionmark.com/us/perception/ (accessed 10 December 2016).

Lorusso, G.D. (2004) A style guide for effective and consistent formatting of multiple-choice questions, *Pathology Education*, **27** (2), 25–32.

Mennell, J. (2006) The future of forensic and crime scene science Part II. A UK perspective on forensic science education, *Forensic Science International*, **157**, 13–20.

McCoubrie, P. (2004) Improving the fairness of multiple-choice questions: A literature review, *Medical Teacher*, **26** (8), 709–712.

McKeachie, W.J. (1986) *Teaching Tips*, 8th edn, Heath, Lexington, MA.

McKenna, C. and Bull, J. (1999) *Designing Effective Objective Test Questions: An Introductory Workshop*, Computer Assisted Assessment Centre, Loughborough University.

Miller, A.H., Imrie, B.W. and Cox, K. (1998) *Student Assessment in Higher Education: A Handbook for Assessing Performance*, Kogan Page, London.

Nicol, D. (2007) E-Assessment by design: Using multiple-choice tests to good effect, *Journal of Further and Higher Education*, **31** (1), 53–64.

Paxton, M. (2000) A linguistic perspective on multiple choice questioning, *Assessment and Evaluation in Higher Education*, **25** 109–119.

Scantron (2015) Remark Classic OMR. Available at: http://www.scantron.com/software/classroom-testing/remark-classic/overview (accessed 10 December 2016).

Schultheis, N.M. (1998) Writing cognitive educational objectives and multiple-choice test questions, *American Journal of Health System Pharmacy*, **55**, 2397–2401.

Science and Technology Committee, 7th Report: The Forensic Science Service, 2011, House of Commons. Available at: http://www.publications.parliament.uk/pa/cm201012/cmselect/cmsctech/855/85502.htm (accessed 10 December 2016).

Scouller, K. (1998) The influence of assessment method on students' learning approaches: multiple choice questions examination versus assignment essay, *Higher Education*, **35**, 453–472.

Tarrant, M., Knierim, A., Hayes, S.K. and Ware, J. (2006) The frequency of item writing flaws in multiple-choice questions used in high stakes nursing assessments, *Nurse Education in Practice*, **6**, 354–363.

Traub, R.E. and MacRury, K. (1990) Multiple choice vs. free response in the testing of scholastic achievement, in *Test und Tends 8: Jahrbuch der Pddagogischen Diagnostik* (eds K. Ingenkamp and R.S. Jager), Beltz Verlag, Weinheim and Basel.

Walker, D.M. and Thompson, J.S. (2001) A note on multiple choice exams, with respect to students' risk preference and confidence, *Assessment and Evaluation in Higher Education*, **26** (3), 261–267.

Welsh, A.L. (1978) Multiple choice objective tests, in *Resource Manual for Teacher Training Programs in Economics* (eds P. Saunders, A.L. Welsh and W.L. Hansen), Joint Council on Economic Education, New York, pp. 191–228.

Williams, R.L. and Clark, L. (2004) College students' ratings of student effort, student ability and teacher input as correlates of student performance on multiple-choice exams, *Educational Research*, **46** (3), 229–239.

18

The Future of Forensic Science Education

John P. Cassella,[1] Anna Williams,[2] and Peter D. Maskell[3]

[1] *Staffordshire University, Department of Forensic Science and Crime Science, Faculty of Computing, Engineering and Science, Science Centre, Stoke on Trent, UK*
[2] *University of Huddersfield, School of Applied Sciences, Queensgate, Huddersfield, UK*
[3] *Abertay University, School of Science, Engineering and Technology, Dundee, UK*

Introduction

The forensic science education sector has the job of producing the next generation of researchers, practitioners and educators. There is no lack of provision of forensic courses in the United Kingdom and the United States, with the sector developing at an unparalleled rate over the last 20 years (Quarino and Brettell, 2009; Rankin *et al.*, 2012). In the United States, the American Academy of Forensic Sciences website (www.aafs.org) revealed over 100 forensic science programmes leading to a bachelor's degree. In addition, over 50 programmes leading to a masters' level degree in forensic science or a related discipline in the United States alone are listed. In the United Kingdom, the Universities and Colleges Administration Services (UCAS) states that there are 87 providers of degree courses containing the word 'forensic' in the title available for a 2017 start. This rapid expansion of teaching courses has been openly criticised (Rankin *et al.*, 2012) with relevance, suitability and quality of the degree content raised as issues. Courses have suffered from a rapid growth beyond the capability of the academic and technical support staff, the existing resources and indeed existing hard structure facilities, resulting more from a financial need rather than for pedagogical motives. This has caused academic staff to have to hurriedly develop their skills in order to stay 'one step ahead' of the students. Forensic science is a discipline in which the educators have to walk a tightrope between vocational training and theoretical teaching, in order to produce graduates who carry considerable professional responsibility and can demonstrate consistent competence in the workplace. Also integral to the course is instilling an understanding of the statistical power of any data obtained from forensic techniques

Forensic Science Education and Training: A Tool-kit for Lecturers and Practitioner Trainers, First Edition.
Edited by Anna Williams, John P. Cassella, and Peter D. Maskell.
© 2017 John Wiley & Sons Ltd. Published 2017 by John Wiley & Sons Ltd.

and recognition of their implications for the Court. Such issues create problems for educators, who come from a range of backgrounds and perspectives, and who therefore have to align their different priorities and professional requirements with the validation mechanisms of the university. The degrees have had to simultaneously meet the requirements of academia, professional organisations and prospective employers, as well as meet the needs of a disparate and changing student body, including mature students and those that require learning support. Practitioner training also poses challenges to the trainers, from teaching 'old dogs new tricks', deconstructing entrenched processes and methodologies, to contextualising their practice for teaching and assimilation in the classroom.

This forensic science education text is the first of its kind to capture a diverse collection of literature, websites and practitioner experiences and to distil them into a helpful and meaningful toolkit and reflective aid for new academics and practitioner trainers working in today's forensic education. We have included a number of, but by no means an exhaustive range, forensic sub-disciplines. Therefore, this volume contains the collective experiences of forensic practitioners and teachers, and has been designed to offer new lecturers tools to assist in the creation and in the delivery of undergraduate and postgraduate modules and courses in forensic science. We have also aimed to offer practitioners coming into the Higher Education sector an understanding of the HE marketplace, and to facilitate a bridge between professional practice and academia to help demystify the complexities and nuances of academia and how to deliver relevant concepts in pedagogical theory. Implicit in these chapters is an understanding that up-to-date, relevant teaching must be research-led and, as much as possible, interactive. Heavy teaching loads for all academic staff and the increasing administrative requirements coupled with insufficient funding means that research can become, for some, a luxurious aspiration. It is hoped that the experiences offered by the authors in this text will inspire readers to develop research interests, take the questions out of the lecture theatre and the laboratory into research projects that they and their students can investigate and publish. It could serve as a spring board for lecturers to build upon their own research areas, facilitating the generation of ideas and opportunities to apply for funding, ultimately resulting in research that can impact and improve frontline forensic services and also impact on the forensic science teaching in the classroom.

This chapter will consider how we ensure and maintain quality of teaching, learning and assessment, how we manage the currency of competency in academic staff delivering their subject and how they interact with the increasing number of practitioners – both policing and forensic scientists – now working alongside them in HEIs. Also, we will explore the impact and implications of the new Teaching Exercise Framework (TEF) and the future of the Research Exercise Framework (REF) for forensic science education, and consider the changing needs of employers, the prospects for graduates seeking employment with small to medium enterprises (SMEs), the police and government organisations, in the changing face of public funding. We will also consider the current and future for wide-ranging discussions about, and dissemination of, good practice in teaching, learning and assessment in forensic science and related disciplines. A prediction of the next decade of education in light of falling student numbers, increasing university fees and reduced opportunities for funding coupled with a shrinking forensic jobs market will be considered.

The Teaching Exercise Framework and the Research Exercise Framework

Teaching Exercise Framework

The mass expansion of higher education along with the progressive introduction of fees and an ever expanding research agenda have changed the institutional priorities of UK (and indeed international) universities over the past 25 years from teaching and scholarship to research and economic innovation (Forstenzer, 2016). The aim of the incoming Teaching Excellence Framework (TEF) is to rebalance 'the relationship between teaching and research' in universities and place 'teaching at the heart of the system,' by introducing a teaching quality assessment mechanism using core metrics and qualitative evidence. Universities deemed to have 'excellent' teaching will be rewarded with the opportunity to increase undergraduate fees in line with inflation. Therefore, the newly created Teaching Excellence Framework (House of Commons, Business, Innovation and Skills Committee, 2016) will have enormous implications for teaching in the coming decade. It is increasingly reported in the news media that it is not difficult to find students from a range of degree subjects who feel let down by their degree courses. Countless surveys have been published indicating that students don't feel they are getting value for money, while the Universities' Minister has been quoted as saying that the quality of teaching in higher education is 'lamentable.'

To help improve the situation and address these criticisms and to give applicants a better idea of what sort of teaching they can expect at university, the Government will be revealing its new Teaching Excellence Framework (TEF). It's expected that the TEF will use statistics such as student satisfaction scores or the progress made by students from disadvantaged backgrounds, as well as other existing data. Universities that pass the test will be allowed to raise their fees in line with inflation. The key to its usefulness in HEIs will require the metrics to focus on considering how well-thought-out the structure of a programme is and not on an individual teacher or module. A concern is that whilst student satisfaction scores and employability data are already available at a course-specific level, the TEF will measure institutions on a university-wide basis – which might not be that helpful.

Research Exercise Framework

The Research Excellence Framework is a UK Government-level mechanism for assessing the quality of research publications and subsequently apportioning government funding to HEIs for the coming five-year period and beyond. In order to assess research quality and focus the assessment on specific areas, the REF is divided up into 'Units of Assessment' (UoA). Whilst there are Units of Assessments for traditional subjects such as engineering, physics and chemistry, there is no UoA for forensic science, and no current plans to include one in the next REF in 2020. Forensic science, by its very definition, utilises numerous distinct sciences and as such it may easily be included in at least 20 of the current 35 Higher Education Funding Council for England (HEFCE) Units of Assessment in the Research Excellence Framework exercise conducted to assess the quality of UK research. As an analogy, chemistry uses tools developed in engineering, physics, computer science and mathematics. However, clearly, it would be inappropriate to submit mainstream chemistry research for scrutiny under any of the UoA relating to these other disciplines. To do so would inevitably skew the types of research conducted within chemistry so as to better fit the demands of those UoAs. Also, it would fragment chemistry research teams such that the work of individual members of such teams would be examined under different units. Finally, it would mean that chemistry would be assessed out of context. It is difficult to see, for example, how high quality synthetic organic chemistry research could be rationally assessed as good quality physics — even if a chemist were asked to conduct this assessment.

Yet this is the current position that forensic science finds itself in and it is a widely held contention that this is damaging development in this crucial field. One consequence of this situation of pitting oranges against apples is the on-going poor success rate to receive funding through the established bodies such as the Higher Education Funding Council for England and the Research Councils UK.

In recent years there have been significant national reviews and changes within the forensic industry giving forensic science a significantly higher profile specifically as a distinct subject. This has led to a chink of light in forensic research, with the funding by the Leverhulme Trust of the Leverhulme Centre for Forensic Science at Dundee University for ten years.

This suggests that high quality forensic research, published in journals with a high impact factor, will have little or no contribution to the financial outcome of the REF exercise. This lowers the perceived value of forensic research, both by universities delivering forensic science, the grant awarding bodies and the academic community themselves. In the current situation, academics find their research having to be submitted as part of the REF under the auspices of other Units of Assessment, which may not necessarily be the most appropriate. For example, forensic anthropology articles have been included in the biological sciences UoA. Researchers should consider, early in the research process, how their research will fit into existing UoAs, rather than retrospectively attempting to shoehorn their work into this current REF structure. However, the boundaries and definitions of the UoAs for the upcoming 2020 REF are yet to be published. It is still extremely unlikely that forensic science will have its own UoA.

The global issue of research opportunities and research funding is nowhere more obviously suffering than in the arena of forensic science. The impact of assisting to solve crime and facilitate an early and secure conviction (or release of the innocent) is absolute. Despite the lack of a UoA for forensic science in the REF, there is still therefore a societal need to conduct research. This is driven by the requirement for robust data to present to the courts, as well as scientific development and indeed confirmation of new techniques and processes. Whilst securing research funding is challenging, the opportunity exists to use postgraduate and indeed undergraduate students as researchers, as part of their development and assessment during their degree programmes. Quarino and Brettell (2009) comment that the development of forensic science doctoral programmes would greatly benefit the profession. Doctoral level research can be performed not only on the application of existing technologies to forensic science problems, but on addressing those aspects of forensic science that have been widely anecdotally accepted but not rigorously scientifically proven, such as bite mark and shoe wear analysis. For instance, greatly needed research into the development of statistical models to unequivocally prove the uniqueness of fingerprints, handwriting, or footprint evidence can be facilitated within doctoral programmes. The validity of long-held concepts, such as the Locard's Exchange Principle, could also be empirically examined. The development of doctoral programmes may also influence public sources of funding and to provide lobbying power and hence more financial support to forensic science research.

Whilst ostensibly the REF may be seen as a limiting factor to teaching delivery, as it diverts staff attention and effort from the classroom and student support, it drives the creation of new knowledge for publication, and will ultimately benefit teaching and learning.

Accreditation of Forensic Science Providers

One aspect that will define forensic practice and education over the next decade and beyond is accreditation of not only forensic sciences education but also of practitioners and forensic science providers.

The UK Forensic Science Regulators recommendation to the industry is for providers of forensic services to obtain United Kingdom Accreditation Service (UKAS) accreditation so that the end-user of their information may be absolutely confident of the information supplied to the Criminal Justice System. The two most common accreditation standards are ISO17025 (for testing laboratories, i.e. DNA testing and toxicology testing) and ISO17020 for 'inspection bodies' such as searching crime scene and postmortem investigations. Although there have been concerns, such as at a meeting of forensic practitioners and legal professionals at Leeds University School of Law in 2012 (NUCFS, 2012), that 'accreditation will help establish mutual trust in the validity of the basic analytic methods used. However, accreditation does not state which method to use, only that the method used has to be suitable for its purpose.' The nature of the ISO accreditation addresses the possible variability that might exist between forensic science providers. A part of the requirement for validation is that accredited providers take part in external proficiency testing schemes that allow comparisons between providers and require the providers to undertake corrective actions in the event of the expected deviation from the expected result. An up-to-date list of accredited forces and private companies can be sourced via the UKAS website (www.UKAS.org).

Accreditation of Academic Forensic Courses

The academic content, nature of delivery, incorporation of expertise from practitioners and relevance to real world forensic science has developed within UK HEIs. Central to this has been the Quality Assurance Mechanisms in place in UK HEIs, the involvement of the university subject-specific External Examiner System and of course the Chartered Society of Forensic Sciences (CSoFS) accreditation processes. The CSoFS accreditation service is for those Higher Education Institutions delivering courses that contain forensic components. The courses intended for accreditation are normally at bachelors' degree with honours level or indeed a postgraduate qualification, such as a taught masters' degree with forensic elements. The CSoFS scheme (CSoFS, 2016) establishes and maintains standards of education within forensic science and involves major employers and professional interests. Accreditation is based upon a series of 'Component Standards.' The standards address specific areas of forensic practice and are intended to augment underlying scientific knowledge of the forensic components. The component standards form a substantial part of the Quality Assurance Agency (QAA, 2012) benchmark statement for forensic science. All forensic courses have a core Interpretation, Evaluation and Presentation of Evidence (IEPE) Component Standard. General forensic science degrees are covered by two further component standards; Crime Scene Investigation and Laboratory Analysis. Additional specialist areas have their own component standards in addition to the IEPE. The National Occupational Standards (NOSs) are applicable to various employment roles whilst the CSoFS Component Standards address the educational and development needs pertaining to relevant roles in the forensic field. The outcome of this process has been to bring into line the basic elements of the delivery and content to ensure appropriateness and currency for the profession.

The quality of HEI forensic science courses has undergone some scrutiny in the media but the work reported by Welsh and Hannish (2011) demonstrated that, in the United Kingdom, the Quality Assurance Agency (QAA), which safeguards the public interest in sound standards of Higher Education qualifications and informs and encourages continuous improvement in the management of the quality of Higher Education, is 'satisfied.' The QAA conducts institutional audits of Higher Education Institutions. The QAA has reported 'broad confidence' in the soundness of all of the universities that offer Forensic Science and Crime Scene degrees in the United Kingdom, current and likely future management of the quality of its academic programmes and the academic standards of its awards; broad confidence is the highest confidence judgment the QAA can give.

Accreditation of Forensic Science Practitioners

There are currently two routes for the 'accreditation' of forensic practitioners in the United Kingdom: that of accreditation of the practitioner by their professional body (e.g. Forensic Pathologists and Forensic Anthropologists) and also by the Chartered Society of Forensic Science (CSoFS). The CSoFS accreditation model has been designed for Small to Medium Enterprises and sole traders who do not currently have formal accreditation to the appropriate ISO standards. The assessment of competence is a direct route to being held on the CSoFS's formal register, providing that other necessary criteria are met. The ongoing development of competencies in a range of forensic disciplines is an iterative development and the CSoFS continues to announce assessment events for different disciplines on the Society's website. Elements of the assessment process are be externally endorsed by various UK universities depending on the discipline involved. The register of competent companies and forensic science providers is intended to provide confidence to the public and assurance to the Courts that the competent presentation of expert evidence is an important part of an individual's role.

The Court will, quite rightly, continue to have the final say with regards to who can present evidence, whether accredited or not – and if they meet the reliability tests for an expert witness. Barristers may well consider the reliability criteria and have an input in this area before engaging with an expert.

One issue that pervades current forensic education within HEIs is the separation that still exists between education and the practitioner. Whilst the *ad hoc* systems have facilitated some involvement and innovative educational practices for those HEIs that have formed a liaison with their regional police service and forensic providers, there is no national or structured systematic activity across institutions and organisations. This is becoming increasingly more important in order to ensure graduates who are fit for practice. Issues such as competency and accreditation are sporadic within the industry and one mechanism to drive forward a consistent approach in the United Kingdom will be to embed these practices into the education of undergraduates, so that they expect them to be part of their eventual employment.

Employers in the Next Decade

Currently, there are a number of private forensic service providers who function through tendering for services from police forces around the United Kingdom. The volume and scope of these tenders has changed significantly since the closure of the Forensic Science Service (FSS), who previously did the majority of the work. The closure of the FSS means that there are fewer forensic jobs available for graduates. Forensic science graduates are therefore highly reliant on the 'transferable skills' gained through their degrees. An outcome of this will undoubtedly be a reduced need for forensic graduates and potentially the demise of forensic science degrees in some universities.

The future of forensic science in Higher Education is challenging for a number of reasons. The national level changes in the forensic and policing landscapes in the last few years is testament to how rapidly situations can change. The closure of the UK Forensic Science Service, the increase in the numbers of independent forensic companies and the developing role of the UK Forensic Regulator, are all evidence of these profound changes. Thus far, there have been no high profile miscarriages of justice reported in the media, however such an event would undoubtedly send ripples for a requirement of immediate change through the industry, just as they have done previously. The UK based *New Scientist* magazine (Geddes, 2012) reported that the 75% of UK forensic scientists who responded to a *New Scientist* survey believed that the closure of the UK's Forensic Science Service (FSS) would lead to an increase in miscarriages of justice. Most forensic scientists also believed that switching to private and in-house police labs would reduce impartiality in interpretation, and therefore accuracy, of evidence.

However, 78% of forensic scientists surveyed did not feel confident that the regulator has sufficient resources to ensure that standards are adequate and consistent between providers.

Quarino and Brettell (2009) state that it 'stands to reason' that professionals who have academically studied forensic science may be more inclined to view an employment position as a 'career' rather than simply as a 'job.' These individuals may be open to engage in opportunities beyond their typical job duties, such as research, and become actively involved in professional organisations or policy groups. A better-educated workforce may allow laboratories to go beyond task completion and become more focused on problem solving, but clearly this will be based upon and balanced by the economic pressures of a profit-oriented company.

Whilst it has been suggested in many forms by many different stakeholders that forensic science education within Higher Education Institutions had a shelf-life and that, for the most part, programmes were of variable quality and of limited use to the practitioner industries they served (the Forensic, the Policing and the Criminal Justice System), it now appears that more than ever before those industries wish to have a meaningful dialogue and develop relationships with HEIs.

The Future of Forensic Science Education and Practitioner Training

It is clear that forensic science education in 2017 remains as challenging as it did nearly 20 years ago when the explosion of undergraduate courses occurred in the United Kingdom. In fact, with the changes in the industry, the challenges are even greater. The closure of the UK's Forensic Science Service, the expectations of accreditation by the International Organisation for Standardisation (ISO) and developing quality standards and competency testing across the industry place pressures on an already stretched workforce. Public service cuts will undoubtedly continue into the next decade and clearly have an effect on the number of staff, the nature of the work undertaken and the technology that will underpin both. These industry level changes are inexorably bound up with the educational landscape. With courses already bursting at the seams with academic content, there is the expectation that the elements mentioned here should also be included and their understanding and applications assessed within degree courses if the graduates are to be fit for the modern forensic workplace and indeed the Court of Law.

There have been a number of very positive developments in terms of the nature of the educational provision. The closure of the Forensic Science Service in 2012 and the 30-year retirement rule in the police force has resulted in more former forensic scientists and former police officers now working as part of the full-time academic teams throughout UK HEIs. There are greater and indeed stronger links between the forensic and police practitioners and academia. There have been numerous UK and international conferences over the past 15 years that have facilitated networks to develop, grow and share good practice across the industry. The role of organisations, such as the UK Chartered Society of Forensic Sciences, the American Academy of Forensic Sciences, and the involvement of educational bodies such as the UK-based Higher Education Academy and the UK Quality Assurance Agency have all served to develop, refine and improve the quality and diversity of forensic science educational provision. The development of research frameworks still has to be further developed but the progress so far has allowed trickle-down of newly created research knowledge into the lecture theatre and laboratory.

The Educational and Industry Forum offers the opportunity for accredited universities, forensic suppliers, providers, other universities and stakeholders to meet and discuss current developments within the forensic arena on an annual basis.

The contribution to on-going public safety makes research, development and innovation within forensic science a key area, which has been recognised by the UK Home Office Technology Strategy Board and its 'Special Interest Group in Forensic Science'. The utility of forensic science and the probity that can be achieved are key to the UK Criminal Justice System and to public safety. Such research stems from the work conducted in universities by academic and research funded staff but there is also the contribution from the research project work conducted by masters' and indeed undergraduate students. This level of fundamental, yet robust, work can offer a significant contribution to the existing knowledge base and thereby be of use to the Criminal Justice System in answering questions that would otherwise not be investigated due to the lack of staff, time and indeed funding in the forensic research arena. Such basic forensic research, often conducted as the first piece of significant, independent research by an undergraduate or a masters' level student, is now being viewed by forensic practitioners and legal advocates to be a previously un-mined resource of information of appropriate quality to be of use.

Conclusions

Looking forward, it is clear that forensic science educators and practitioner trainers have to adapt to the changing landscape and stakeholder requirements. University students are consumers who are mainly motivated by employment prospects and, in the tough job markets of today and tomorrow, they need reassurance of employment opportunities. Forensic science degrees need to appeal simultaneously: to those who want a good quality science degree that allows them to keep their employment options open; to those who want to a generalised background to forensic science; and to those who want to specialise in a particular field of forensic science. Universities, departments and course providers are under increased pressure to provide high quality, stimulating content that is directly relevant to practitioner and employment experience, that utilises a wide range of multimedia and advanced technology, appeals to a variety of learning types and that doesn't break the bank. This is an enormous task and a delicate balancing act for educators that does not appear to be diminishing in the foreseeable future.

Academics, researchers and teachers need to adapt the focus of their research in line with available grants, and demonstrate that their teaching is research-led. The competing pressures of the REF and TEF mean that wholesale changes are necessary across the forensic science educational landscape.

For practitioners, there is a real need for measures to reduce bias in UK laboratories and to raise the standards of forensic science as a whole, regardless of the decision to close the FSS. A vast majority, 81%, of *New Scientist* magazine survey respondents felt that more independent research was needed to overcome current weaknesses in forensic science in the United Kingdom — something many feel will now no longer get done.

Although the forensic science education sector faces significant challenges, the future is bright for forensic education with the opportunity to embrace change and to give even better services to the forensic sector in terms of training, education and research in the next decade.

References

Chartered Society of Forensic Science (CSoFS) (2016, ongoing) Component Standards: the Creation of a Professional Body with Component Standards for Education. Available at: http://www.forensic-science-society.org.uk/Accreditation/Component (accessed 12 December 2016).

Forstenzer, J. (2016) The Teaching Excellence Framework: What's The Purpose? Available at: http://www.crickcentre.org/wp-content/uploads/2016/01/TEF-Whats-the-Purpose-booklet-Josh-Forstenzer.pdf (accessed 3 August 2016).

Geddes, L. (2012) Forensic failure: Miscarriages of justice will occur. *New Scientist*, **2851**, 10–12.

House of Commons Business, Innovation and Skills Committee (2016) The Teaching Excellence Framework: Assessing quality in Higher Education Third Report of Session

2015–16. Available at: http://www.publications.parliament.uk/pa/cm201516/cmselect/cmbis/572/572.pdf February 2016 (accessed 28 July 2016).

NUCFS (2012) Celebrating the Second Century of the School of Law. Symposium at the University of Leeds, in collaboration with the Northumbria University Centre for Forensic Science Forensic Evidence: Expertise; Ethics; and Effectiveness, 23 July 2012, University of Leeds.

QAA (2012) *Subject Benchmark Statement: Forensic Science,* Available at: http://www.qaa.ac.uk/Publications/InformationAndGuidance/Pages/Subject-benchmark-statement-forensic-science.aspx (accessed 18 July 2016).

Quarino, L. and Brettell, T. (2009) Current issues in forensic science higher education. *Analytical and Bioanalytical Chemistry,* **394** (8), 1987–1993.

Rankin, B. Taylor, G. and Thompson, T. (2012) Should higher education respond to recent changes in the forensic science marketplace? *New Directions,* **8,** 27–32.

Welsh, C. and Hannis, M. (2011) Are UK undergraduate Forensic Science degrees fit for purpose? *Science & Justice,* **51** (3), 139–142.

Further Reading

Gilmore, M. (2012) Foreword, in *Live-time Forensics. Harnessing Science and Innovation for Forensic Investigation in Policing.* ACPO, 4f. Available at: https://connect.innovateuk.org/documents/3144739/3824722/Live-time Forensics brochure%28draftv6LR%29.pdf (accessed 23 March 2015).

Jamieson, A. and Moenssens, A. (Editors-in-Chief) (2009) Wiley Encyclopaedia of Forensic Science (five volume set). Wiley-Blackwell, ISBN: 978-0-470-01826-2.

National Institute of Justice (1999) Forensic Sciences: Review of Status and Needs, Washington DC. Available at: https://www.ncjrs.gov/pdffiles1/173412.pdf (accessed 2 September 2015).

Silverman, B. (2011) Research and Development in Forensic Science: a Review. (Silverman Review). Available at: https://www.gov.uk/government/uploads/system/uploads/attachment_data/file/118916/forensic-science-review-report.pdf (accessed 14 August 2016).

The Science and Technology Committee (2011) The Forensic Science Service. Seventh Report of Session 2010–12, Available at: http://www.publications.parliament.uk/pa/cm201012/cmselect/cmsctech/855/855.pdf (accessed 31 October 2015).

Index

Forensic Science Education and Training: A Tool-kit for Lecturers and Practitioner Trainers, First Edition.
Edited by Anna Williams, John P. Cassella, and Peter D. Maskell.
© 2017 John Wiley & Sons Ltd. Published 2017 by John Wiley & Sons Ltd.